岑

COLOR ATLAS & TEXTBOOK OF HISTOPATHOLOGY

SIXTH ENGLISH EDITION

with 11 Tables and 597 illustrations, including 464
color photomicrographs
and 65 electron photomicrographs

Color Atlas & Textbook of
Histopathology

by Professor WALTER SANDRITTER

Director of the Pathological Institute,
Freiburg University

and

Professor CARLOS THOMAS

Pathological Institute,
Freiburg University

with the assistance of

N. BÖHM, N. FREUDENBERG, M. HAGEDORN,
U. N. RIEDE and K. H. SALFELDER

Translated and edited by

WILLIAM B. WARTMAN, M.D.

Formerly Morrison Professor of Pathology,
Northwestern University;
Professor of Pathology, University of Virginia

YEAR BOOK MEDICAL PUBLISHERS, INC.

CHICAGO · LONDON

Library of Congress Cataloging in Publication Data

Sandritter, Walter.
  Color atlas & textbook of histopathology.

Translation of Histopathologie.
  Second-5th ed. published under title: Color atlas &
textbook of tissue and cellular pathology.
  Bibliography: p.
  Includes index.
  1. Histology, Pathological. I. Thomas, Carlos,
joint author. II. Wartman, William B. III. Title.
  [DNLM: 1. Histology. 2. Pathology. QZ4.4 S219h]
  RB25.S2513 1978   616.07   78-23170
  ISBN 0-8151-7552-3

International Standard Book Number: 0-8151-7552-3

This book is an authorized translation from the German edition published and
copyrighted © 1965, 1967, 1968, 1971, 1975 and 1977 by F. K. Schattauer Verlag
GmbH, Stuttgart, Germany. Title of the German edition: Histopathologie. Lehrbuch und Atlas für Studierende und Ärzte.

What is hardest of all to do?
What seems to you most easy:
To see clearly with your own eyes,
What your eyes lay before you.

GOETHE

To the memory of

LUDWIG ASCHOFF

October 1, 1866–June 24, 1942
Director of the Pathological Institute of the University of Freiburg
1906–1936

ARNOLD LAUCHE

September 14, 1890–September 29, 1959
Director of the Pathological Institute of the University of Frankfort on the Main
1943–1959

GEORG HERZOG

November 4, 1884–April 2, 1962
Director of the Pathological Institute of the University of Giessen
1926–1954

"In learning we develop the requisite process of thinking, and this training is not lost as long as we are possessed of our full mental vigor."

THEODOR BILLROTH

Preface to the English Edition

Thirteen years have passed since Professors Walter Sandritter and Julius J. Schorn, of the Justus-Liebig University, published their little book "Histopathologie." Ten years later the first English edition, with the new name "Color Atlas and Textbook of Tissue and Cellular Pathology," was published. Today, there are seven editions in German, six in English, two in Spanish, four in Japanese, one in Italian and one in French—an uncommon record to establish in only a baker's dozen of years. Professor Schorn, who was responsible for the beautiful photomicrographs in the first edition, died in an automobile accident before the book came out, and, until this edition, Professor Sandritter has been the primary author.

The original idea for the book was to consider pathology from the point of view of the microscopic signs of disease and to arrange these findings in an atlas. This was a reasonable approach, since much new and useful knowledge in both experimental and diagnostic pathology has come to us by way of the light and electron microscopes. Naturally, this approach has limitations, but the authors discovered ways to avoid some of the difficulties by adding short accounts of general pathology and gross pathology, along with some of the experimental and clinical aspects of disease. Subsequently, Professor Sandritter and Dr. C. Thomas wrote "Makropathologie," in which they gave a fuller account of gross pathology. Professor W. H. Kirsten, of the University of Chicago, translated the work into English under the title "Macropathology." This was followed by the publication of Sandritter and G. Beneke's "Allgemeine Pathologie," which in short order became a highly respected account of general pathology that has yet to be translated into English.

From the start, the beautiful color photomicrographs and the clear diagrams of the pathogenesis of a great number of the disease processes have been the chief attractions of all these books, particularly "The Color Atlas and Textbook of Tissue and Cellular Pathology," and they have accounted largely for the general appeal of the books. The care with which representative lesions have been selected, the expertness with which they have been photographed, and the beauty of the reproductions all contributed to the books' success. These works are clearly important additions to the writings in pathology.

New material has been added to each new edition of "Histopathology." For example, discoveries made with the electron microscope and chapters on the skin, blood and bone marrow, and fungi and parasites were added to the second edition; in the fifth edition, chapters on the kidney, specifically the account of glomerulonephritis, and on lymph nodes, the alimentary system and bones and joints were completely revised to reflect new knowledge about these diseases.

This new sixth edition (German seventh) has been the most thoroughly revised of all. In fact, it may be said that it is a new book, a fact that became clear to me as I made the translation again and discovered the extent of the changes and the amount of work needed to make them. There are now 372 pages and 597 illustrations, in comparison to 308 pages and 497 pictures in the previous edition. Much of the text has been rewritten. There are new accounts of the tumors, lymph nodes, blood and bone marrow, new sections on lesions of the breast, skin, gallbladder, oral cavity and genitalia, and an expansion of the discussion of cytodiagnosis. The tables and diagrams have been redesigned in color.

The result of all these additions and changes is a book that gives the student a clear and wide-ranging account of the facts of microscopic pathologic anatomy. So once again, as Ben Jonson put it, "Come forth thou bonny, bouncing book" and may your readers reward you with their approval.

William B. Wartman

Charlottesville and Christmas Cove
Summer 1977–78

Preface to the Seventh German Edition

One of the major purposes of a textbook of pathology is to utilize the accumulated empirical and experimental knowledge of this specialty to introduce the student to the field of clinical medicine. Of the many ways of doing this, there are clear advantages to one based on a visual or optical approach such as histopathology, or the microscopic pictures of diseased tissues. The "typical" histological structure thus becomes a continuing guide for the student during his clinical years and gives him a solid base on which to build his increasing knowledge of the complexities of disease. From this point of view, a textbook of pathological histology complements works of clinical medicine and general pathology and should be used along with them. Needless to say, no book can replace the study of actual histopathological preparations.

In order to achieve the purposes of this book, the material has been organized around the principles of special or systemic pathology; this should facilitate the correlation with clinical cases and enlarge the student's knowledge of general pathology. The comments on general pathology in the Introduction and the corresponding illustrations provide a useful review of the subject. This section was included for the special benefit of the beginner in order to guide him in understanding the photomicrographs in the latter part of the book. Similarly, the brief technical comments will help the student to use the microscope and to become familiar with the methods of preparation and staining of histopathological material.

The book is intended chiefly for medical students and young residents and assistants in pathology. However, as every experienced pathologist will recognize, there is such an abundance of material that careful selection is necessary to best serve these readers. We have taken pains to give special weight to representative and important lesions—a difficult task in view of the great number of disease illustrations. Diagrams have been inserted in an attempt to clarify and explain the course of the pathological events in didactic fashion.

The illustrations in this book are the central point of departure. The explanations supplied for them have been kept as concise as possible and placed on facing pages so that illustrations and text can be readily compared. Although the arrangement of the book in the form of an atlas has imposed certain limitations, we feel that the gains far outweigh the few losses that result from shortening the text. As far as possible the text has been arranged so that a general principle or short definition is given first, followed by an explanation that applies to the accompanying illustration and also describes possible variations. Short notes on the macroscopic appearance and often on the pathogenesis have been inserted where they seem important for an understanding of the microscopic findings. A short list of references to the literature, including both original and review papers and arranged according to subject, should make possible more intensive study of areas of special interest to the reader.

The above comments were written in 1964, for the preface to the first edition of this book. Since that time there have been widespread changes in the curricula of medical schools that seemingly have altered our teaching. But actually the course content has remained much the same; it has merely been served up in a different form. Knowledge of the fine tissue changes that occur in disease is still an essential part of medical learning, and the ability to "see with his eyes" is still one of the most important skills for a physician to acquire.

In the preparation of the seventh edition of this book, we have carefully taken into account many of the recent advances in medical knowledge. Fully 30% of the book is entirely new and the rest has been extensively revised and rewritten. There are new chapters on the pathology of the breast, skin, gallbladder, oral cavity and genitalia. The chapters on blood, bone marrow, spleen and lymph nodes, as well as the one on parasites, are now in accord with the newer classifications. In the chapter on tumors special attention is given to precancerous lesions, with discussions of others such as fibromatosis and pseudosarcoma. The tumors of the different organs are now discussed under the appropriate organ systems. The tumor nomenclature of the World Health Organization (WHO) is used throughout the book.

Today it is quite clear that cytodiagnosis has taken a position of ever increasing importance in the diagnostic armamentarium of physicians. Because almost every organ can be sampled by needle biopsy and such samples examined both histologically and cytologically, the usefulness of cytodiagnosis has been greatly extended. It is of great diagnostic value not only in gynecology (investigation of the menstrual cycle, early detection of cancer) but also in other areas such as the prostate, breast, thyroid, liver and kidney. As a result of all these advances, every physician must have a basic understanding of the principles, the proper use, and the limitations of the method.

It is important for both medical students and young physicians to keep in mind constantly that, despite all the recent advances in laboratory diagnosis, histopathology has better than 90% reliability and that many diseases can be diagnosed only by biopsy. For example, there is no comparably reliable chemical test for cancer. For this reason it is important for physicians to have a sound knowledge of the histopathological changes that occur in diseased tissues, as well as an understanding of the language of the pathologist. Painstaking pathological work will be of little value if the physician attending the patient does not correctly interpret the pathologist's opinion.

The diagrams have been completely redesigned for this edition, a task for which we are specially indebted to Dr. U. Riede. He has also supplied the various codes used in the diagrams (e.g., red = inflammation). Mr. Tschörner, the artist for the publisher, has expertly redrawn the original rough sketches. Our thanks also go to numerous colleagues who have so freely given us light and electron microscope photographs. As always, the publisher has been a helpful partner. In particular we thank Professor Matis and Director Reeg.

W. Sandritter, C. Thomas

Freiburg i. Br.
Summer, 1977

Contents

Introduction–General Pathology

A certain amount of practical knowledge and skill, particularly with respect to use of the light microscope, is desirable on the part of the reader if he is to get the most good from reading a textbook of histopathology. Profitable use of the microscope requires knowledge of its construction and of the interrelations of its individual parts. Furthermore, it is only possible to interpret a histological slide after one is informed as to how the tissue has been prepared for cutting and how it has been stained. A solid foundation in normal Histology and General Pathology goes without saying, for the principles of General Pathology are used constantly in Special Pathology.

Preliminary Technical Remarks

Use of Microscope

The light source, the lens system with its diaphragms and the eye must all be correctly aligned with one another in order to obtain optimal information from a histological section. Artificial light, which consists predominantly of yellowish red light rays, can be corrected by a blue filter so that it will approximate daylight. Köhler's principle is commonly used to adjust the light source, since by using this principle it is possible to illuminate only the object area that is to be examined and that entirely uniformly. With a microscope with a built-in light source, swing in the front lens of the condenser. Focus the microscope on the specimen and stop down the *field diaphragm*. Rack up the condenser as far as possible and then lower it slowly, thus focusing the field diaphragm within the specimen area.

Center the condenser with the two centering screws if necessary (the condensers of many student microscopes are permanently centered so that this step may be omitted). Open the field diaphragm until its shadow disappears from the field of view. The field diaphragm should always be adjusted so that its image just disappears behind the edge of the eyepiece stop. Adjust image contrast and, if necessary, sharpness–but not image brightness–with the *condenser (aperture) diaphragm* by opening it entirely and then closing it down just far enough to remove glare from the specimen. Unstained objects can be seen best when the condenser diaphragm is closed as far as possible or with a phase contrast microscope. With blurred images, reducing the condenser diaphragm will increase the contrast.

The microscopic image is produced by diffraction of the light by the structures in the histological preparation in the focal plane at the back of the objective (primary image). The secondary image, which is the one observed in the ocular, arises from magnification of the primary image.

Objective and ocular must be properly matched. In usual histological practice, an ocular with a $10\times$ magnification is used with the following objectives, in which the first number gives the magnification and the second the numerical aperture of the objective, which is a measure of its resolving power:

1. *Scanning lens:* objective 2.5 to 5.0 − magnification $25 - 50\times$.
2. *Low magnification:* objective 10/0.25–magnification $100\times$.
3. *High dry magnification:* objective 40/0.65 − magnification $400\times$.

For still higher magnification, especially for examination of smears of cells (blood, lymph node), oil immersion objectives (100/1.25) are available with a magnification up to $1,000\times$.

When using the microscope, the following suggestions will prove helpful. With a monocular microscope, always keep both eyes open, since the adjustment for distance obtained in this way prevents rapid eye fatigue due to constant accommodation.

The lowest magnification should always be used before going to the other objectives because it is easier to orient the various structures under low magnification.

If the image is blurred, you should think of the possibility of the slide being upside down with the cover-slip resting on the stage of the microscope.

Preparation and Staining of Histological Sections

Sections are prepared from blocks of tissue measuring about 2 × 2 cm. The selected tissue is usually hardened and fixed in formol (ordinary 40% commercial formalin diluted with water 1:9 so that the resulting solution is about 4%). The *hardening* results from coagulation and denaturation of protein, while the *fixation* arrests autolysis and bacterial decomposition. In order to prepare sections 5–10 micra thick, the tissue must have a consistency suitable for cutting. To obtain this, the tissue may either be frozen (at −20°C.) with carbon dioxide snow and cut on the frozen-section microtome (this method is used particularly for demonstrating fat or for rapid diagnosis of biopsy specimens at the time of surgery) or the tissue can be processed through a series of alcohols (from 70 to 100%), methyl-benzoate, and benzol into paraffin with a melting point of 56° C. Liquid paraffin at 60° C. penetrates the finest tissue spaces and produces a good cutting consistency. After cutting on a microtome, the sections are mounted on microscopic slides and stained, after first being deparaffinized with xylol.

Note: Frozen sections permit demonstration of neutral fat–in paraffin sections, the fat is dissolved by alcohol and the droplets of fat appear as optically empty spaces in the tissue.

The methods used for *histological staining* have been developed empirically and the physical-chemical basis for them is not exactly known except in a few cases. Electrostatic binding, among other factors, plays a principal role. Negatively charged groups, for example, nucleic acids (phosphate groups) or proteins ($-COOH$ groups) or the mucopolysaccharides ($-COOH.SO_4$), bind with the basic dye groups, which behave as cations. Acid dyes (e.g., eosin) with electron negative charges bind predominantly with positively charged protein groups (NH_2-groups). Excess and easily soluble dye in the tissue is removed after staining by differentiation in water, alcohol or weak acid. Finally, the water is removed with 70 and 96% alcohol, the section immersed in a clearing agent (xylol), mounted in Permount or Canada balsam and covered with a cover-slip.

For further details on histological techniques, see Davenport, Lilly, Humason, etc.

Histochemistry deals with specific and sometimes quantitative identification of chemical substances in tissues, such as nucleic acids, certain proteins, carbohydrates, enzymes, etc. (see Pearse, 1960).

Artifacts in histological sections are caused chiefly by improper fixation, embedding (cracks or tears) or staining (transparent, unstained flaws).

Table 1 reviews the features of some commonly used stains. *Fluorescence microscopy,* in which tissues are stained with fluorescing dyes and examined under ultraviolet light, allows detection of certain substances, e.g., immunologically active proteins, because the ultraviolet light rays (e.g., 350 Mμ) liberate secondary rays in the visible range (compare p. 220). Some substances show self fluorescence, e.g., lipids, porphyrins and elastic fibers.

Table 1. **Staining Methods**

Method	Results		Remarks
Hematoxylin-eosin (H & E)	**Blue** *Hematoxylin* Basophilic cytoplasm, nuclei, bacteria, calcium	**Red** *Eosin* Cytoplasm, connective & all other tissues	p. 40
van Gieson (v. G.)	**Yellow** *Picric Acid* Cytoplasm, muscle, amyloid, fibrin, fibrinoid	**Red** *Fuchsin* Connective tissue, hyalin	**Black** *Iron Hematoxylin* Nuclei p. 52
Elastic stain	**Black** *Resorcin-fuchsin* Elastic fibers	**Red** *Nuclear fast red* Nuclei	p. 70
Elastic-van Gieson (E.v.G.)	used in combination		p. 62
Azan	**Red** *Azocarmine* Nuclei, erythrocytes, fibrin, fibrinoid, acidophilic cytoplasm, epithelial hyalin	**Blue** *Aniline blue, Orange G* Collagen fibers, basophilic cytoplasm mucus	p. 160
Silver stain	**Black** *Ammoniacal AgNO₃* Reticulum fibers, nerve fibers		Collagen fibers brown
Fat stain	**Red** *Sudan III, Scarlet Red* Neutral fat	**Blue** *Hematoxylin* Nuclei, cytoplasm	p. 38
Congo red	**Red** *Congo red* Amyloid	**Blue** *Hematoxylin* Nuclei	p. 164
Weigert's fibrin stain	**Blue** *Lugol's solution, Crystalviolet* Fibrin, bacteria	**Red** *Nuclear fast red* Nuclei	Not specific for fibrin p. 100
Berlin-blue reaction	**Blue** *Calcium ferrocyanide* Hemosiderin, Fe^{III}	**Red** *Nuclear fast red* Nuclei	p. 82
Giemsa (May-Grünwald-Giemsa)	**Blue** *Methyl violet* Nuclei, all basophilic substances	**Red** *Azur-eosin* Eosinophils, cytoplasm & its granules, collagen fibers	Metachromatic: Mast cells violet Melanin green p. 238
Ladewig	**Blue-greyblue** *Aniline blue* Parenchyma Mesenchyma	**Orange red** *Acid fuchsin-gold-orange* Muscle Fibrin	**Black** *Iron hematoxylin* Nuclei p. 248
Mason-Goldner	**Orange red** *Azofuchsin* Parenchyma Fibrin	**Green** *Light Green* Mesenchyma	**Black** *Iron hematoxylin* Nuclei p. 166

3

Table 1. **Staining Methods** (con'd)[1]

Method	Results		Remarks
Spielmeyer's myelin stain	**Blue-black** *Iron-alum hematoxylin* Myelin, erythrocytes		p. 280
Ziehl-Neelsen	**Red** *Carbofuchsin* Acid-fast rods, Tb bacilli, lepra bacilli	**Blue** *Hemalum* Nuclei	
Periodic Acid-Schiff Reaction (PAS)	**Red** *Schiff reagent* Adjacent hydroxyl groups and amino-alcohols		Neutral and acid polysaccharides p. 180 Demonstration of Fungi, parasites
Levaditi	**Black** *AgNO₃-reduced* *Pyrogallic acid* Spirocheta pallida Listerella mono-cytogenes		p. 318
Thionine, Toluidine Blue	**Blue** Basophilic cytoplasm	**Blue** Nuclei	Mucus, mucin, lipids are metachromatic p. 270

[1]See pp. 12 and 317, for other special stains.

Histological Interpretation and Diagnosis

A famous physician (FRANZ VOLHARD) once said: *"The Gods have put diagnosis before therapy— man must put careful observation and interpretation before diagnosis." Analysis must precede synthesis* as it does in all other branches of knowledge. Analysis begins with the examination of the subject with a clear-cut objective in mind. *Careful observation* of similarities and dissimilarities, the separation of the typical and the atypical, the general from the special, all contribute to the desired knowledge of the subject. The arrangement, color, size and form of the tissue elements and their relations to one another all help to determine the essential characteristics of the various structures under consideration. As such observations cannot be obtained without adequate preparation, a thorough theoretical grounding and a certain amount of experience become essential.

The beginning student will find it helpful in getting exact histological details either to make drawings or to set down his observations in abbreviated, outline form. The student is thus forced to emphasize the essential features and to de-emphasize unessential ones.

After first carefully making the necessary observations, it is then possible to take the second step, that is, to synthesize the observations and make a diagnosis. On the other hand, hasty, careless examination will often lead to an incorrect opinion. In order to arrive at a *diagnosis,* the histological observations need to be classified in some logical manner, usually one which has been reached through a compromise of experience and hypothesis. But, by its very nature, no diagnosis can be considered final, since it can change with the progress of scientific knowledge. Thus, it is understandable that an exact description retains its validity indefinitely, even when the interpretation and diagnosis of a section have already been revised.

The student will therefore be well advised to put his chief effort into a careful description of a microscopic section. In examinations, this is always graded higher than a diagnosis unsupported by accurate description.

4

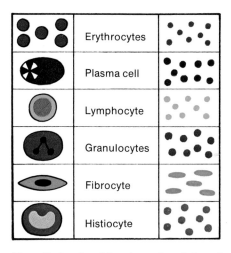

	Inflammation Necrosis		Hyalin
	Exudate Edema		Fibrin, Fibrinoid Thrombus
	Pus		Fatty degeneration Fat
	Collagen Fibers Scar		Vascularization (granulation tissue)
	Nucleus		Cytoplasm Parenchyma, Muscle

	Erythrocytes		
	Plasma cell		
	Lymphocyte		
	Granulocytes		
	Fibrocyte		
	Histiocyte		

Fig. 1. Explanation of the colors and symbols used to depict lesion components and pathological processes.

In practice, the first step in examining a histological preparation is to look at the section with the *unaided eye*. The shape and the various components of the tissue structures—easily recognized by differences in staining—often provide essential topographical information and have an important influence on the next step in the analysis of the section. An inverted ocular used as a scanning lens will provide an over-all view of the tissue at very low magnification. Ordinary *low-power magnification* can then be used to examine in greater detail the structures already seen with the inverted ocular. In this way, a rough over-all picture of the essential elements of the lesion is formed. Further details can also be distinguished with *low magnification*, such as the size and position of the nuclei and the structure of the cytoplasm. This magnification is probably the most useful of all, for at a magnification of about one hundred-fold, all the essential structures are well seen without losing the over-all architectural relationships. A drawing at this stage of the examination will fix the typical findings firmly in mind. Practically all histological preparations can be diagnosed with low magnification. *Higher magnification* is used only to clarify individual details, such as the shape and division of nuclear chromatin, mitoses, and so forth.

Such a methodical approach is an essential prerequisite for profitable observation and correct diagnosis. In studying histopathological slides the student gets the knowledge required to separate essential from nonessential observations—knowledge that a physician uses at the bedside.

5

Notes on General Pathology[1]

These brief, almost stenographic, introductory remarks about general pathology are intended only as a means of making it easier to understand the complexities of special pathology. Reference to the appropriate illustrations of the book permits its use as a guide to the principles of general pathology.

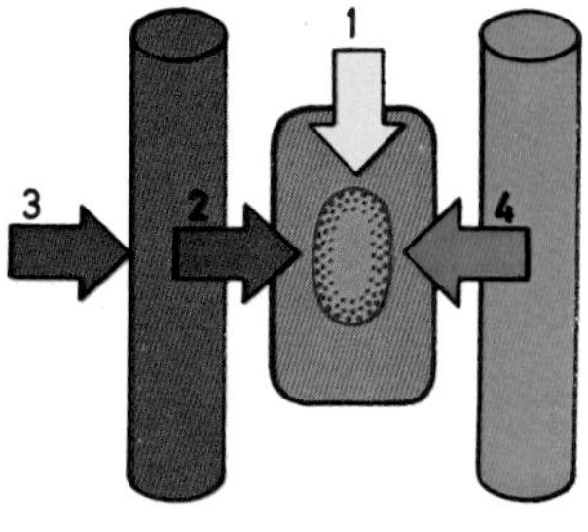

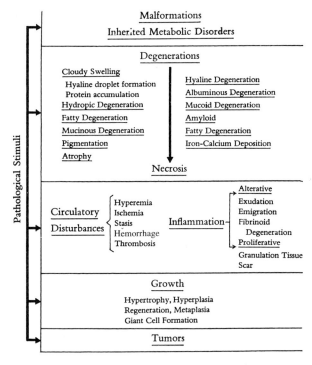

Fig. 2. See text for explanation.

In the schematic diagrams and tables the same symbols and colors are used for similar pathological processes throughout the book (Fig. 1). The individual components of a lesion or process are indicated by colors or symbols based, unless otherwise noted, on the gross (e.g. pus-greenish yellow) or microscopic appearance (e.g., collagen fibers-curly lines).

A knowledge of general pathology is an excellent foundation for the study of disease. The knowledge so obtained can be applied in nearly all special situations, since *the host in reacting to the many different pathological stimuli that may affect it has only a limited number of possible responses available*. These originate essentially from either transient or permanent increase *(anabolism)* or decrease of metabolism *(catabolism)* or from *work failure*. In addition, complex tissue responses occur in *circulatory disturbances*, the various forms of *inflammation* and in *tumors*.

In theory, pathological stimuli can reach the cells and tissues in various ways (Fig. 2):

1) *directly* (e.g., trauma, radiant energy). 2) by way of the *blood stream* or the *lymphatics* with resultant direct cell injury (e.g., toxins, alterations of the vascular contents as in thrombosis). 3) *indirectly*, when the stimulus acts on the *vessel walls*, a secondary circulatory disturbance then causing the cell injury (e.g., nervous derangement of permeability). 4) the pathological stimulus can come from the *alimentary tract*. Finally, primary (e.g., inborn) defects of metabolism may cause secondary cellular reactions.

The following diagram sets out the possible reactions of the organism to pathological stimuli in simple fashion (Fig. 3).

Fig. 3. Schematic survey of possible host reactions to pathological stimuli.

---

[1] For a more detailed treatment of the subject see the textbooks of Anderson, Boyd, Florey, Montgomery, Muir-Cappell, Perez-Tamayo and Robbins, Walter and Israel, Sandritter and Benecke: Allgemeinen Pathologie (Schattauer-Verlag, 1974).

Malformations: Inherited Metabolic Disorders

Malformations or *metabolic disorders* can develop in the embryonal (up to the third month of pregnancy) and fetal periods (after the third month) either because of inborn errors in the genetic material or of the action of pathological stimuli (e.g., teratogens). These manifest themselves, for example, either in *agenesis* (absence of enzymes, e.g., galactosemia; defective organ formation) or *aplasia* or *hypoplasia* (faulty development of existing organs). A great number of different manifestations can be produced in this way.

Degenerations

The different sorts of *degeneration* are morphological manifestations of metabolic disturbances either of cells (left-hand column of Fig. 3) or of intercellular substances (right-hand column of Fig. 3).

Cloudy swelling and hydropic degeneration (Fig. 4) result from disturbance of the metabolic systems that maintain the ionic environment of cells (so-called ion pumps). When these regulatory mechanisms fail, then sodium and water flow into the cells and potassium leaves them. As a result, the mitochondria swell and the cytoplasm appears to be filled with fine "protein granules" *(cloudy swelling)*. The resulting cloudiness is due to increased scattering of light *(Tyndall effect)*. The mitochondria may also be transformed into water-filled vesicles *(hydropic transformation* of mitochondria). The water may accumulate in the ground substance or cause widening of the cisternae of the endoplasmic reticulum (hydropic degeneration). Compare p. 160 (light photomicrograph) pp. 16, 45 (electron photomicrographs).

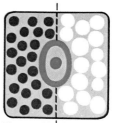

Fig. 4. Cloudy swelling (left), hydropic degeneration (right).

Nuclei may also show swelling *(degenerative nuclear swelling)*. This must be distinguished, however, from physiological or *functional nuclear swelling*, which is often accompanied by enlargement of the nucleolus and is a reflection of increased metabolic work.

Hyalin droplet degeneration (protein accumulation) should be distinguished from cloudy swelling (Fig. 5). The microscopical appearances of the two conditions can be similar, but in hyalin droplet degeneration active work is performed by the cell (anabolism) with accumulation of protein (cytoplasmic coacervation), for example, the reabsorption of protein in the renal tubules. Such reabsorption of material is accomplished by pinocytosis, in which small vesicles are formed by constriction of the cell membrane. Phagocytosis, on the other hand, is the process by which the cytoplasm takes up large, formed materials, such as bacteria (see pp. 10, 21).

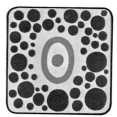

Fig. 5. Hyalin droplet degeneration (protein reabsorption).

See p. 160 *(light photomicrograph) and p. 168 (electron photomicrographs)*.

The term *fatty degeneration* (perhaps better called fatty change or fatty metamorphosis) describes the appearance of microscopically visible fat, either in the form of fine (Fig. 6, right) or large (Fig. 6, left) droplets. The size of the droplets depends upon the proportion of neutral fat (large droplets contain little phospholipid). Normally, fat is taken up in the form of fatty acids, which is accomplished through pinocytosis. The fatty acids are synthesized to triglycerides, bound to phospholipids and proteins, and delivered to the blood as lipoproteins. Any disproportion between the amounts of triglycerides (e.g., increased alimentary supply) or of phospholipids (e.g., choline deficiency) or failure of energy coupling (oxygen or enzyme deficiencies) leads to accumulation of fat, i.e., to fatty degeneration.

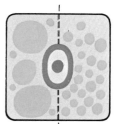

Fig. 6. Fatty degeneration. Large droplet form (left), fine droplet form (right).

See p. 38 *(light photomicrograph) and p.* 163 *(electron photomicrographs)*.

Fat phanerosis may develop in *necrobiosis* (perceptible, slow cell death) in which structurally intact fat tissue is broken down into microscopically visible droplets.

In disordered carbohydrate metabolism, glycogen droplets may appear (e.g., in the kidney in diabetes), or mucinous degeneration develop (production of mucopolysaccharides but without secretion) as, for example, in mucinous carcinoma (signet-ring cells, Fig. 7).

See p. 303

Alteration of the character of mucin secretion may also result in obstruction of excretory ducts (e.g., cystic fibrosis of the pancreas).

Fig. 7. Signet ring cell.

See p. 130

Glycogen storage disease is caused by an *inborn error* of carbohydrate metabolism.

Pigments are naturally colored materials that are laid down in either diffuse or granular fashion. They usually have as the chief component either *protein* (e.g., melanin), *lipid* (lipopigments, e.g., lipofuscin) or derivatives of *hemoglobin* (hemosiderin or siderin, hematoidin, bile pigment). In addition, a number of *exogenous pigments* may be seen.

See the following Figures:

Lipofuscin, pp. 9, 35

Melanin, p. 223

Hemosiderin or siderin, pp. 132, 244

Hematoidin, pp. 9, 244

Bile pigment, p. 132

Malaria pigment, p. 132

Exogenous pigments, pp. 9, 244

Table 2 gives the most important differential characteristics of the different pigments.

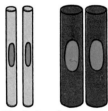

Atrophy of cells (Fig. 8) results from inactivity or chronic metabolic deficiency, is manifested by reduction in cell size *(simple atrophy)* and eventually results in reduction of cell number *(numerical atrophy)*.

Degeneration of the connective and supporting tissues affects chiefly the *ground substance*. It may result in unsheathing of the fibers, infiltration of fat and mucin and deposition of foreign substances.

Fig. 8. Atrophy, hypertrophy.

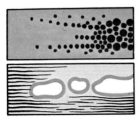

Albuminous or granular protein degeneration and mucoid degeneration of the connective tissues (Fig. 9) result from disintegration of the ground substance with precipitation of protein in cartilage or other tissues having a low metabolic rate. Protein complexes appear in the ground substance, or there is an increase in mucopolysaccharides. The collagen fibers are exposed in the process and finally destroyed, with the result that cysts are formed *(muco-cystic degeneration,* e.g., in a meniscus). *See p.* 270.

Fig. 9. Albuminous or granular protein degeneration (above), muco-cystic degeneration (below).

Table 2. **Pigments**

Substance	Components	Location	Iron Reaction	Fat Stain	H$_2$O$_2$	Acid	Base	PAS[1]	Ag NO$_3$[2]	Fluorescence[3]	Gmelin Test
Lipofuscin p. 9	unsaturated oxidized fatty acids	Parenchymal cells	–	(+)	(+)	–	–	+	+[4]	+	–
Ceroid	unsaturated oxidized fatty acids	intracellular (mesenchymal)	–	+	–	–	–	+	±	+	–
Melanin p. 223	tyrosine derivatives	intracellular	–	–	+	–	(+)	–	+[5]	–	–
Siderin Hemosiderin pp. 132, 244	iron glycoprotein	intracellular	+	–	–	+	–	+	+	–	–
Hematoidin p. 244	bilirubin	extracellular	–	–	–	+	+	–	–		+
Bile Pigment p. 132	bilirubin biliverdin	intra- and extracellular	–	–	–	+	+	–			+
Malarial Pigment p. 132	hemoglobin derivative	intracellular	(+)	–	+	+	+		–		
Formalin Pigment p. 132	protoporphyrin	extracellular	–	–	–		+			–	
Exogenous Pigments p. 246	e. g., carbon, silver, etc.	intra- and extracellular	–	–	–				–		–

1 Periodic acid-Schiff reaction for demonstration of polysaccharides (α glycol).
2 Reduced silver.
3 Primary fluorescence without staining.
4 Brown.
5 Black.

Fig. 10A. Distinguishing Characteristics of "hyaline" Hyaline, Fibrinoid, Amyloid Light microscope: eosinophilic, homogeneous, strongly light refractive

Kind	Light microscopic structure	Electronmicroscopic structure	Characteristics	Occurrence
Epithelial hyaline	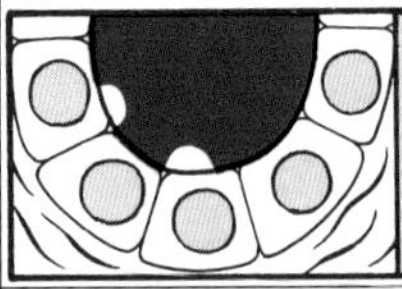	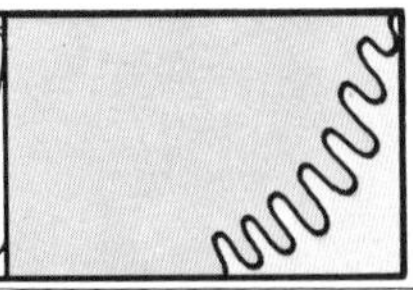	H & E, Azan-red. V.G.-yellow. Protein produced in cells and secreted into extracellular spaces (e.g. gland lumens).	Thyroid colloid. Prostatic secretion. Parotid mixed tumor.
Cellular & hematogenous hyaline	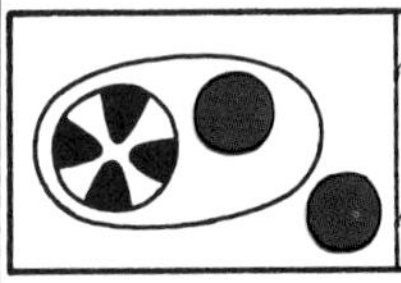	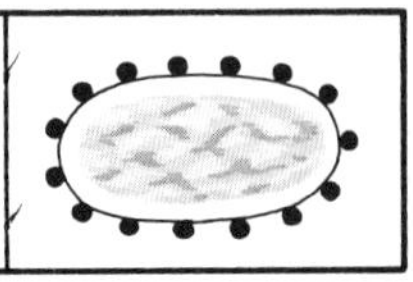	H & E, Azan-red. V. G.-yellow. Protein produced in cells (e.g. plasma cells) intracytoplasmically or after cytolysis of extracellular deposits.	Mallory bodies. Russel bodies.
	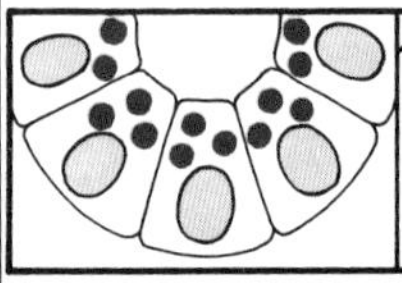	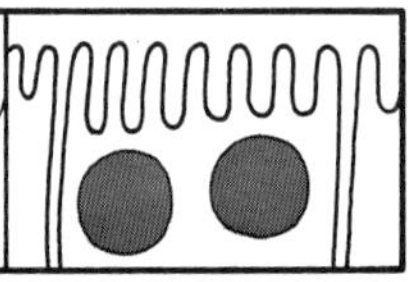	H & E-red, V. G.-yellow. Heterophoyocytosis of protein with intracytoplasmic storage in lysosomes	Hyaline droplets. Protein storage in renal tubule cells.
	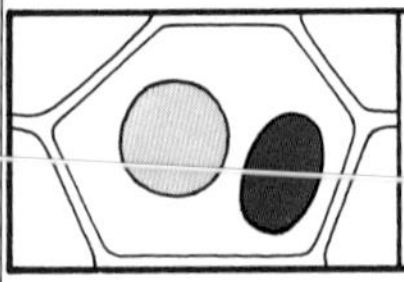	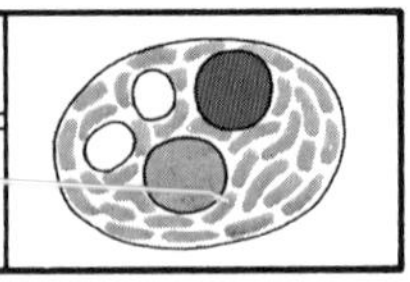	HE-red, V. G.-yellow Necrotic cellular material. Hyaline thrombi. Blood plasma. Fibrin.	Councilman bodies. Shock lung. Kidney. Hyaline kidney casts. Lung edema. Lung hyaline membrane.
Connective tissue hyaline	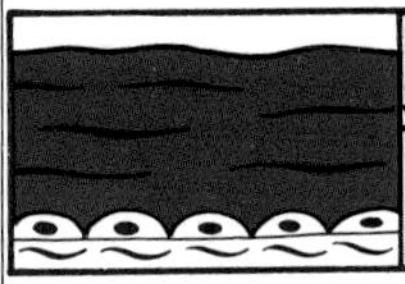	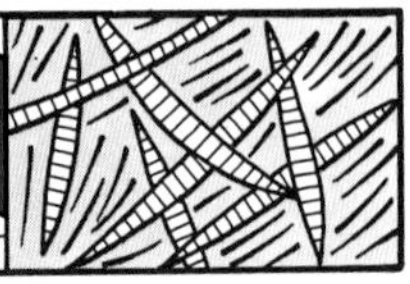	V. G.-red. Azan-blue. Quaternary structure of the collagen due to disturbed fibrillo-genesis. Tangled arrangement of fibrils with deposition of acid mucopolysaccharide between them + non-collagenous protein.	Pleural hyaline. Capsular hyaline of spleen (sugar icing).
Vascular hyaline	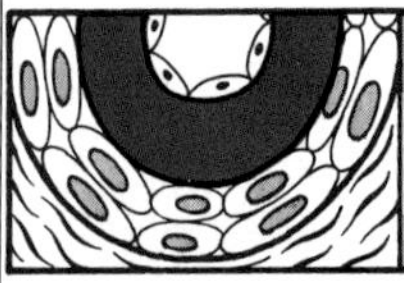	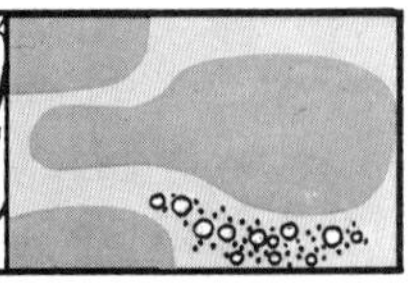	V.G.-red yellow. Blood protein. Lipoproteins & immune precipitates and cell detritus. On glomerular mesangial matrix + basal membranes.	Hyalinization of arterioles. Kimmelstill-Wilson hyaline in glomeruli.
Amyloid	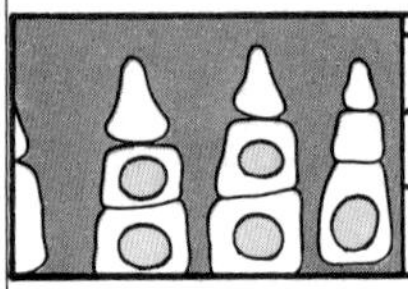	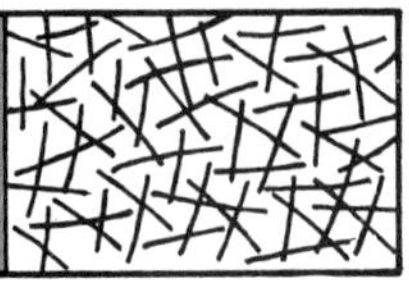	V. G./yellow. Congo-red-red. Cellular synthesis of glycoproteins and immunoglobulins (light chain). Intra- and extracellular aggregates and rod-shaped proteins.	Amyloidosis

Fig. 10B. Distinguishing Characteristics of Fibrinoid

Kind	Light microscopic structure	Electronmicroscopic structure	Characteristics	Occurrence
Fibrinoid swelling	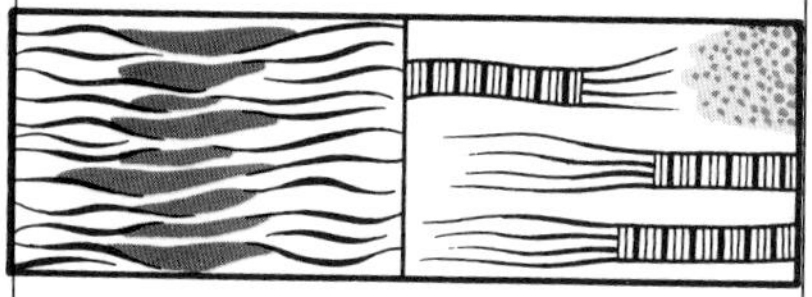		V. G.-yellow. Quaternary structure of the collagen focally destroyed. Partial protofibrillar degeneration. Therefore greater solubility. Blood protein deposits and collagen antibodies often not visible.	Aschoff bodies. Gastric ulcer.
Fibrinoid precipitation	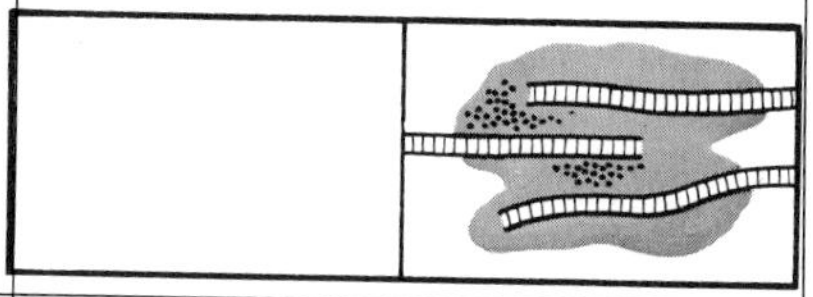		V. G.-yellow. Quaternary structure of collagen mostly intact. Fibrils crowded on each other and coated with immune precipitates	Rheumatic nodules. Chronic primary polyarthritis.
Fibrinoid necrosis	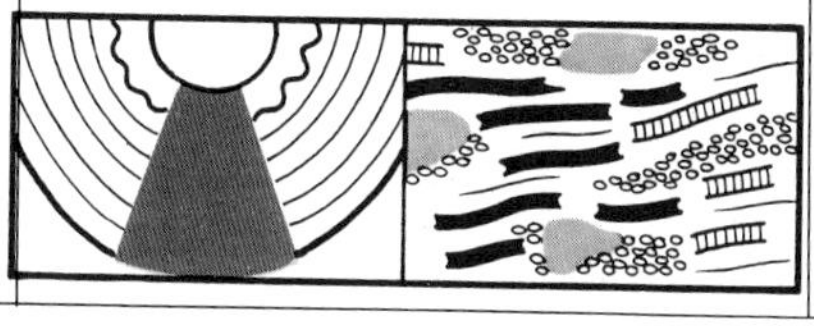		V. G.-yellow. Total lysis of collagen and elastica. Cellular debris of necrotic myocytes and fibrocytes + fibrin + immune precipitates.	Fibrinoid necrosis in panarteritis nodosa. Malignant hypertensive vasculitis. (Malignant nephrosclerosis.)

Hyalin

"Hyalin" is a catch all word used to describe a variety of lesions of diverse causes and development that have a similar appearance when examined with the light microscope. Hyalin was first observed and described in the mid-nineteenth century when only the light microscope was available for examination of diseased tissues and since the lesion appeared homogeneous and was highly light refractive, in this respect resembling the microscopic appearance of hyalin cartilage, it was called "hyalin." Because the word was convenient it has continued to be used to indicate any alteration in either tissues or cells that stains red with eosin, is homogeneous in appearance and has a high refractive index. Hyalin has various sites of localization and recent electronmicroscopic and biochemical studies have shown that the structure and chemical composition of hyalin may be different in different sites and under different conditions. The following sorts of hyalin are recognized: *epithelial hyalin* produced by epithelial cells, e.g. colloid. *Cellular hyalin* resulting from retention of cellular secretion, e.g. retention of antibodies in plasma cells, the so-called Russel bodies, or the Mallory bodies in liver cells of alcoholics, or the hyalin droplets of reabsorbed protein in renal tubules. In a wider sense of the word, the large homogeneous areas of eosinophilic necrosis found for example in myocardial infarcts or in the isolated necrotic cells sometimes found in liver and known as Councilman bodies, are also described as hyalin. Other examples are hyalin casts formed in proteinurea, hyalin membranes in the lung, hyalin thrombi in shock, which are sometimes called hematogenous hyalin. *Connective tissue hyalin* has a porcelain white gross appearance, e.g. hyalinization of the pleura or capsule of the spleen. The lesions result from a little understood disturbance of formation and orderly deposition of collagen fibers. In *vascular hyalin* (hyalinization of arterioles—a special form of arteriosclerosis) the hyalin material lies between the intima and atrophic media and consists of blood proteins, lipids, immunoglobulins (Ig G, Ig M), necrotic medial muscle and mucopolysaccharides (Gupta et al., 1972). Glomerular hyalin is produced by the mesangial cells (mesangial matrix).

Amyloid is a hyalin substance that stains specifically with Congo Red dye and when examined with the electron microscope is found to be composed of fibers lacking periodicity (Figs. pp. 246, 248). Recent studies show that amyloid is produced by cells of the reticuloendothelial system and is deposited extracellularly. The usual sites of deposition are spleen, liver, kidney, adrenal and intestines. (See Figs. on pp. 134, 164, 202, 208, 246.)

The different sorts of fibrinoid cannot be separated histologically since all appear homogeneous and eosinophilic. In contrast to connective tissue hyalin, fibrinoid is invariably accompanied by an inflammatory reaction in the tissues, as for example in Aschoff nodules, or the extra-cardiac nodules of rheumatic fever or panarteritis. In Aschoff nodules the collagen fibrils are split and show loss of cross-striations (fibrinoid swelling), in the extra-cardiac nodules of rheumatic fever accumulations of blood protein and fibrin lie between the fibrils (fibrin stains are positive, *fibrin precipitation*). In panarteritis there is necrosis of blood vessel walls or of adjacent tissues with fibrolysis of collagen bundles which are splintered and no longer show cross-striations (*fibrinoid necrosis*).

Table 3. **Distinguishing Characteristics of Hyalin, Amyloid, Fibrinoid and Fibrin**

Stain	Hyalin	Amyloid	Fibrinoid	Fibrin	Remarks
Hematoxylin Eosin	**red** homo-geneous	**red** homo-geneous	**red** homo-geneous	**red** fine fibers or homo-geneous	
van Gieson	**red**[1]	**yellow**	**yellow**	**yellow**	
Congo Red	–	**red**	–	–	
Methyl Violet	–	**red**	–	–	metachromatic red
Azan	**blue**[2]	**red**	**red**	**red**	
Weigert's Fibrin Stain	–	–	±	±	depending on the fixative used and on the age of the fibrin
Digested by Trypsin Pepsin	– –	– –	+ –	+ –	
Tissue Reaction	–	occasional giant cells	slight acute in-flammation, granulation tissue, histiocytes	granula-tion tissue	

Note: Hyalin–no tissue reaction. *Fibrinoid*–almost always a tissue reaction: granuloma, e.g., Aschoff nodules (p. 48), or granulation tissue (panarteritis, p. 69). [1] Epithelial hyalin: yellow. [2] Epithelial hyalin: red.

Necrosis

Necrosis (focal death of tissue) is recognized morphologically by destruction of cell nuclei (pyknosis = nuclear shrinkage, karyolysis = nuclear dissolution, karyorrhexis = fragmentation of nuclei, Fig. 11, and p. 20), homogenization of the cytoplasm and distinctly increased eosinophilia. (See also pp. 40, 45.)

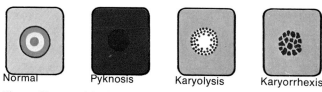

Fig. 11. Diagram of the different manifestations of nuclear destruction.

In the early or acute stages, denaturation of proteins occurs and evokes a leukocytic reaction. Later, the necrotic tissue is resorbed by granulation tissue and finally a scar is formed. There are, however, various other paths that differ from this ordinary sequence of events, as shown in Figure 12. In occasional cases, regeneration occurs with complete restitution of tissue integrity (e.g., liver, especially in young persons).

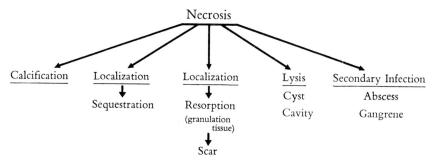

Fig. 12. Sequelae of necrosis. *(See pp. 40, 42.)*

Electron Microscopy

The advances in the field of electron microscopy have added a new dimension, that of ultrastructure, and it is essential to consider the significance of this fact with respect to general pathology. The advancing edge of this new dimension is closing the large gap between light microscopy and biochemistry. Electron microscopy, and in particular histochemical electron microscopy, is making visible for the first time those cellular structures that are the morphological bases of metabolic processes. This new knowledge has greatly increased our understanding of disease. Structure and function are no longer to be conceived of as antagonists, but rather as parts of a whole (see LaVia and Hill; 1975).

The electron micrographs that follow on the next pages have to do with certain angles of general pathology. Those illustrating special pathology are placed under the sections on the respective organs.

In attempting to present the electron microscopic basis of general pathology in tabular form (pp. 16, 17), it is realized that the brevity of the tabular form imposes severe restrictions. Only the barest outline of the alterations of cell organelles can be indicated. However, the juxtaposition achieved in the table makes it clear that at the level of ultrastructure, as well as at the level of light microscopy, there are no *specific* cellular lesions and the most widely different injurious agents may call forth quite similar reactions.

---

[1] The rule shown in the electron micrographs is one micron in length unless otherwise indicated.

Ultrastructure of a Normal Liver Cell

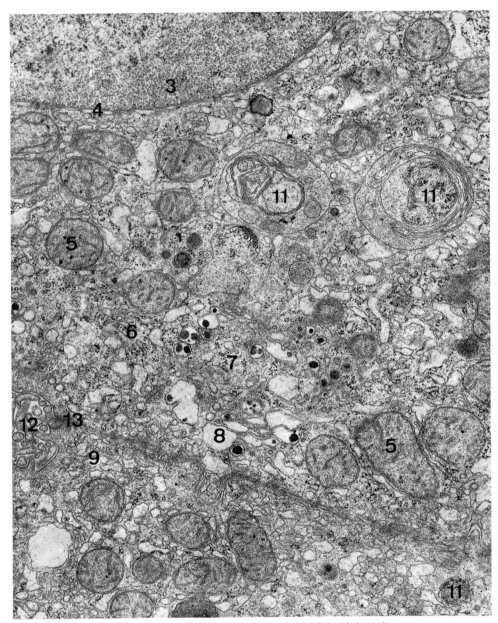

Fig. 13. Normal liver cell of the mouse. Electron photomicrograph (Dr. Schroeder). 20,600x.

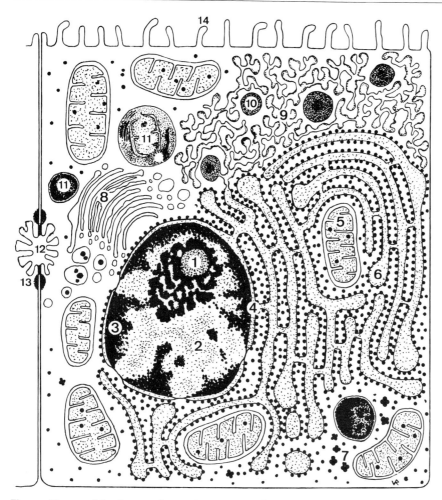

Fig. 14. Diagram of the electron microscopic appearance of a normal bipolar liver cell (the same legend numbers are used in Fig. 13). 1. *nucleolus* (formed of ribosomes and transfer–RNA) with pars amorpha and nucleoluema. 2. *loose chromatin* (euchromatin: synthesis of messenger RNA). 3. *dense chromatin* (heterochromatin: genetic building block). 4. *perinuclear, cistern with nuclear pore*, transition to rough endoplasmic reticulum. 5. *mito-chondria* with cristae (citric acid cycle, respiratory enzymes, part of fatty acid synthesis) and *matrix granules* (lipoprotein with cations, calcium depot). 6. *rough endoplasmic reticulum* (RER) with outer border of *ribosomes*. Transformation of rough endoplasmic reticulum (RER) into smooth endoplasmic reticulum (SER). 7. Protein is synthesized on the ribosomes and *polysomes* with the help of messenger–RNA. In the cisternae of the RER protein transport occurs. The *Golgi apparatus* (8) serves as a condensation and packaging station. 9. *smooth endoplasmic reticulum* (SER). Tubular cisternae without ribosomes. The RER and SER together form a membrane system [the *endoplasmic reticulum* is the same as the biochemist's microsome fraction] with organ specific enzymes (Staudinger, 1962). SER contains organ specific enzymes such as glucose-6-phosphatase (glycogen metabolism) hydroxylase, demethylase, etc. for detoxication. 10. Peroxysoma. These contain catalase and counteract internal storage of peroxidase. 11. Lysosomes with absorbed organelle constituents. They contain acid hydrolases such as acid phosphatase, β glucuronidase, cathepsin, collagenase, etc. 12. Bile capillary with microvilli. The fragments of disintegrating lysosomes are excreted here. The apical or biliary pole of the cell. 13. Desmosomes: these bind the liver cells to each other. 14. Microvilli on the surface of the liver cell extending into the space of Disse. Basal or vascular pole of the cell.

Table 4. **Pathological Alterations of Cell Organelles**

Normal	Pathological	Remarks
(1)	a) Swelling mitochondria Normal (1) Matrix type Crista type (2)	**Swelling:** *histologically* this is the matrix type of cloudy swelling. The crista-type is unremarkable histologically. Swelling may progress to degeneration of cytoplasm. *Causes:* O_2 deficiency. Uncoupling of oxidative phosphorylation. Toxins. Substrate deficiency. *Metabolic Effect:* reduced oxidative phosphorylation.
(2)	b) Structural changes 	**Structural Changes:** *Histologically* – no equivalent. Giant mitochondria can appear deceptively like Mallory bodies. Structural changes accompanied by hyperplasia of mitochondria cause cytoplasmic oxyphilia (oxyphile cells in hyperthyroidism). *Occurs with:* hypovitaminosis, chronic alcoholism, disturbance of protein synthesis. *Metabolic effect:* disturbance of citric acid cycle and/or oxidative phosphorylation.
(3)	c) Membrane changes (3)	**Membrane Changes:** No *histological* equivalent. Myelin-like degeneration of external membrane. Proliferation of cristae. *Causes:* Chronic O_2 deficiency. Increased CO_2 or O_2 tension (lung), muscular exercise, tumors, cholestasis.
(4)	d) Matrix changes (4)	**Matrix Changes:** Amorphous thickening of mitochondrial matrix. *Causes:* Malnutrition, hypovitaminosis, methylcholanthrene application, alcoholism. Dense matrix aggregates (with calcium). *Occurs with:* tissue necrosis, nephrocalcinosis. Loss of matrix granules. *Occurs with:* calcium deficiency, ischemia and necrosis. Crystalline inclusions: *Occur with:* alcoholism, Wilson's disease, polymyositis, lipid nephrosis, cholestasis, dehydration and hypovolemic shock.
(5)	**Rough endoplasmic reticulum** a) Vesiculation b) Lysis of ribosomes c) Vacuolation d) Ballooning electron microscope reversible / light microscope	**Rough endoplasmic reticulum:** *Histologically* the first sign is vacuolization and ballooning. *Occurs with* ischemia, toxins and end stages of many different cell injuries.
(6)	 (6)	**"Finger print" degeneration:** *Occurs* in chronic intoxication (hydrocarbons), excessive regeneration, carcinogenesis, disturbed protein metabolism. Frequently manifested *histologically* by basophilic nodules (so-called cytoplasmic "nebenkerne").
	 e) f)	**Collapsed cisternae (e):** manifestation of membrane injury by peroxidation (e.g. CCl_4). Reduced synthetic output (hypothyroidism). **Blocked cisternae (f):** with accumulation of products of synthesis. *Occurs in:* plasma cells as Russel bodies, in cartilage cells in chondrodystrophy.

Table 4. (continued)

Normal	Pathological	Remarks
 (7)		**Ribosomes** Polysomes (aggregates of 80 S-ribosomes) disappear. 50 S- and 30 S-ribosomes appear. *Histologically:* swollen, basophilic cytoplasm (RNA). Diffuse basophilia. *Occurs* with: CCl_4 poisoning, antibiotics, nutritional deficiency, carcinogenesis, ischemia. *Metabolic effect:* decreased protein synthesis.
 (8)		**Smooth endoplasmic reticulum** **Hyperplasia and proliferation.** *Histologically:* cells appear milky (milk glass)—hyperplastic cells with hyalinized cytoplasm. *Causes:* barbiturate, antiepileptic, antidepressant drugs. Resorcin. Hydrocarbons. Carcinogens. Alcoholism. Jaundice. Virus hepatitis B. **Vacuolization and ballooning** similar to that in rough endoplasmic reticulum.
 (9)		**Golgi apparatus** a) hypertrophy due to swelling. *Occurs* in: Oxygen deficiency, Vitamin E deficiency b) intracisternal accumulation. *Occurs* in various sorts of secretory disturbances.
 (10)		**Peroxysomes:** *Function:* degradation of toxic cell peroxidases (catalase). a) Hypoplasia in necrosis, malignant change in a tumor (hepatoma). b) Hyperplasia due to antihyperlipidemic agents, salicylates, antihistamines.
 (11)		**Lysosomes:** *Autolysosomes:* Absorption and digestion of cellular cytoplasmic constituents (organelles, glycogen etc.) = autophagocytosis. *Occurs* in all cells with a moth eaten appearance in sublethal cell injury. Hunger, atrophy of inactivity, senile involution of organs. Product of degradation = lipofuscin granules. *Heterolysosomes:* Absorption and digestion of foreign bodies by phagocytosis. Digested materials: fibrin in Shwartzman phenomenon, hemosiderin from hemorrhage, bacteria and viruses in infections. Protein or hemoglobin. Nuclear fragments, mononuclear cells in typhus. Cellular fragments in Kupffer cells in hepatitis (= Councilman bodies).
 (12)	 a b	**Hyaloplasm** a) *Amyloid* (special stains). b) *Fatty degeneration:* Histologically there are cytoplasmic fat droplets.

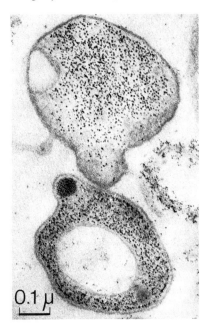

Fig. 15. Macrophage resulting from injection of iron and showing siderosomes with both large particles (siderin) and finely granular ones (ferritin, 55Å). 50,000×. (Jones-Williams).

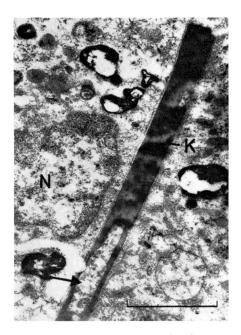

Fig. 16. Hematoidin crystal (K) contained in a macrophage and surrounded by invaginated cell membrane (→). N = nucleus. 25,000× (Gieseking.)

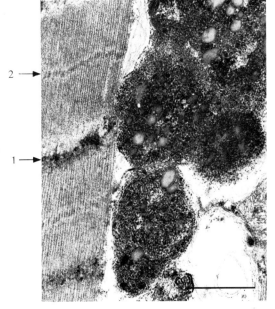

Fig. 17. Lipofuscin in hypertrophied heart muscle (human). 1→, Z bands; 2→, M bands. 30,000×.

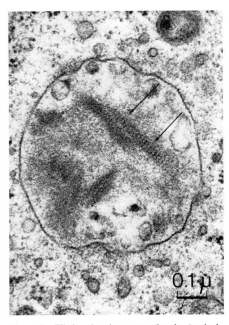

Fig. 18. Fibrin showing cross bands (typical periodicity →) lying in a cytoplasmic vacuole in a Kupffer cell following administration of endotoxin ("fibrin-clearing" mechanism in the Shwartzman phenomenon). 71,000× (Prose).

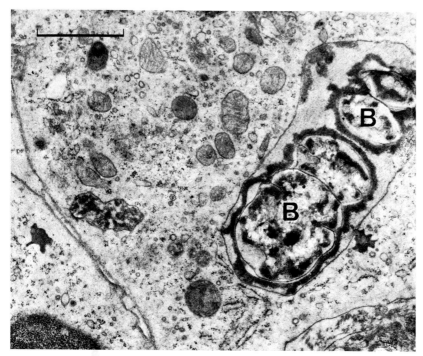

Fig. 19. Phagocytosis of bacteria in the blood by a macrophage. 24,000× (Staubesand).

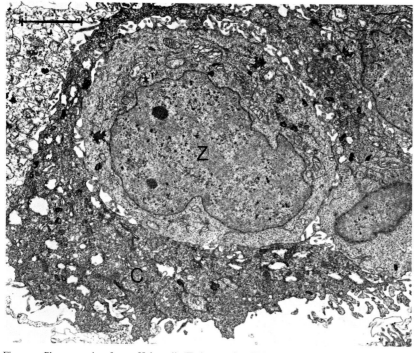

Fig. 20. Phagocytosis of one Hela cell (Z) by another Hela cell. The cytoplasm (C) of the phagocytizing cell has completely surrounded the other cell. 8,000×. (Staubesand and Wittekin.)

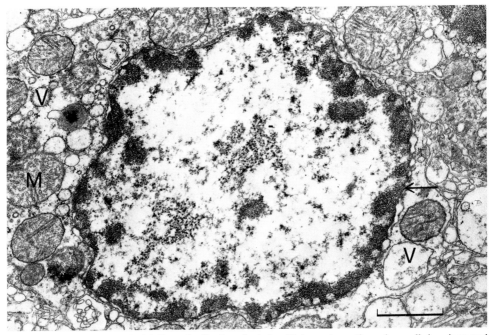

Fig. 21. Ischemic necrosis of epithelium of a distal renal tubule with hyperchromatic nuclear wall, i.e., increased margination of chromatin on the nuclear membrane plus pallor of the interior. V = vacuole in ER (vacuolar degeneration), M = swollen mitochondria. 17,000× (Torovic).

Cell Necrosis

Depending on the severity of an injury and the length of time that it acts, different sorts of cellular necrosis are observed (Fig. 22). If the injury is short acting (i.e. acute) and lethal, coagulation necrosis occurs. This starts with damage to membranes and leakage of fluid so that the cells become hydropic with marked swelling of mitochondria and leads to total disintegration of the cellular constituents and break-up of the cell. As a rule coagulation necrosis involves groups of cells.

If the injury is long acting (i.e. chronic) and sublethal, the affected cells appear much shrunken (shrinkage necrosis). Nuclei and cytoplasm are mostly shriveled and dense. In the initial stages, mitochondria remain intact both morphologically and functionally. This sort of necrosis as a rule involves single cells (e.g. in viral hepatitis). In the liver, such shrunken necrotic cells are frequently phagocytosed by other cells (hepatocytes, Kupffer cells) and with light microscopy are seen as eosinophilic hyaline bodies, the so-called Councilman bodies. After being completely broken down by lysosomes they are eliminated by the cell (Sandritter and Riede, 1975).

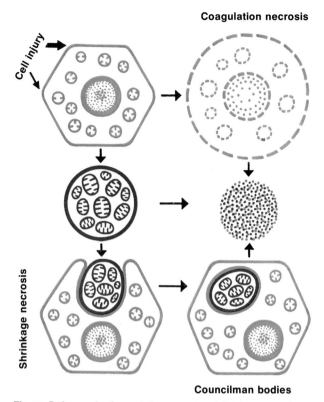

Coagulation necrosis

Cell injury

Shrinkage necrosis

Councilman bodies

Fig. 22. Pathogenesis of coagulation necrosis and shrinkage necrosis.

Circulatory Disturbances

The *circulatory disturbances,* like inflammation, involve complex processes in a variety of tissues. These processes take place in the terminal circulatory channels, the arterioles, meta-arterioles, capillaries and venules. Even under normal conditions, there is a changing interplay of hyperemia (in activity) and anemia (at rest), which, under pathological conditions, change to *passive* (stasis of blood) or *active hyperemia* or to *ischemia. Stasis* indicates stagnation of the blood current with hemoconcentration. If the stasis persists, necrosis will result. Depending upon local factors, there will develop either an *anemic infarct* (coagulation necrosis: in organs supplied with end-arteries, e.g., heart, kidney, spleen, etc.) or a *hemorrhagic infarct* (necrosis and hemorrhage, e.g., in lung, intestine).

Hemorrhage may occur for various reasons (e.g., injury of capillary walls, deficiency of platelets, deficiency of fibrinogen). Derangement of the coagulation mechanism together with slowing of the blood stream and endothelial injury results in formation of a thrombus which either breaks off *(embolus),* becomes organized, calcified or softened interiorly *(putrid softening)* or is dissolved *(fibrinolysis).*

See the following Figures:

Inflammation

Inflammation consists of a series of complex reactions by vascular and connective tissue elements to a tissue injury. In the acute phase, there is *hyperemia, fluid exudation* (if chiefly blood serum=*serous inflammation;* if chiefly fibrinogen = *fibrinous inflammation;* if accompanied by hemorrhage = *hemorrhagic inflammation)* and *emigration* of leukocytes *(purulent inflammation).*

Fig. 23 shows the intensity of the response of some tissue reactions in both acute and chronic stages of inflammation.

Intensity

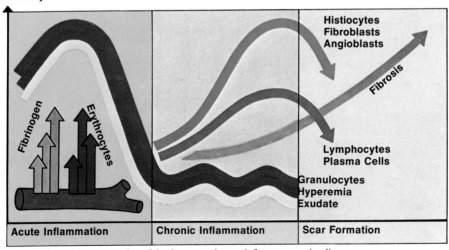

Fig. 23. Schematic representation of the tissue reactions to inflammatory stimuli.

See the following Figures:

In the *chronic stages,* proliferation of connective tissue cells, histiocytes and capillaries predominate *(granulation tissue).* Different morphological appearances and functional disturbances are produced, depending upon the duration of the injury, the amount of denatured protein (necrotic tissue, fibrin) deposited or the presence of foreign bodies in the tissue. Essentially, there is proliferation of *fibroblasts,* young connective tissue (fibrosis → scar), *histiocytes* (phagocytic function) [now thought to come from blood monocytes! (LEDER, 1967)] and *new capillaries* (nutritional function). There are also varying numbers of lymphocytes, plasma cells, mast cells and polymorphonuclear leukocytes.

On the basis of the cell type, some authors separate a *cellular form of proliferating granulation tissue,* which is rich in lymphocytes and histiocytes, from *granulation tissue in a narrow sense* (only capillary twigs and fibroblasts), and from an *infiltrating form of granulation tissue* which appears between the local tissue elements and may be transformed into them.

Among the chief functions of granulation tissue the following may be mentioned:

1. *resorption,* e.g., the resorption of necrotic tissue, thrombi or fibrin (p. 43);
2. *tissue replacement,* e.g., replacement of defects in the skin or mucous membranes (p. 217);
3. *localization,* e.g., walling off of an abscess (p. 321).

The result is always the formation of a *scar* to replace the defect caused by loss of local parenchymatous tissue.

See pp. 42, 55, 121, 202, 231
Macroscopic: Immature granulation tissue: red. Scar tissue: white, glistening, fibrous and tough.

Fibrinoid degeneration or necrosis (Fig. 24) develops after severe acute disturbance of vascular permeability with subsequent sudden leakage of blood plasma into the vessel wall and the surrounding connective tissue. Because of this, the vascular tissues are either obscured or destroyed (see Table 3 and p. 12). The blood plasma proteins combine chemically with collagen or the tissue mucopolysaccharides (BE-NEKE, 1963). Fibrin is often demonstrable with both the light and electron microscopes. A slight, fleeting leukocytic reaction or secondary proliferation of histiocytes (e.g., Aschoff nodules in rheumatic fever) or granulation tissue (e.g., in periarteritis nodosa) may follow, with consequent resorption of the fibrinoid (see pp. 67, 69).

Circumscribed nodules of granulation tissue are seen in granulomatous inflammation (histiocytic granuloma, e.g., Aschoff nodules; foreign body granuloma; epithelioid granuloma of tuberculosis, etc.).

See pp. 106, 214, 236

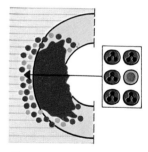

Fig. 24. Fibrinoid necrosis in an artery.

By the term "specific inflammation" is meant a tissue reaction distinguished by a characteristic (specific) morphological appearance that suggests the etiologic agent, e.g. tuberculosis, which shows a typical arrangement of cells and tissues (often with necrosis). It should be noted, however, that such lesions are specific only in a limited sense, since epithelioid cell granulomas, for example, may occur in diseases of different causes (tuberculosis, syphilis, brucellosis, histoplasmosis, sarcoid, etc.).

See the following Figures: Tuberculosis, pp. 56, 106; Syphilis, p. 138

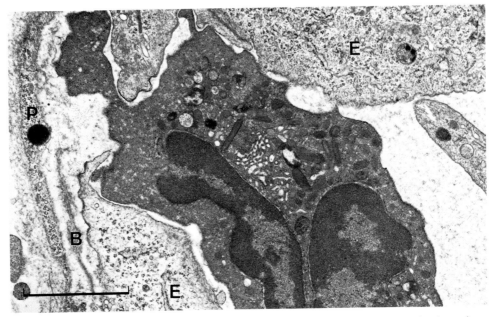

Fig. 25. Early stage of leukocyte emigration from a venule in acute inflammation of rat omentum. A polymorphonuclear leukocyte has pushed between two endothelial cells. B-basement membrane. P-cytoplasm of a pericyte. 27,500×. (I. Joris)

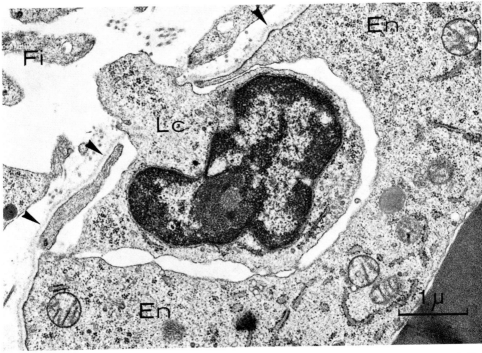

Fig. 26. Lymphodiapedesis, post capillary venule in the lymph node of a normal fetus 165 mm crown- length. Endothelial cell (En), lymphocyte (Lc), process of a fibroblast (Fi), erythrocyte in the venule lumen. Note the defect in the basement membrane (arrows), which is continuous elsewhere, and the place of egress of the lymphocyte. About 19600×. (G. Kistler)

Acute Inflammation

In *serous inflammation*, fluid leaks from the blood vessels. Figures 25 and 26 show what happens. The tight adhesion between the endothelial cells (normally desmosomes) is lost. Through these pores (0.1 to 0.8 μ) blood serum escapes and collects under the basement membrane or the pericytes (Figs. 25 and 27). *Leukocytes, lymphocytes, monocytes* and *erythrocytes* also pass through these pores (Fig. 25). Exudation of *fibrinogen* is thought to take place in a similar fashion. Once outside the vessels, it poly-merizes to fibrin. Because a thick layer of fibrin may be deposited on and be bound to the collagen fibers, a homogeneous, eosinophilic microscopic appearance results that is referred to as *fibrinoid swelling* or *degeneration*. Lysosomal enzymes and the acid pH of the inflamed area cause the collagen fibers to loosen (tuft-like splintering, Fig. 35). In addition, fibrin may be deposited between the proto-fibrils *(fibrinoid necrosis)*. Leukocytic proteolytic enzymes often cause tissue liquefaction (abscess), during which process the collagen fibers disintegrate (Fig. 35) and probably can form hyalin. (Fig. 35, *reconstituted hyalin*).

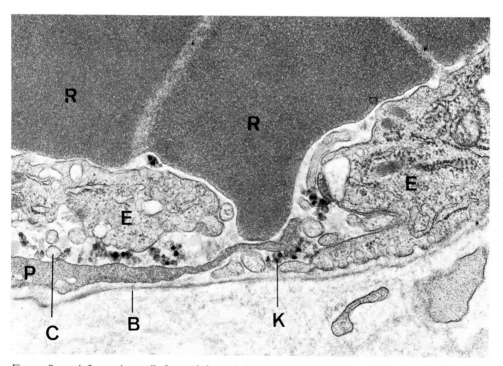

Fig. 27. Serous inflammation: wall of a venule in rat skeletal muscle. Local injection of histamine and carbon. A gap has formed between endothelial cells (E) through which carbon (K) as well as chylomicrons (C) from the blood have passed. Part of an erythrocyte (R) has also passed through the gap. The erythrocytes are tightly packed—a sign of blood stasis. P-cytoplasmic process of a pericyte, B-basal lamina. 47500×. (I. Joris)

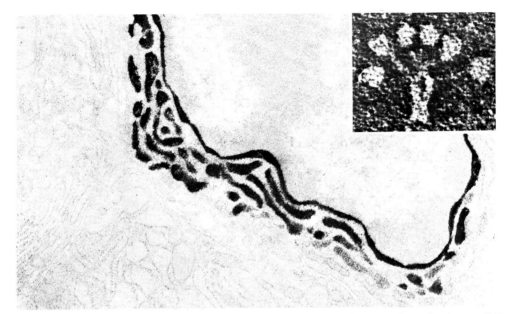

Fig. 28. Site of specific antibody formation (antihorseradish peroxydase) in the ergostoplasm of a plasma cell (6 days after first injection) (Cottier). 24000×. Insert: above right, human complement factor C with 6 binding sites. 1100000×. (Villiger).

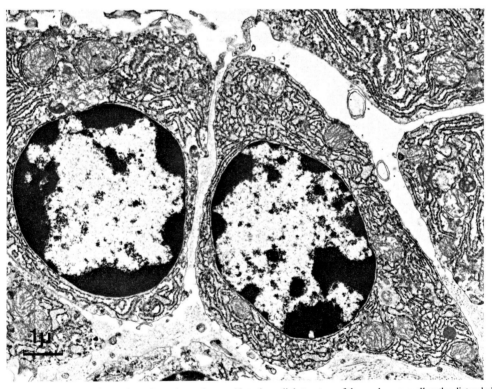

Fig. 29. Plasma cell from a bronchogenic carcinoma. Note the radial structure of the nucleus as well as the distended rough endoplasmic reticulum. About 105000×. (Kistler).

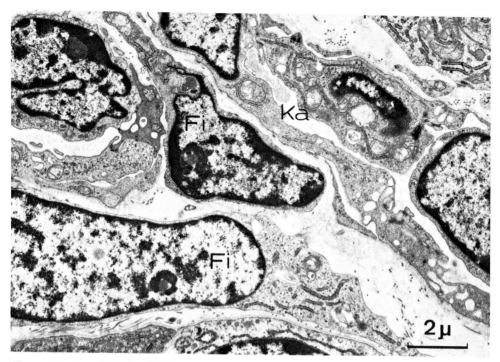

Fig. 30. Fibroblasts (Fi) and capillaries (Ka) in the interstitial tissue of a fetus 180 mm length from crown to rump. About 8500×. (Kistler).

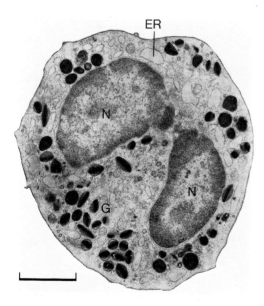

Fig. 31. Eosinophilic granulocyte from rat bone marrow. G = eosinophilic granules with crystalline inclusions (lysosomes); N = lobulated nucleus; ER = endoplastic reticulum. 7000×. (Staubesand).

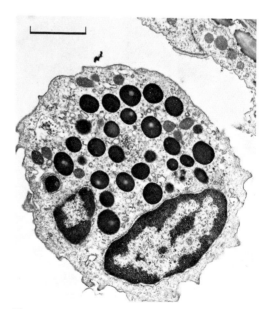

Fig. 32. Mast cell (rat) with intracytoplasmic granules containing histamine and serotonin. 13000×. (Staubesand).

27

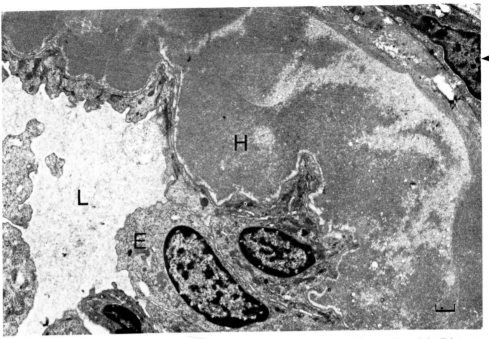

Fig. 33. Hyalinized afferent arteriole of renal glomerulus (human) in hypertension. L-lumen of arteriole. E-intact endothelium. H-amorphous hyaline material. → necrotic muscle of media. 8500×.

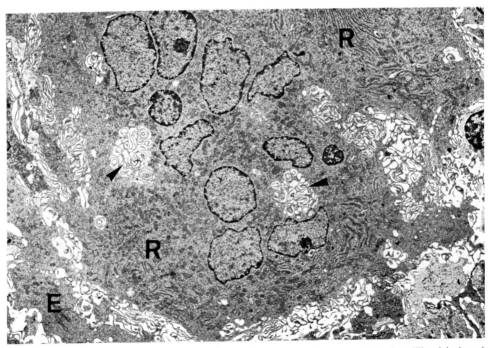

Fig. 34. Langhans' giant cell (R) in a lymph node. Note the numerous cell processes with microvilli and the invaginations of membranes (arrow). Epithelioid cells (E). About 1700×. (Kistler).

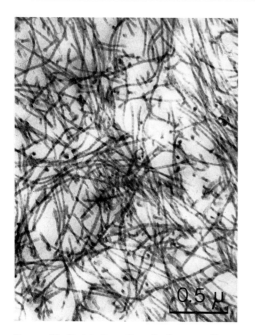

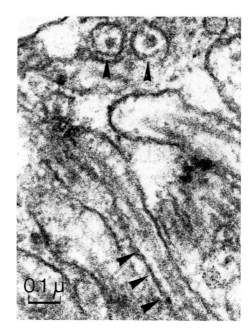

Fig. 35. Hyalin transformation of collagenous fibrous tissue showing cross striations (reconstituted hyalin). 30000× (Gieseking).

Fig. 36. Persistent chronic hepatitis B in a 38-year-old person with a kidney transplant. Smooth endoplastic reticulum (arrow) of a liver cell shown in longitudinal and cross sections. Hepatitis B surface antigen. About 11500×. (Kistler).

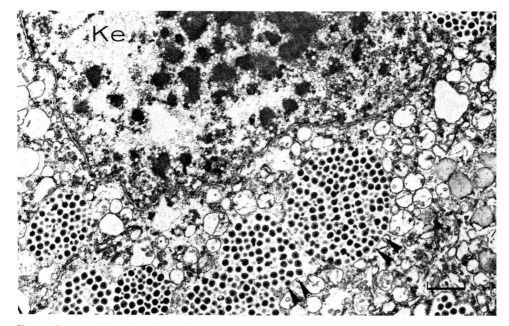

Fig. 37. Cytomegalic inclusion disease of the newborn. Epithelial cells of renal proximal tubule showing immature virus particles in the nucleus (KE) and vacuolar swelling of the endoplasmic reticulum with mature (encapsulated) cytomegalic viruses (arrows). About 10700× (Kistler).

Growth and Tumors

Increase in metabolic work finds morphological expression in enlargement of cells and nuclei (hypertrophy, Fig. 8) or in increased numbers of cells (numerical hypertrophy or hyperplasia). See p. 37. Formation of equivalent specific organs and tissues is called regeneration. In addition, one sort of tissue can be transformed to another sort, e.g. ciliated epithelium to squamous epithelium, a process called metaplasia. The basal cells of the epithelial tissue in this example have differentiated to epithelium that is foreign to the site (see p. 192). Tumors (see p. 287).

Giant cells appear under various conditions and in a variety of forms (Fig. 39). Frequently, they are the result of the increased work of resorption (e.g., Langhans' giant cells, foreign body giant cells, osteoclasts). They can also result from fusion of cells or from nuclear division without cytoplasmic division (amitotic division). In many cases, giant cells develop from capillary twigs (e.g., giant cells in an epulis). Touton giant cells are found in chronic resorbing inflammation in fat tissue.

See the following Figures: foreign body giant cell, p. 214; Langhans' giant cell, p. 106; giant cells in an epulis or brown tumor, p. 110; giant cells in an Aschoff nodule, p. 48; Touton giant cells, p. 214; Hodgkin and Reed-Sternberg giant cells, p. 239; osteoclasts, p. 266; placental giant cell, p. 199; tumor giant cell, p. 310.

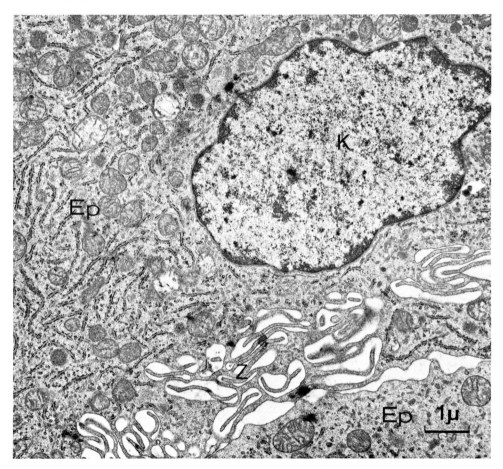

Fig. 38. Epithelioid cell (EP) from a hilus lymph node in pulmonary tuberculosis. Large ovoid nucleus (K) with scanty marginal heterochromatin. The cytoplasm is rich in mitochondria and has well developed rough endoplasmic reticulum. The number of cytoplasmic processes (Z) is noteworthy. 12000-×. (Kistler).

Giant Cells

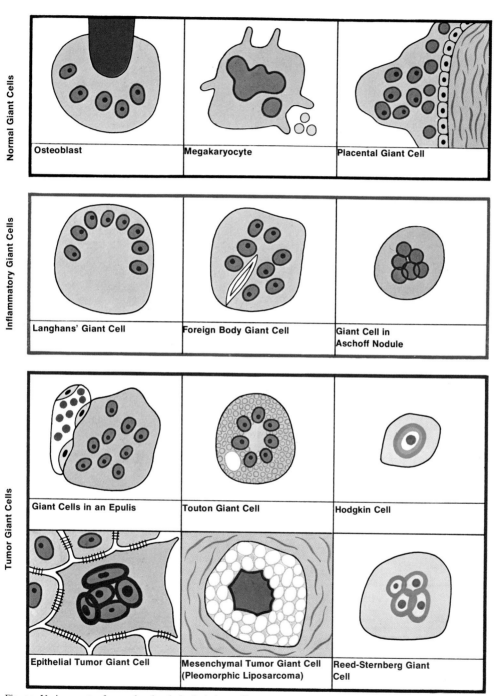

Fig. 39. Various sorts of normal and pathological giant cells.

Addendum

The student and young physician can easily forget that the pathologist has an important function to play in the preservation and care of the state of health. In practice, this function is often manifestly concerned with the examination of *biopsy material,* since frequently the decision between life and death for the patient depends upon the pathologist's diagnosis. An *unequivocable histological opinion* can lead the clinician to a single, simple diagnosis. In many cases, the correct interpretation of the histological appearance is suggested by the clinical findings, being dependent upon such things as the site from which the biopsy specimen was taken and the age and sex of the patient. This information is often essential for pathological diagnosis. For this reason, it is important that the form accompanying the request for examination of an important biopsy specimen be completely filled out by the person submitting it. Likewise, the fixation of the biopsy specimen must be just right (aqueous 40% formalin diluted 1:9, the ratio of specimen to volume of fixative at least 1:20, thickness of tissue block not more than 1 cm.). As to the biopsy itself, it is essential that *both normal and diseased tissue be removed,* so that the two can be compared in the histological preparation. In the case of polyps and papillomas, the tissue in the deepest part of the biopsy should be most carefully examined in order to discover possible invasion.

The use of frozen sections, which can be cut on the cryostat and stained in a few minutes, enables the pathologist to make a quick diagnosis during a surgical operation. This allows the surgeon to plan his operation, for example, in a case of suspected carcinoma of the breast–to decide the necessity of removing the axillary lymph nodes. The accuracy of a diagnosis made from a frozen section by a competent pathologist is almost as good as from a paraffin section. But there are limitations to the use of rapid frozen sections for diagnosis and certain questions cannot be answered. The method is only rarely helpful in diagnosing the different diseases of lymph nodes.

Every piece of tissue removed from a patient should be examined histologically–a requirement that the physician in his own best interests should never neglect, even when the macroscopic appearances seem ever so plain.

If a physician takes to heart these simple rules, he cannot fail to help his patients.

Systemic Pathology

1. Heart

The brief introductory remarks about the normal microscopic anatomy of each of the organs discussed in the rest of the book are based on standard textbooks, such as MAXIMOFF and DEMPSEY and PORTER.

Heart muscle shows cross-striations, centrally placed oval nuclei and a syncytial arrangement of the fibers with slender anastomoses. By comparison, *skeletal muscle* shows no such anastomoses between fibers, and the nuclei lie at the periphery of the cells, whereas *smooth muscle,* although showing centrally located nuclei, lacks cross-striations. The cross-striations depend upon the presence of myofilaments with isotropic and anisotropic bands. The intercalated disks are bright, narrow bands that demarcate the longitudinal limits of individual heart muscle cells (see p. 37). Between the muscle fibers there is a small amount of connective tissue containing capillaries and larger vessels.

The *endocardium* is made up of a single layer of endothelium lying on a bed of loosely arranged elastic and collagen fibers.

The *leaflets of the heart valves* are avascular, covered with endothelium and contain collagen and elastic fibers.

Epicardium and pericardium are both covered with flattened cells.

In evaluating *pathological changes* in heart muscle, attention should be paid to the width of the fibers, foreign materials in the sarcoplasm (fat, glycogen, etc.), the cell nuclei, and the cellular constituents of the interstitial tissue. In looking at the valves, pay particular attention to vascularization and, of course, to thickening of the valve substance and to surface deposits. The epicardium and pericardium frequently show a coating of fibrin in pathological conditions.

Polypoidy may be seen in the heart muscle of aged persons or in hypertrophied hearts (Figs. 1.1 and 1.2). Until age 9–12 years diploid nuclei usually predominate (Fig. 1.2 lower right), in adult life tetraploid nuclei are usual (Fig. 1.2 middle). In cardiac hypertrophy nuclei appear with a DNA content of 8_c, 16_c and 32_c (8_c = upper portion of Fig. 1.2). Thus the DNA content may be as much as 16 fold greater than in diploid nuclei (2_c). Polypoidy also occurs in children with cardiac failure. It seems probable that polypoidy is due to increased function.

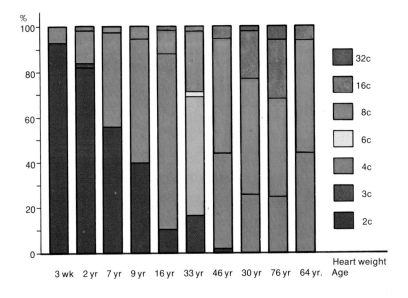
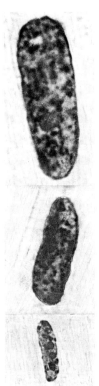

Fig. 1.1 (Above). Pattern of development of polypoidy in human heart muscle.
Fig. 1.2 (right side). Heart muscle nuclei (Feulgen reaction to show DNA). Below, a diploid nucleus (2_c), in the middle a tetraploid (4_c) and above an octoploid nucleus (8_c), 1200X.

34

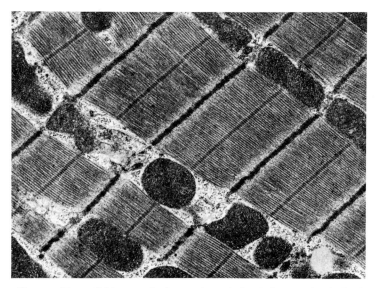

Fig. 1.3. Myocardial hypertrophy in experimental chronic hypertension in the dog. Thick bundles of myofibrils with large mitochondria rich in cristae (Knieriem).

In **atrophy of heart muscle** the natural brown color of **lipofuscin pigment** is best brought out by using hematoxylin alone, since it stains only the cell nuclei (Fig. 1.4, p. 9). The brown pigment lies at the poles of nuclei in the form of granules of different sizes. This zone is without myofilaments. The pigment is made up chiefly of unsaturated fatty acids (brown color of rancid fat) and may occur normally in heart muscle (waste pigments of cellular "wear and tear" → lysosomes).

The differentiation of lipofuscin from other pigments is given on page 9.

Macroscopically, the organs in brown atrophy are shrunked and brown.

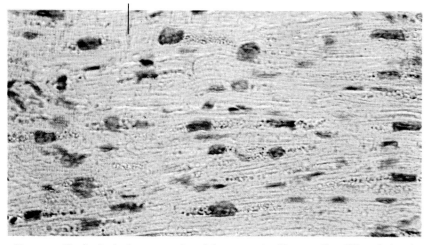

Fig. 1.4. Lipofuscin in brown atrophy of heart muscle; Hematoxylin, 600×. (→) points to an intercalated disk.

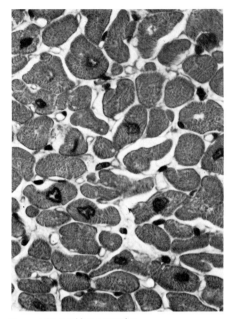

Fig. 1.5. Normal heart muscle;
H & E, 600×.

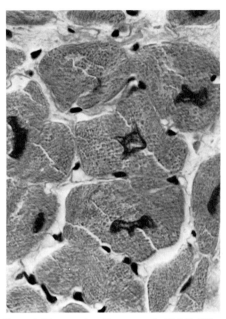

Fig. 1.6. Hypertrophy of heart muscle; H & E, 600×.

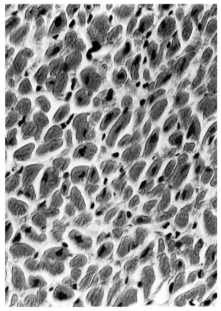

Fig. 1.7. Atrophy of heart muscle;
H & E, 600×.

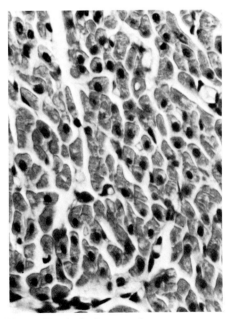

Fig. 1.8. Developing heart muscle;
H & E, 600×.

Cardiac Hypertrophy—Cardiomyopathy

The four accompanying photomicrographs have been taken at the same magnification in order to permit comparison of the changes in diseased heart muscle with the normal. The changes can be easily appreciated by comparing the *width of the muscle fibers,* the *size and shape of their nuclei* and the *number of nuclei* per section. Compared with **normal heart muscle** (Fig. 1.5), the myocardial fibers in **cardiac hypertrophy** (Fig. 1.6, heart weight 650 Gm.) are about three times as thick (in the photograph, normal fibers measure 0.8 cm., and hypertrophied fibers 2–3 cm.). Because of this, the number of nuclei per unit area of the section appears to be decreased. Likewise, the nuclei are nearly double the normal size; their DNA content corresponds to an octoploid value (see Figs. 1.1 and 1.2). The nuclei also show bizarre changes in configuration. Some observations suggest that an increase in number of fibers also occurs (normal: 2 million; 800 Gm. heart: 4 million. Sandritter and Adler 1971). In the sarcoplasm the thickening of transversely cut myofilaments can be clearly seen and, in comparison to normal myocardium, they are increased both in number and transverse measurement. Notice that normal or even atrophic fibers may appear next to hypertrophied ones.

In **atrophy of heart muscle** (Fig. 1.7, heart weight 200 Gm.), a relative increase in number of nuclei occurs; that is, a greater number of cell nuclei are seen in a unit area of the section. The fibers are clearly smaller (0.5 cm.) than in normal or hypertrophied hearts and often are also decreased in number *(numerical atrophy).* In **developing heart muscle** (Fig. 1.8, 6-year-old child), we likewise find an apparent nuclear increase. The fibers are even smaller than in atrophy (0.4 cm.) and, by comparison, the nuclei are round and deeply stained.

Cardiomyopathy (Cardiomegaly) is a disease syndrome recognized clinically by functional manifestations and enlargement of the heart. Two sorts are recognized: **secondary cardiomyopathy** due to known causes (cardiac enlargement due to endocrine disturbances such as acromegaly, hyper- and hypo-thyroidism, infectious diseases, collagen diseases, sarcoidosis, alcoholism etc.) and *primary cardiomyopathy* (due to unknown causes, idiopathic cardiomyopathy). In the **hypertrophic form** (Fig. 1.9) both parts of the ventricular septum are very thick (greater than 1.5 cm.), especially in the upper portion of the septum. Hypertrophied ventricular septum functions like a *subaortic stenosis.* Histologically the myocardial bundles have a disorderly pattern due to loss of their normal parallel arrangement and form a tangled network of fibers *(congenital, no hypertension).* The second type is manifested by *dilatation of all cardiac chambers* with relative mitral insufficiency *(dilatation type* of cardiomyopathy). There is no clear morphological correlation (Roberts and Ferrans, 1975; Knieriem and co-authors, 1975).

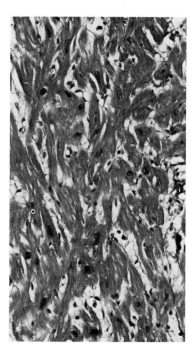

Fig. 1.9. Non-obstructive hypertrophic cardiomyopathy (10-year-old child). Note the tangled arrangement of the myocardial bundles; H & E, 180× (Knieriem).

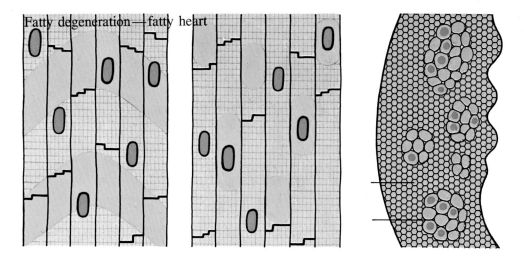

Fig. 1.10. Fatty degeneration–fat infiltration of heart.

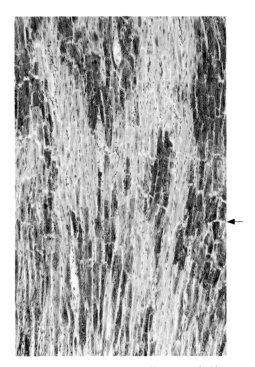

Fig. 1.11. Fatty degeneration of heart muscle (tigering); Sudan—hematoxylin, 82×.

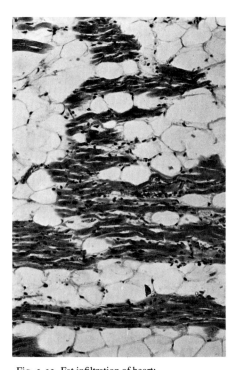

Fig. 1.12. Fat infiltration of heart; H & E, 148×.

Fatty Degeneration–Fat Infiltration

Fatty degeneration (fatty metamorphosis) of heart muscle must be clearly separated from *fat infiltration* or fatty heart (Fig. 1.10).
Fatty degeneration appears in two forms:
1. A *band or streak-like form* in which segments of myocardial fibers containing fat alternate regularly with unchanged fibers so that an appearance like that of a tiger's skin results. The fatty streaks lie next to the venous limbs of capillaries. The cause of this form of fatty degeneration is generalized, deficient oxygenation of the heart muscle.

It is seen frequently in aplastic or pernicious anemia, in massive blood loss or so-called *anemic anoxia* and less frequently in leukemia. This sort of fatty degeneration can likewise be caused by generalized oxygen lack due to disturbances of lung ventilation *(asphyxic anoxia).*

2. A *disseminated focal form,* affecting irregular areas of the heart, in which there is fatty degeneration of single fibers or portions of fibers, usually in association with other degenerative changes of heart muscle such as clumping of sarcoplasm (see p. 46). These changes appear at the edges of myocardial infarcts, after toxic injuries of heart muscles, such as diphtheria or interstitial myocarditis, and after poisoning, for example, with phosphorus, arsenic chloroform, ether and fungi.

Macroscopically, the heart is dilated and shows small, speck-like, grayish yellow spots.

In **fatty degeneration of the myocardium** (tigering), the essential changes can be seen at a glance (Fig. 1.11). In sections stained with Sudan or scarlet-red, the striped pattern of the fatty myocardial fibers clearly contrasts with the unaltered fibers which are stained faintly blue by the hematoxylin. The resemblance to the skin of a tiger is very striking, since the stripes vary in width and often do not run exactly parallel through the entire section of tissue, but branch frequently. High magnification shows that the fat is in the form of fine droplets laid down between the myofilaments (see p. 45). Notice the segmentation of the heart muscle fibers in both the right-hand ($\rightarrow$) and left-hand parts of the picture.

Macroscopically, the heart likewise shows a pattern resembling a tiger's skin with parallel yellow lines alternating with reddish brown muscle. It is especially well seen in the papillary muscles of the left ventricle.

In **fat infiltration** or fatty heart (Figs. 1.10., 1.12) there is both *infiltration of heart muscle with fat, such as occurs elsewhere in obesity, and transformation of connective tissue cells into fat cells.* Even with the unaided eye, one can see that the muscle bundles have been separated by finely distributed fat tissue, which extends into the musculature in tongue-like processes. The amount of subepicardial fat is also increased and, microscopically (Fig. 1.12, medium magnification), fat can be seen replacing interstitial tissue. The cell nuclei are pressed to the periphery by the fat droplets and the cytoplasm is reduced to a thin membrane. Since the fat content of the cells is dissolved by the process of paraffin embedding, in which alcohol and xylol are used, only optically empty spaces are seen in the section.

Macroscopically, fat infiltration is most pronounced in the right ventricle. The cut surface shows yellow, streak-like infiltration of the myocardium. Frequently, there are also islands of fat beneath the endocardium. In estimating the weight of the heart, especially in cardiac hypertrophy, allowance must be made for the amount of fat tissue. *Clinically,* marked obesity may cause the so-called Pickwick syndrome with elevated diaphragm, hypoventilation, cyanosis, polycythemia and cor pulmonale. Cause of death is usually pulmonary embolism. NOTE: Obesity increases the risk factor for myocardial infarction.

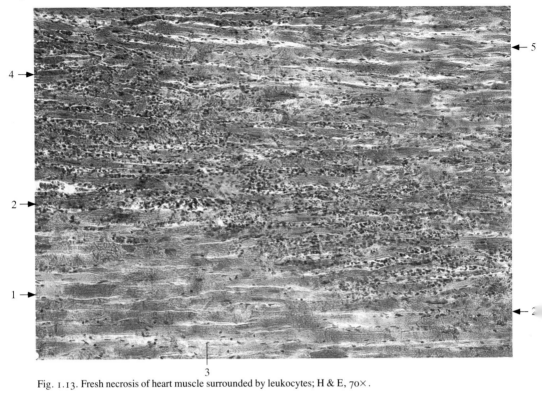

Fig. 1.13. Fresh necrosis of heart muscle surrounded by leukocytes; H & E, 70×.

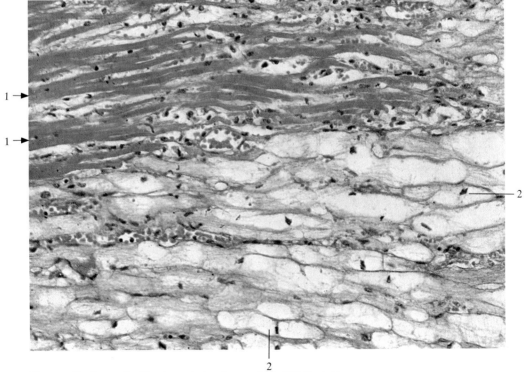

Fig. 1.14. Fresh necrosis of heart muscle showing sarcolysis; H & E, 225×.

Infarct of the Heart

*Infarcts of the heart show ischemic coagulation necrosis resulting from lack of oxygen due to obstruc-
tion of the coronary arteries (arteriosclerosis, thrombosis, which are common, or embolism, which is
rare, or narrowing of the orifices of the coronary arteries by syphilis).*
Table 1.1 shows the *time sequences* of the macroscopic and microscopic changes and of some of
the clinical events.

Table 1.1. **Time Sequences of Events in Heart Infarcts**

Time	Macroscopic	Microscopic	Other Changes
15 sec.	—	—	ECG changes (experimental)
30–60 min.	—	Edema of fibers	Electron microscopic changes (pp. 44, 45) H_2O uptake
2 hrs.	—	Hyalinization of fibers (homogeneous, eosino-philic)	Calcium loss up to 24 hours
3 hrs.	—	Clumping of sarcoplasm Fatty degeneration	Increased sodium content. Decreased enzymes of the citric acid cycle in infarct
4 hrs.	TTC-reaction negative	Necrosis	Infarct enlarging and CPK
6 hrs.	Slight pallor	Leukocytic reaction	
9 hrs.	Yellow, dry, firm	Fully developed necrosis	
18–24 hrs.	Yellow, dry, firm	Fully developed necrosis	Increased enzymes in serum
2–3 wks.	Red granulation tissue	Granulation tissue	
5 wks. 2 mos.	Scar White, firm, fibrous	Scar tissue	

Legend: TTC-Reaction = triphenyltetrazolium chloride reaction (for detection of succinic dehydrogenase).
CPK = creatinine phosphokinase (Galen, 1975)

Figure 1.13 shows a **new infarct** with fresh muscle necrosis that is about 8 hours old (→ 1) and bordered by a broad zone of leukocytic infiltration (→ 2). At the edge of the infarct, in adjacent myocardium, there is a zone of recent hemorrhage (→ 4), beyond which the myocardium is normal (→ 5).
Muscle fibers in the necrotic area lack nuclei and have homogeneous cytoplasm. Notice that the nuclei
of the interstitial connective tissue are preserved (→ 3).
Fresh Myocardial Necrosis Showing Sarcolysis. Microscopic examination of the necrotic myocardium with high magnification shows very clearly the homogenization of the sarcoplasm (Fig. 1.14 and
p. 45) and the absence of cross-striations (→ 1). The depth of staining with eosin is also noteworthy.
Myocardial nuclei have disappeared, although nuclei of the interstitial connective tissue cells are still
present. The illustration also shows advanced sarcolysis, or dissolution of necrotic sarcoplasm, leaving
only the empty shells of the sarcolemma (→ 2) (myocarditis in diphtheria). Essentially the same process, but with clumping of the sarcoplasm, is seen in Figure 1.22. Capillaries, some collapsed and
others dilated, can be recognized in the interstitial tissue. Remnants of the sarcolemma may persist in
the scar of an infarct for long periods.

Macroscopic appearance: a circumscribed, lemon yellow, dry, firm area.

Complications of Myocardial Infarcts: rupture of the ventricle with pericardial tamponade, rupture of a papillary muscle (mitral insufficiency may develop), mural thrombosis with arterial embolism, fibrinous pericarditis, acute or chronic ventricular aneurysms, cardiac shock.

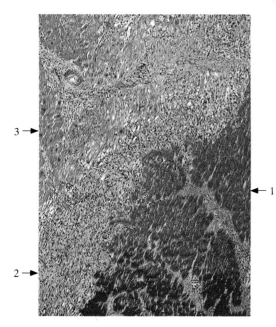

Fig. 1.15. Organization taking place in a somewhat older myocardial infarct;
H & E, 41×.

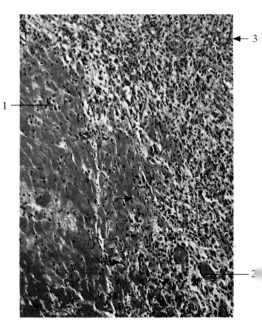

Fig. 1.16. Organization taking place in a somewhat older myocardial infarct (detail);
H & E, 120×.

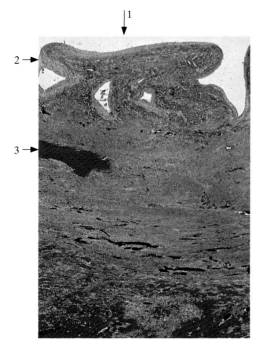

Fig. 1.17. Subendocardial myocardial scar;
H & E, 15×.

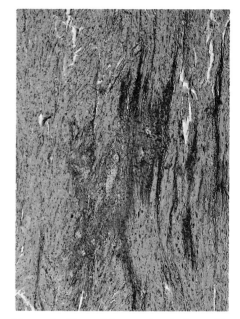

Fig. 1.18. Myocardial scars due to incomplete coronary artery insufficiency;
van Gieson, 39×.

Necrotic heart muscle will largely be reabsorbed by granulation tissue during the course of 2–3 weeks, depending upon the size of the infarct. In such an **organizing infarct** (Fig. 1.15), examination of a microscopic section with the unaided eye or at low magnification shows an irregularly shaped, intensely red area which is the *necrotic zone* (→ 1), a richly cellular layer (blue appearing) bordering the necrotic zone *(granulation tissue* → 2)*, bordered in turn by the less deeply eosin-stained *normal heart muscle* (→ 3). Medium magnification reveals the essential alteration, namely necrotic muscle fibers that have lost their nuclei. Higher magnification shows the loss of cross-striations. The cytoplasm of the myocardial fibers is homogeneous and eosinophilic. In addition, the nuclei of the interstitial tissue have nearly completely disappeared. In adjacent granulation tissue, capillaries can be seen with medium magnification as small, empty, round or ovoid spaces between which there are round cells (lymphocytes, histiocytes, see p. 24), fibroblasts and connective tissue fibers having a distinctive smooth, straight shape. The cellular infiltration seen in the granulation tissue extends only slightly into the uninjured myocardium in which well-preserved nuclei can be clearly seen.

Macroscopic: Red granulation tissue intermixed with remnants of yellow necrotic tissue.

Figure 1.16 is a detail under higher magnification of another somewhat **older infarct in the process of organization** showing the line of division between necrosis and granulation tissue. In the necrotic zone on the left-hand side of the picture are seen once again anuclear muscle fibers with homogeneous, intensely red eosinophilic sarcoplasm. The nuclei of the interstitial connective tissue are partially preserved, and in some places wandering histiocytes can already be seen (→ 1). The granulation tissue is richly cellular and contains dilated capillaries (→ 2). The earliest wandering cells to infiltrate the granulation tissue (→ in picture) are histiocytes with large round to oval nuclei and basophilic cytoplasm. In the upper right-hand part of the figure (→ 3) the granulation tissue is less cellular. A delicate background of fine collagen fibers has appeared between the small rod-shaped nuclei of the fibroblasts.

Compare this picture with the granulation tissue shown on page 54. Notice the similar structure: *wandering histiocytes*–the highly cellular *middle zone* with capillaries, angioblasts, histiocytes, lymphocytes and fibroblasts–and an *outer zone* in which fibrous tissue is being formed.

The final outcome of a myocardial infarct is a **scar of the heart muscle**. Figure 1.17 is from a section of myocardium taken perpendicular to the endocardium, so that the trabeculae (→ 1) of the inner ventricular surface can be seen. The endocardium is thickened by connective tissue (→ 2) and beneath it the muscle fibers are for the most part preserved, since they are nourished from inside the heart chambers. Next to the myocardium there is a broad layer of practically acellular collagenous tissue: the scar. At the lower margin of the picture, normal myocardium can be seen interspersed with small islands of scar tissue. Within the large scarred area there is a red area (→ 3): fresh necrosis of a surviving remnant of myocardium (recurrent infarct).

Macroscopic: White scar tissue, sometimes intermixed with yellow areas of necrosis.

Myocardial Scars in Coronary Insufficiency (Fig. 1.18) *Coronary insufficiency* (BÜCHNER) *develops because of a disproportion between the amount of oxygen needed by the myocardium and the amount of oxygen available to it* (for example, in cardiac hypertrophy or coronary arteriosclerosis with obstruction insufficient to cause massive infarction but sufficient to cause an oxygen deficiency). The essential difference from a myocardial infarct can be seen on naked-eye examination. Instead of a large necrotic area or a large scar in the heart muscle, there are small disseminated, fleck-like scars which in sections stained by van Gieson's method are colored bright red. Heart muscle stains yellow.

Macroscopic: Firm, fibrous, glistening, white scar tissue.

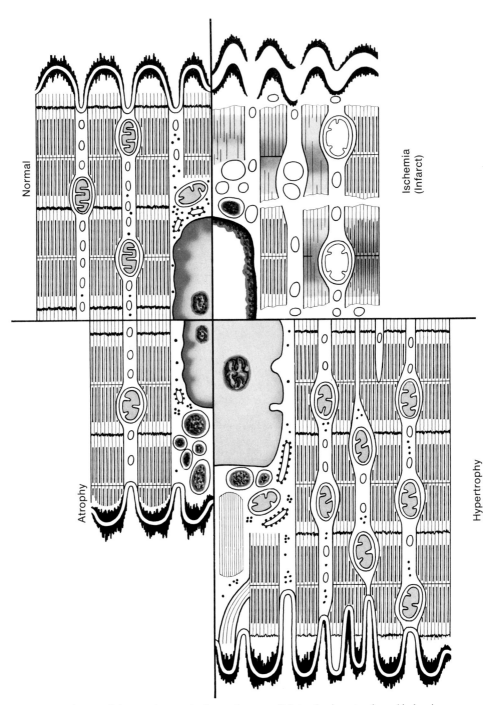

Fig. 1.19. Diagram of electronmicroscopic changes in myocardial atrophy, hypertrophy and ischemia.

Fine Structure of the Myocardium

In *myocardial hypertrophy* all myocardial cells are enlarged. Elementary fibrils are numerous, but not thickened and usually appear to be normally branched. Because of the enlargement of cells, the number of mitochondria is increased. At the nuclear poles there are accumulations of rough endoplasmic reticulum and lipofuscin granules as well as newly formed myofibrils (without sarcomere formation). Both nuclei and nuceoli are enlarged (polyploidy). The intercalated discs (cell boundries) are more separated than normal (increased electrical resistance. Altered transmural irritability).

In *cardiac atrophy* the number of myocardial cells is decreased and the number of normal sized elementary fibrils is reduced. Lipofuscin (= waste pigment) accumulates adjacent to the small sized nuclei.

In a fresh *myocardial infarct* the sarcomeres are broken (light microscopy shows fragmentation of myocardial cells) and the myofibrillar pattern is erased because of clumping of the filaments. Mitochondria become vacuolated and irreversibly injured. The nuclei show the typical hyperchromatic nuclear walls of necrosis. Contact between cells is lost due to rupture of the intercalated discs.

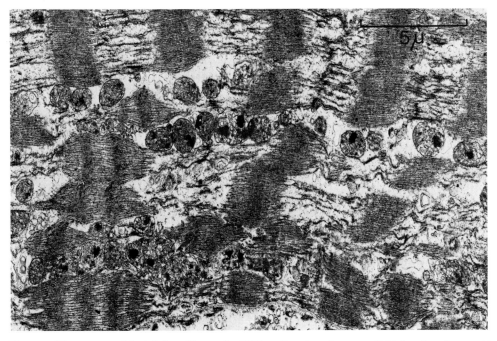

Fig. 1.20. Ultrastructure of fresh infarct 6 hours after ECG confirmation of a myocardial infarct in a 67-year-old man. Clearly recognizable sarcolysis with beginning clumping of myofilaments. Some mitochondria show dense matrix aggregates. Autopsy material. 7500×.

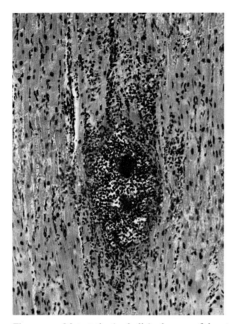

Fig. 1.21. Metastatic (embolic) abscess of heart muscle;
H & E, 141×.

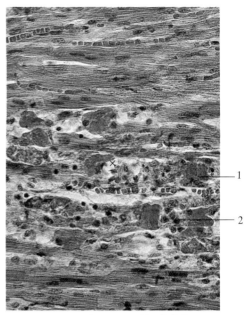

Fig. 1.22. Diphtheritic myocarditis; H & E, 315×.

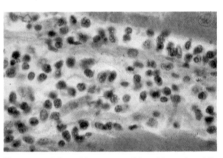

Fig. 1.24. Idiopathic myocarditis with eosinophils;
H & E, 592×.

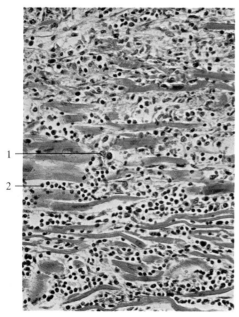

Fig. 1.23. Interstitial myocarditis in scarlet fever;
H & E, 255×.

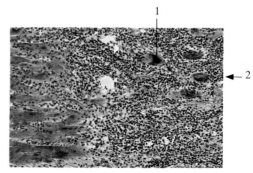

Fig. 1.25. Idiopathic myocarditis with giant cells;
H & E, 110×.

Myocarditis

Inflammations of the heart muscle may be grouped as follows:
1. *serous myocarditis,*
2. *purulent myocarditis,*
3. *non-purulent interstitial myocarditis:*
    a) degenerative or parenchymatous inflammation *(diphtheria, dysentery);*
    b) lympho-histiocytic form *(scarlet fever, infection, hypersensitivity);*
    c) granulomatous myocarditis *(idiopathic myocarditis* of Fiedler; active *rheumatic fever* with Aschoff nodules).
4. *necrotic myocarditis* (chiefly viral. Coxsackie virus). Histologically focal necrosis and exudate similar to scarlet fever.

Serous myocarditis is manifested by inflammatory edema of interstitial tissues (e.g., in thyrotoxicosis and burn injury among others, see the electron micrographs of serous inflammation, p. 25).

Purulent myocarditis originates mostly from metastatic colonies of bacteria or from septic arterial emboli (pyemic abscesses, for example, in thrombo-ulcerative endocarditis; see also kidney p. 182). Figure 1.21 shows a **metastatic abscess of the heart muscle** with centrally situated bacterial colonies (globular, dusky heart), destruction of tissue (abscess) and great infiltration of polymorphonuclear leukocytes. Neighboring tissues are sparsely infiltrated with polymorphs.

Non-purulent, diphtheritic myocarditis (Fig. 1.22) always shows *degenerative changes of the parenchymatous cells,* and the ordinary features of inflammation are not pronounced (parenchymatous or alterative inflammation). In Figure 1.22, different stages of myocardial injury can be recognized: homogenization and clumping of sarcoplasm ($\rightarrow$ 1) progressing to sarcolysis (X), so-called toxic myolysis. See also p. 40. At higher magnification, the injured fibers stain intensely red and have irregular shapes. In addition, some myocardial fibers show focal fatty change (see p. 38). Histiocytes have mobilized around degenerated fibers ($\rightarrow$ 2), to remove dead and dying debris. In addition, there are occasional polymorphonuclear leukocytes. Healing results in the formation of many small focal scars.

Macroscopic: Dilation of the heart with either small, poorly defined, grayish yellow foci or small scattered scars.

Interstitial myocarditis may occur during the course of scarlet fever. There is *infiltration of lymphocytes and histiocytes* (Fig. 1.23) and a less conspicuous degenerative component. Between the widely separated muscle fibers there is a sparse infiltration of histiocytes ($\rightarrow$ 1), lymphocytes ($\rightarrow$ 2), fibroblasts and occasional plasma cells and considerable interstitial edema. Some muscle fibers are intact, others are degenerated and some are necrotic. Develops in the third week of infectious fevers.

In some cases of myocarditis of unknown cause **(idiopathic myocarditis with eosinophils),** the myocardium is either diffusely or focally infiltrated with eosinophils (Fig. 1.24) (Allergic origin?) In addition, granulomatous inflammation **(idiopathic giant cell myocarditis)** (Fig. 1.25) may occur with a richly cellular infiltration of lymphocytes, fibrocytes and plasma cells and complete destruction of foci of heart muscle. In such cases, the inflammatory exudate contains giant cells having clumped nuclei, the so-called muscle giant cells ($\rightarrow$ 1 and 2). In sarcoidosis epithelioid cell granulomas develop.

Macroscopic: Dilatation of the heart. The cut surface shows numerous small, poorly circumscribed, grayish red or grayish yellow fleck-like foci.

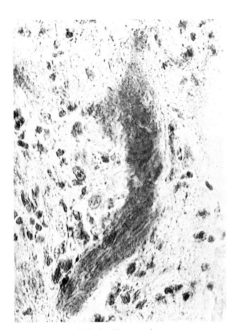

Fig. 1.26. Fresh fibrinoid necrosis.
H & E, 480×.

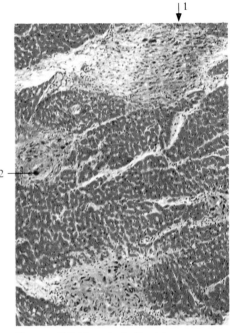

Fig. 1.27. Full-blown Aschoff nodules.
H & E, 120×.

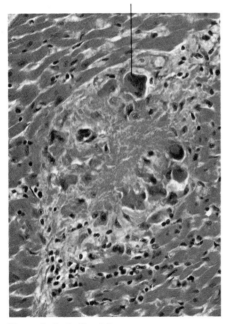

Fig. 1.28. Aschoff nodule.
H & E, 330×.

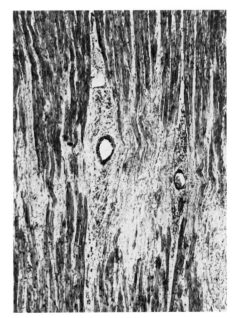

Fig. 1.29. Rheumatic scar.
H & E, 56×.

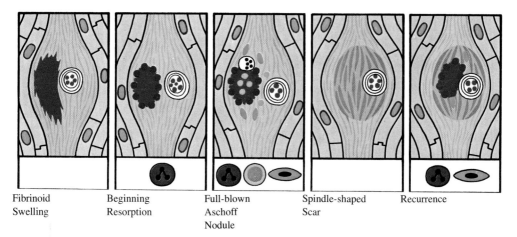

| Fibrinoid Swelling | Beginning Resorption | Full-blown Aschoff Nodule | Spindle-shaped Scar | Recurrence |

Fig. 1.30. Diagram to show the time relationships in rheumatic myocarditis. Note that the symbol for leukocytes is incorrect – it should be histiocytes.

Figure 1.30 shows the *course of rheumatic myocarditis* in active rheumatic fever. Similar changes take place in the aorta, peritonsillar tissues, heart valves and joints. *The illness begins with fibrinoid swelling (necrosis) of the perivascular connective tissue* (see also p. 11). *The body reacts by producing a histiocytic granuloma containing giant cells which is called an Aschoff nodule* (ASCHOFF, 1904). The histiocytes remove the fibrinoid material (phagocytic function of the histiocytes). *The end stage is a perivascular scar of connective tissue* in which histiocytes have been transformed into fibroblasts and have formed collagen fibers (p. 24). *Recurrences* localize preferentially in old scars.

In examining the tissue microscopically, attention should be directed to the large interstitial spaces. Figure 1.27 was taken at medium magnification and shows many **full-blown Aschoff nodules** (→ 1) with compact accumulations of histiocytes and giant cells (→ 2). High magnification shows the early change of **fresh fibrinoid necrosis** (Fig. 1.26) consisting of bright red, homogeneous material which completely obscures the connective tissues. The host reaction commences immediately with mobilization of histiocytes, which can be recognized by their large, chromatic nuclei, large nucleoli and poorly demarcated, faintly basophilic cytoplasm. A few lymphocytes are also present. Figure 1.28 shows an **Aschoff nodule** at a somewhat more advanced stage. In the center of this nodule there is fibrinoid material. At the margins there are histiocytes as well as giant cells derived in part from muscle cells (→), since in this case the inflammation has involved the myocardium.

At the termination of the acute inflammatory phase, the histiocytes become oblong in shape and form collagen fibers. As a result, perivascular **rheumatic scars** develop (Fig. 1.29). These scars appear as elongated and pointed bright red areas. In the illustration, a few solitary histiocytes are still embedded in the scar tissue.

Macroscopic: Dilatation of the heart; small, white focal scars in the healed stage. Almost always accompanied by active or subsiding rheumatic valvulitis.
Occurs in inflammatory rheumatic disorders (rheumatic fever, primary chronic polyarteritis, osteoarthritis and most commonly in rheumatism of soft tissues).

Endocarditis

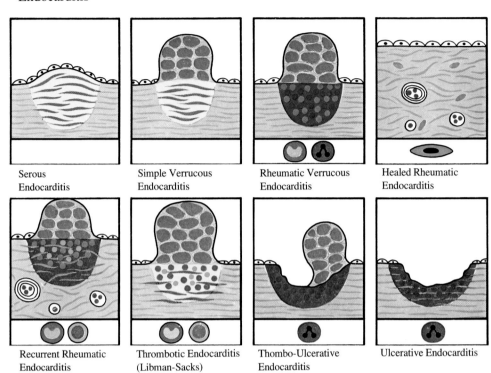

| Serous Endocarditis | Simple Verrucous Endocarditis | Rheumatic Verrucous Endocarditis | Healed Rheumatic Endocarditis |

| Recurrent Rheumatic Endocarditis | Thrombotic Endocarditis (Libman-Sacks) | Thombo-Ulcerative Endocarditis | Ulcerative Endocarditis |

Fig. 1.31. Diagrammatic representations of different sorts of endocarditis.

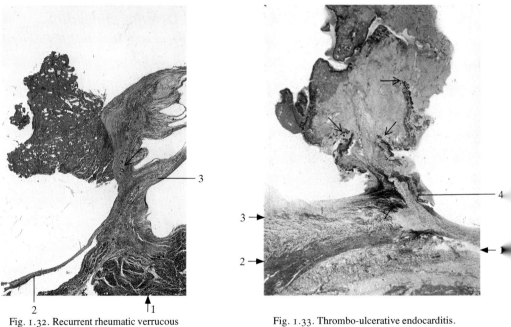

Fig. 1.32. Recurrent rheumatic verrucous endocarditis.
H & E, 10×.

Fig. 1.33. Thrombo-ulcerative endocarditis.
H & E, 11×.

Endocarditis

Endocarditis is an inflammation of the heart valves and is characterized not only by conspicuous fluid and cellular exudation in the connective tissues of the leaflets or cusps, but also by superimposed thrombosis. The changes occur chiefly at the line of closure of the valve.

The aortic cusps and mitral leaflets are preferentially affected.

There are 5 different sorts of endocarditis. 1. The mildest and most fleeting sort, and perhaps also the precursor of all other forms of endocarditis, is **serous endocarditis** (Fig. 1.31), in which blood serum proteins exude into the connective tissue of the valves and cause swelling of the fibers and interstitial edema (macroscopic: slight, glistening swelling). 2. **Simple verrucous endocarditis** (Fig. 1.31) is distinguished from rheumatic endocarditis only by the intensity of the edema and cellular reaction. A break develops in the valvular endothelium which is then overlaid by a thrombus consisting almost exclusively of blood platelets, although a small amount of fibrin is also usually present. Frequently seen in shock (deposits of aggregated platelets along the line of closure, MITTERMAYER et al., 1971). 3. **Rheumatic endocarditis** (Fig. 1.31) has almost the same microscopic appearance. However, fibrinoid swelling is marked, and correspondingly there is a more pronounced inflammatory reaction of polymorphonuclear leukocytes and histiocytes. Healing (**burned-out rheumatic endocarditis,** Fig. 1.31) is accompanied by vascularization and scarification with deformity of the valve. Recurrent attacks of rheumatic endocarditis are frequent (**recurrent rheumatic endocarditis,** Fig. 1.32).

Macroscopic examination reveals grayish white, glistening, easily wiped-off warty growths on the valve surfaces.

4. **Thrombotic endocarditis** (Libman-Sacks) is a non-bacterial endocarditis with soft, coarse thrombi formed of platelets and fibrin. There is marked fibrinoid degeneration of the valvular tissue and a decided inflammatory reaction (Fig. 1.31). The lesions are found frequently in *acute disseminated lupus erythematosus* along with renal involvement (wire loop glomerular lesions).

5. **Thrombo-ulcerative and ulcerative endocarditis** (also called endocarditis lenta or subacute bacterial endocarditis, Fig. 1.33) are in contrast to verrucous endocarditis, bacterial infections of the valves, usually Strep. viridans. Staphylococci and other infectious agents also are common. There is usually marked leukocytic infiltration and destruction of the valves.

Macroscopically, there are valvular deformities and polypoid thrombi. *Complications of endocarditis:* 1. in nonbacterial endocarditis: arterial emboli, valvular defects; 2. in bacterial endocarditis: valvular deformities, metastatic pyemic abscesses, focal embolic glomerulonephritis (Löhlein).

In **recurrent rheumatic endocarditis** (Fig. 1.32), low magnification shows thickening of the mitral leaflet due to a superimposed broad layer of red-staining eosinophilic material. Heart muscle (→ 1) is seen at the lower margin of the photograph, and the endocardium of the left ventricle at → 2. Medium magnification shows connective tissue thickening of the valve leaflet and numerous capillaries (→). The chordae tendinae show fibrous thickening (→ 3). The thrombus consists of eosinophilic material (blood platelets). From the fact that capillaries are present in the ground substance of the valve, it can be concluded that there was a previous episode of endocarditis.

Thrombo-ulcerative endocarditis (Fig. 1.33) *is a form of bacterial endocarditis with destruction of valve leaflets and superimposed, bacteria-laden thrombi.* Both low and medium magnification show aortic media (→ 1), and left ventricular myocardium (→ 2) covered by endocardium (→ 3) that has been thickened by fibrous connective tissue. Remnants of valvular tissue are still plainly seen (→ 4). A thrombus, composed of fibrin and platelets and containing bacterial colonies (→), sits on top of the valve. Calcification of the connective tissue fibers (×) at the base of the leaflet indicates that there had been previous inflammation with subsequent scarring.

Pericarditis

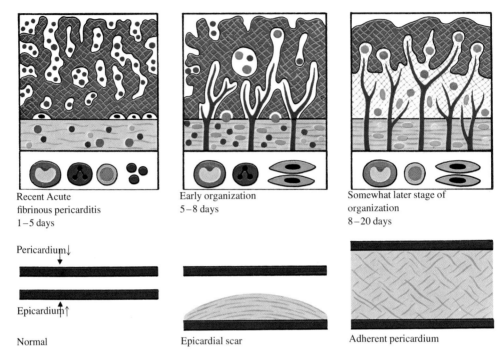

Recent Acute
fibrinous pericarditis
1–5 days

Early organization
5–8 days

Somewhat later stage of
organization
8–20 days

Pericardium↓

Epicardium↑

Normal

Epicardial scar

Adherent pericardium

Fig. 1.34. Diagram of the essential features and time sequences in pericarditis.

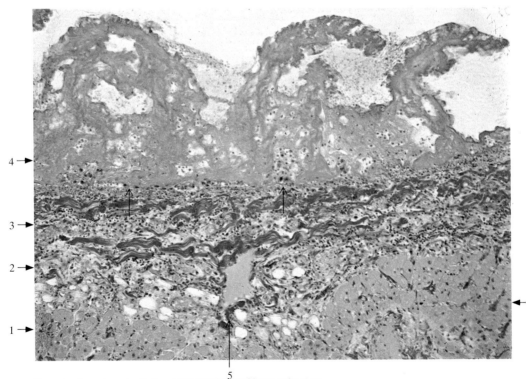

Fig. 1.35. Recent, acute, fibrinous pericarditis; van Gieson stain, 62×.

Pericarditis

Pericarditis is an inflammation of the serous coverings of the heart, including both the visceral or epicardial, and the parietal layers. All variants of the inflammatory reaction may occur (serous, fibrinous, purulent, hemorrhagic, chronic, granulomatous, etc.). *It can arise by metastasis,* for example, in sepsis or infectious diseases; *by direct extension,* for example, from the lung, pleura or esophagus; or as a *toxic response,* for example, in uremia; or as a result of *myocardial infarction.*

Any inflamed serosal surface (pleura, peritoneum, pericardium) will show the same histological changes and the same end results.

Figure 1.34 illustrates the **chief changes and the time sequence in fibrinous pericarditis.** The black areas are fibrin.

Recent acute fibrinous pericarditis (1–5 days): Fibrinogen and serum proteins have leaked from the pericardial capillaries and immediately polymerized to fibrin fibers. Irregularly shaped, tangled masses of fibrin are present on the surface of the pericardium (Fig. 1.35). The lining endothelial cells are in part destroyed and in part preserved, although swollen by irritation.

Early organization of acute fibrinous pericarditis (5–8 days): At this stage, granulation tissue (capillaries, histiocytes, fibroblasts) has begun to grow in from the epicardium and pericardium (Figs. 1.36 and 1.37), leading to destruction of the fibrin and its partial reabsorption by proteolytic enzymes of the histiocytes.

Later stage of organization of fibrinous pericarditis (8–20 days): Proliferation of granulation tissue has progressed, and increasing numbers of collagen fibers are forming from the fibroblasts in the deeper parts (Fig. 1.36).

In the end, a **pericardial scar** of collagenous tissue develops (eventually forming flat hyalinized fibrous plaques in the epicardium, known as soldier spots). If the inflammation has involved both the epicardial and parietal surfaces, the pericardial sac may be obliterated (*adhesive pericarditis, synechia pericardii,* see pp. 52, 55).

Under certain conditions (possibly activation of fibrinolytic mechanisms), the fibrin is dissolved completely and the pericardium is restored to normal. If a large amount of fluid rich in serum proteins and fibrin is a feature of the inflammation, it is called *serofibrinous pericarditis.* Pericardial adhesions usually do not develop in this form.

Recent fibrinous pericarditis (Fig. 1.35). Examination of the section with either the unaided eye or a hand lens discloses three layers: a broad, compact layer of *heart muscle* stained yellow with van Gieson's stain (→ 1), a loose layer of *subepicardial fat tissue* (→ 2) and a shaggy outer *layer of fibrin* (→ 4). With medium magnification, the details can be better seen: the layer of muscle fibers, the layer of loosely arranged connective tissue (van Gieson red, → 3) and fat showing the usual round, optically empty spaces, and occasional infiltrated granulocytes and lymphocytes. The over-lying fibrin is colored yellow with van Gieson's stain and appears as compact masses between which stretches a fine network of fibrin threads, which is seen especially well at the surface. A few leukocytes and erythrocytes are enmeshed in the fibrin network together with a pale yellow-stained, homogeneous, proteinacious material. Notice that only an occasional enlarged cell of the surface endothelium (mesothelium) can be seen (→). A small vein in the fat tissue shows plasma stasis (homogeneous yellow in the van Gieson stain, → 5).

Macroscopic: The surface is dull and shaggy (shaggy heart, cor villosum).

Note: Fibrinous inflammation commonly undergoes fibrous organization resulting in *fibrous adhesions.* For a surgeon, this is important. With fibrinous exudate he must look for the cause of the inflammation: fibrous adhesions indicate a healed lesion.

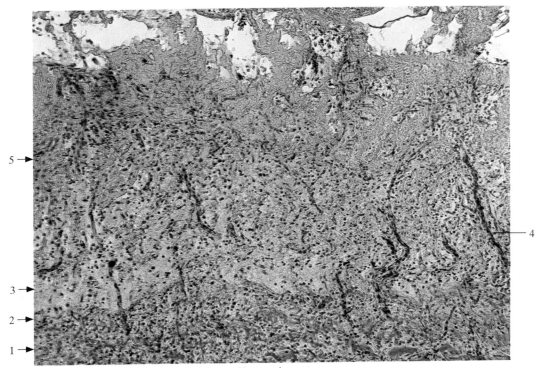

Fig.1.36. Organizing fibrinous pericarditis; van Gieson stain, 99×.

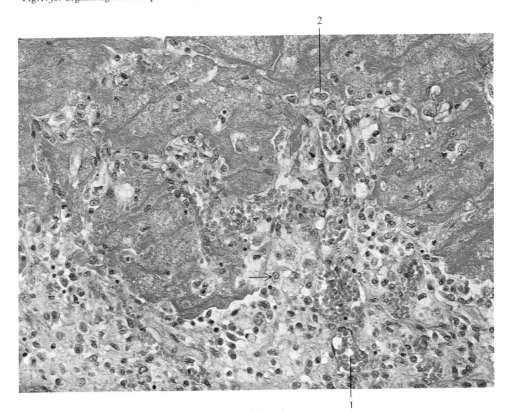

Fig.1.37. Organizing fibrinous pericarditis (detail); H & E, 248 ×.

Organizing fibrinous pericarditis (Fig. 1.36). After about 5 days, granulation tissue begins to invade the fibrin. Examination of a microscopic preparation with a hand lens still shows preservation of the three layers (muscle, fat tissue, superficial layer of fibrin) the subepicardial fat tissue is not clearly demarcated and is densely infiltrated with cells and permeated with collagenous fibrous tissue. With medium magnification and a van Gieson preparation (Fig. 1.36), interlacing of the red-stained epicardial fibers can be seen (→ 1) as well as the infiltration of histiocytes, fibroblasts and lymphocytes (→ 2), which originate from the epicardium. This is followed by the appearance of granulation tissue composed of pale red newly formed connective tissue fibers (→ 3). The vascular sprouts in the connective tissue (→ 4) can be seen clearly to have their origin in the pericardium and from there to course perpendicularly to the surface. The granulation tissue shows fibroblast nuclei (cut longitudinally) and occasional lymphocytes. In the upper portion of the section, the remaining strands of fibrin (→ 5) resemble tongue-like projections into granulation tissue. In many places, lacunae of various shapes have formed in the fibrin, where the histiocytes have brought about resorption.

Macroscopic: Surfaces covered with a grayish white, firmly adherent shaggy layer.

Figure 1.37, **organizing fibrinous pericarditis,** shows the boundary between the fibrin and the connective tissue at high magnification. In the lower portion of the figure, loosely arranged fibrin is being replaced by granulation tissue. Histiocytes (→, also see Fig. 27), lymphocytes and solitary fibroblasts can be seen (also see p. 24), as well as dilated capillaries filled with erythrocytes (→ 1). In the path of the advancing granulation tissue, wandering histiocytes are also found lying in spaces free of fibrin (resorption lacunae → 2).

Pericardial adhesions (Fig. 1.38) may be the end result of fibrinous pericarditis. In our illustration, heart muscle (→ 1) is seen at the bottom of the photograph, overlaid by a thin remnant of subepicardial fat tissue. Above it there is loosely arranged and richly vascularized new connective tissue which fills the space between the two layers of the pericardium. The compact connective tissue of the parietal layer (→ 2) and the mediastinal fat tissue (→ 3) occupy the upper half of the photograph. Mesothelial cells line clefts between the strands of connective tissue so that adenomatous structures may form, which must not be mistaken for metastases of an adenocarcinoma (also peritoneal and pleural adhesions).

Adhesions always carry the possibility of *obliteration* of the pericardial space. However, in most cases, fibrinous pericarditis is inconsequential and only scattered, delicate, easily freed fibrous adhesions are formed.

In *recurrent pericarditis,* additional new granulation tissue is laid down and cicatrized so that eventually a thick, tough, fibrous scar is formed which may sometimes become calcified (armored heart). Pleuritis or peritonitis may have a similar outcome (flat, hyalinized or calcified pleural scars; exuberant peritoneal fibrosis).

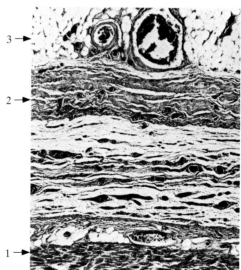

Fig. 1.38. Pericardial adhesion; H & E, 30×.

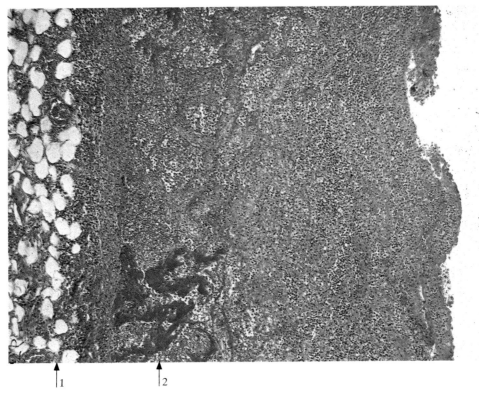

Fig.1.39. Fibrinopurulent pericarditis; H & E, 90×.

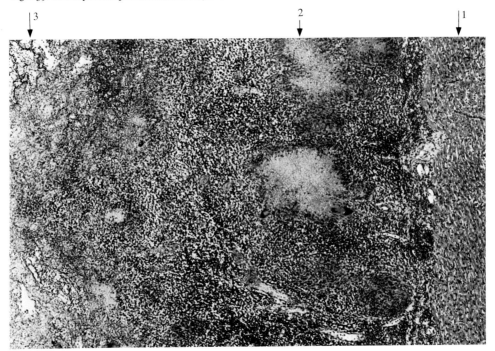

Fig.1.40. Tuberculous pericarditis; van Gieson stain, 42×.

Fibrinopurulent Pericarditis (Fig. 1.39). As has been mentioned for other forms of pericarditis, naked-eye examination of a microscopic slide shows three distinct layers—heart muscle, subepicardial fat tissue and a layer of fibrinous exudate. The figure which does not include heart muscle, shows subepicardial fat (→ 1) covered with fibrin. Just as in non-purulent fibrinous pericarditis, examination with a hand lens shows that the fibrin layer on the surface has a distinctly bluish cast and the network-like structure of the fibrin is largely absent. This is because of dense infiltration of the fibrin with cells which, under high magnification, are seen to be polymorphonuclear leukocytes with typical lobulated nuclei. For the most part, the cytoplasm of these cells is poorly demarcated from surrounding fibrinous exudate. In this particular preparation, only a few clumps of deeply eosinophilic fibrin lie directly on the epicardium (→ 2). The superimposed, more homogeneous, red-staining masses in which the leukocytes are enmeshed consist of coagulated blood plasma, fibrin and erythrocytes. The loosely arranged fibro-adipose tissue of the epicardium on the left-hand side is likewise infiltrated with leukocytes.

Macroscopic examination shows a shaggy heart just as in fibrinous pericarditis, except it is usually not grayish white but rather grayish yellow. Creamy, cloudy, or flocculent exudate fills the pericardial sac (specific gravity in excess of 1018).

Tuberculous Pericarditis (Fig. 1.40). As in fibrinous pericarditis, pericarditis caused by specific infections, such as tuberculosis, is remarkable for the degree of cellular infiltration (→ 1). In addition, round or irregularly shaped granulomas are present that have red, eosinophilic, acellular centers (→ 2) and are surrounded by a cellular zone. Medium magnification shows the typical features of such a tubercle (see p. 106ff.):

1. Central *caseation necrosis* with either a homogeneous or finely granular appearance.
2. A zone of radially arranged *epithelioid cells* surrounding the caseous center. The cells are arranged side by side like epithelial cells; therefore, the term epithelioid.
3. *Langhans giant cells* with nuclei arranged in semi-lunar fashion and in such a way that the opening of the half moon is turned toward the necrosis.
4. A marginal zone of *connective tissue* containing lymphocytes which are scanty, however, in the adjacent tissue.

Between individual tubercles there is an exudate of fibrin and serum rich in leukocytes and lymphocytes. Fibrin can be seen to the right in the figure (→ 3). At the myocardial edge (→ 1), which is chiefly subepicardial fat tissue, numerous lymphocytes accompany the advancing granulation tissue, in which are seen empty double-contoured, capillary sprouts. Tuberculous pericarditis usually arises secondarily most commonly by way of lymphatics or blood vessels, and less commonly by direct extension from neighboring structures. Frequently, an adherent tuberculous bronchopulmonary lymph node is the most probable site of origin.

Macroscopically, the appearance is that of fibrinous pericarditis, but the layer of exudate is yellowish gray and caseous nodules are seen on the cut surfaces. Eventually, a dense adherent pericarditis develops, often with obliteration of the pericardial space, calcification and even constriction of the heart (constrictive pericarditis).

Arteriosclerosis

Aorta

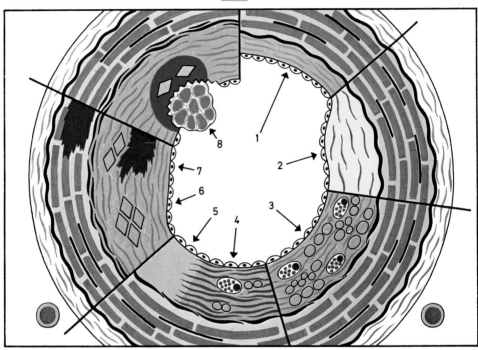

Muscular Arteries

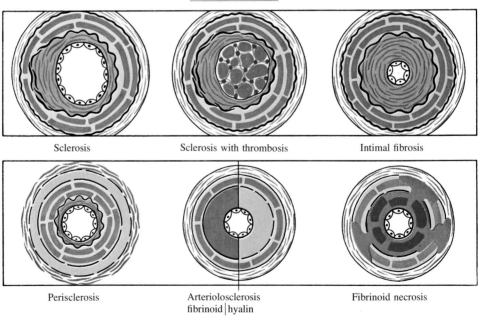

Sclerosis	Sclerosis with thrombosis	Intimal fibrosis

Perisclerosis	Arteriolosclerosis fibrinoid | hyalin	Fibrinoid necrosis

Fig. 2.1. Diagram of various forms of arteriosclerosis.

2. Blood Vessels

In order to evaluate the pathological changes that occur in blood vessels, it is first necessary to be clear as to the kind of blood vessel that is involved–arteries, veins or capillaries. **Arteries of elastic type** (e.g., aorta, subclavian and iliac arteries, etc.), the media of which contains elastic membranes and smooth muscle cells, are especially prone to intimal sclerosis and atherosclerosis (perhaps also medial necrosis, syphilitic medial inflammation). Arteriosclerosis in *large arteries* of **muscular type** (e.g., femoral, popliteal and brachial arteries), which have distinct internal and external elastic lamina, may show medial calcification in addition to intimal sclerosis or can present as an endarteritis obliterans (arteries of the legs). In *small arteries of muscular type,* such as the coronary arteries, the arteries at the base of the brain and those in the renal medulla, arteriosclerosis develops chiefly as focal semi-lunar zones of elastosis and sclerosis. In **arterioles,** arteriosclerosis takes the form of hyalin deposition (arteriolosclerosis). The malignant form of nephrosclerosis as well as periarteritis nodosa likewise (involves arterioles.)

Histological examination should take note of the thickness of the intima, alterations of the media (deposits, inflammatory infiltrates, structural changes) and any cellular infiltrate in the adventitia.

Survey of the various forms of arteriosclerosis (Fig. 2.1).

Arteriosclerosis is a chronic, progressive disease of arteries characterized by deposition of pathological metabolic products and accompanied by tissue proliferation and reconstruction of the vessel wall. Recent studies suggest that arteriosclerosis begins with **edema of the intima** (Fig. 2.1 → 1 Normal, → 2 Intimal edema). Because of this, the intima becomes swollen (glassy macroscopic appearance) with faintly homogenous staining protein material and fibrin situated between connective tissue fibers. This stage is fleeting and reversible. More easily recognized grossly are the **fatty flecks and streaks**–lipidosis–(Fig. 2.2, → 3) caused by deposition of fine droplets of fat (lipoprotein) between the connective tissue fibers of the intima and secondary phagocytosis of the fat droplets by macrophages (macroscopically, flat yellow flecks and streaks).

This stage is reversible, but it can also go on to the next stage–a **fibrous or sclerotic plaque** (Figs. 2.1 → 4, 2.3, 2.6). At this stage, there is a great increase in the intimal connective tissue, which frequently is hyalinized, with simultaneous splitting of the elastic lamellae of the internal elastic membrane. The lipids then fuse into larger foci and, at the same time, *necrosis* develops, probably due to pressure from swelling (Figs. 2.1 → 5, 2.3). As a result, anuclear zones develop with typical spear-shaped spaces corresponding to the shape of cholesterin crystals (**atheroma** with macroscopically visible yellowish white masses and glistening cholesterin crystals, Figs. 2.1 → 6, 2.3, 2.4). Occasional phagocytic cells with vacuolated cytoplasm (foam cells) can be seen at the margins of the atheroma as a reaction to the deposition of fat.

An atheroma may ulcerate and a parietal thrombus form secondarily **(atheromatous ulcer with thrombosis** Fig. 2.1 → 8).** Simultaneously with the development of sclerosis and atheromatosis of the intima, fibrous tissue and mucopolysaccharides are increased in the media (increased mucoid ground substances, uncoupling of reactive groups of the mucopolysaccharides) and fine deposits of calcium are laid down (Fig. 2.1 → 7).

Complications: Thrombosis of ulcerated atheromatous plaques and possible arterial embolization; cholesterol crystal emboli, ectasia, aneurysms, intimal hemorrhages.

Medial calcification (p. 64) causes pipe-stem arteries in the extremities (detected by palpation).

Sclerosis of medium and small arteries (e.g., the coronary arteries) results mostly in semilunar narrowing of the arterial lumen and atrophy of the media. Hemorrhage into the atheromatous plaque and secondary thrombosis may develop (see Figs. 2.1, 2.6, 2.7, 2.8).

Hyalinization of arterioles (arteriolosclerosis or arteriolarsclerosis) is characterized microscopically by homogenization of the vessel wall and consequent atrophy of the media (pp. 58, 61). The hyaline material lies between the intima and media (Fig. 2.1, bottom, middle).

Intimal fibrosis (Fig. 2.1) is seen in inflammatory lesions that encroach upon the walls of arteries, e.g. in the margins of gastric ulcers or pulmonary tuberculous cavities (a reactive defense mechanism against hemorrhage).

Perisclerosis (Fig. 2.1) with deposition of hyaline in the adventitia is seen in the retinal arterioles in hypertension.

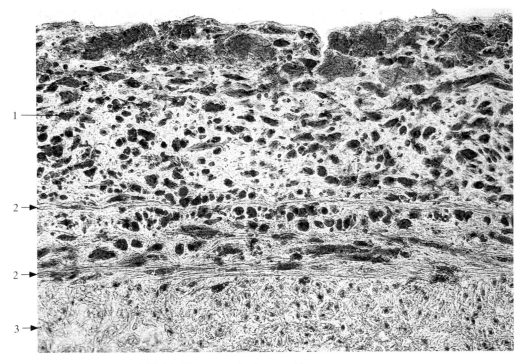

Fig. 2.2. Fatty streak (lipidosis) of the aorta; sudan-hematoxylin, 252×.

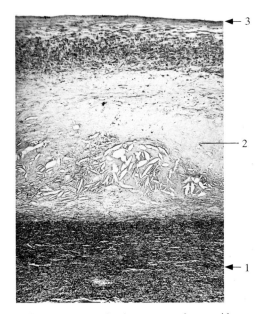

Fig. 2.3. Base of atheromatous plaque with pressure necrosis due to swelling; H & E, 40×.

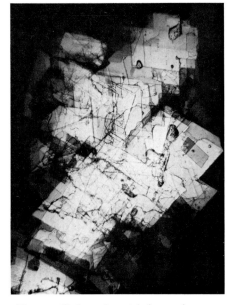

Fig. 2.4. Cholesterol crystals in an atheroma as seen in the polarizing microscope; unstained, 100×.

Arteriosclerosis of the Aorta

Fatty streak (lipidosis) of the aorta (Fig. 2.2). The earliest visible sign of aortic arteriosclerosis is *deposition of lipids and protein material in the intima*. The lipids persist, although frequently they are of no consequence. They can disintegrate or be carried away by the lymph stream (e.g., the so-called aortic milk-streaks of children). Thus, a fatty streak is not necessarily the same as arteriosclerosis. The disease process is initiated first by a mesenchymal reaction in the intima, and only after this is it progressive. Fatty streaks (lipidosis) are thus only an indicator of abnormal permeability of the vessel wall. The less readily visible protein material is probably the chief irritant of the mesenchymal tissues.

In sections stained for fat and examined with a scanning lens, the three layers of the aorta can be easily recognized: adventitia containing nutrient vessels, media which appears as a blue, homogeneous band and intima which shows cushion-like thickening and small, red focal deposits. With medium magnification (Fig. 2.2), the intima, in addition to the red-stained areas of fat, is seen to be stained pale blue and to contain collagen fibers and occasional longitudinally cut nuclei of myocytes. The intima is thickened in the region of the sudan-positive areas. In the uppermost layers of the intima, the lipids form large aggregates, while in the remaining portions of the intima the lipid is in the form of fine droplets contained in round or oval cells with marginally situated nuclei (histiocytes and phagocytes, → 1). These cells were first seen in 1852 by ROKITANSKY and later described more accurately by LANGHANS (1866). Recent studies show these are intimal smooth muscle cells that have acquired phagocytic functions. In Figure 2.2 the internal elastic membrane is already somewhat splintered (→ 2). The media is finely dusted with fatty material (→ 3: muscle cells of the media). With polarized light, doubly refractive material (cholesterol) can be easily demonstrated (Fig. 2.4).

Macroscopic: Yellow, flat lesions, often streak-like.

Base of atheromatous aortic plaque with necrosis due to swelling (Fig. 2.3). The deposition of lipids and protein in the intimal evokes fibroblastic proliferation and collagen fiber production and leads to fibrous thickening of the intima (→ 1 aortic media; → 3 endothelium). The fibroblasts arise from myocytes. When great thickening develops, the intima may well be thicker than the media in some places. Under medium magnification, compactly arranged, eosinophilic, collagenous fibers and a few fibrocytes can be seen. Some areas are completely devoid of cell nuclei. The fibers appear homogeneous, strongly eosinophilic and can no longer be distinguished as separate cells as they fuse into an amorphous substance (necrosis following swelling → 2).

Cholesterol crystals are deposited in such areas and appear as spear-shaped spaces in paraffin sections (Fig. 2.3), whereas in smears examined with the polarizing microscope they appear as doubly refractive rhomboid plates (Fig. 2.4). The media contains increased amounts of mucopolysaccharides (blue staining, chromotropic ground substance) and frequently finely granular calcium deposits.

Macroscopic: Raised lesions which, on sectioning, show glistening cholesterol crystals (atheroma).

In hyaline arteriolosclerosis (Fig. 2.5) deposits of blood proteins and lipids are also seen between the intima and media. The media is much atrophied and only solitary nuclei remain.

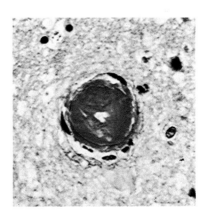

Fig. 2.5. Hyaline arteriolosclerosis in the brain. Azan stain, 200×.

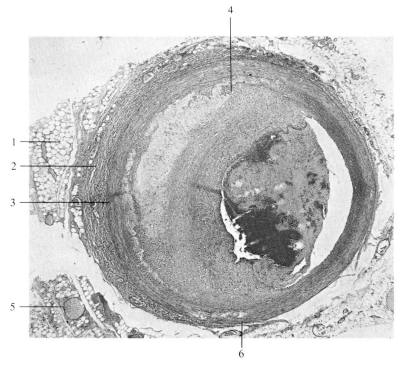

Fig. 2.6. High-grade coronary arteriosclerosis with a recent thrombus; H & E, 26×.

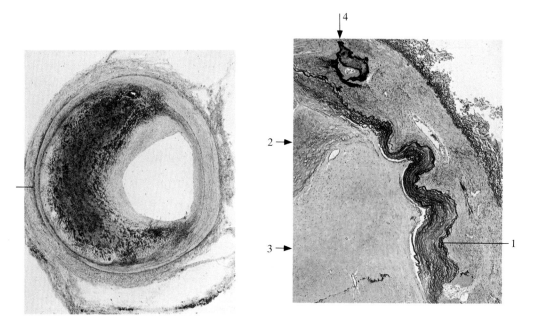

Fig. 2.7. Coronary arteriosclerosis with atheroma formation; suda stain, 14×.

Coronary arteriosclerosis

Among the common diseases of the vascular system, coronary arteriosclerosis and its frequent sequel, a myocardial infarct, takes a foremost place. It arises like the other forms of arteriosclerosis from fat deposition and is followed by sclerosis. Sometimes, marked edema of the intima develops and the artery is suddenly obstructed (a cause of death in young persons). Complications include secondary thrombosis, bleeding in a sclerotic plaque or necrosis from excessive swelling, all of which may lead to sudden narrowing of the lumen of the vessel. Today it is generally thought that coronary thrombosis is the primary event. Hyalinization of small intramural (myocardial) branches is also commonly seen. In discussing the pathogenesis of a myocardial infarct, it is necessary not only to consider the state of the coronary arteries, but also the condition of the myocardium. Hypertrophy and increased cardiac function require increased metabolism. For example, if myocardial metabolism is boosted by adrenalin then a lesser degree of coronary sclerosis can cause necrosis. ATP raises calcium intake, ATPase is activated and ATP consumption is increased resulting in a negative balance (hyperfunctional necrosis, Fleckenstein et al, 1975).

High-grade coronary sclerosis with a recent thrombus (Fig. 2.6). The changes are well shown by examining a cross-section of a coronary artery. The coronary artery is embedded in subepicardial fat tissue ($\rightarrow$ 1). The loosely arranged adventitia ($\rightarrow$ 2) forms an outer mantle. The media appears as a red ring ($\rightarrow$ 3). The intima is thickened by a crescent-shaped layer of fibrous tissue with a lightly stained atheromatous base in which necrosis has occurred as a result of swelling ($\rightarrow$ 4). What remains of the lumen is filled with a preformed thrombus consisting chiefly of platelets, fibrin and erythrocytes (conglutination thrombus, see p. 73). At $\rightarrow$ 5, a small nerve can be seen in the fat tissue. Interference with medial nutrition is suggested by a focus of cystic degeneration ($\rightarrow$ 6) in the media (medial necrosis). Note that the adventitia adjacent to the crescent-like area of intimal sclerosis shows an increase in collagenous connective tissue. Calcium may be deposited secondarily in both the intima and media.

Coronary arteriosclerosis with atheroma formation (Fig. 2.7). Fat stains show clearly the marked deposition of lipid in crescent-shaped areas of intimal thickening. The fatty material is partly within histiocytes and partly lying free in the tissues where it has fused (early atheroma). The inner layer of the sclerotic plaque contains no lipid. Noteworthy is the marked atrophy of the media in the base of the plaque ($\rightarrow$), a finding that is almost always present (disturbed medial nutrition caused by the plaque).

Elastosis of a coronary artery filled with an old thrombus (Fig. 2.8). Sclerosis is always accompanied by more or less marked elastosis, that is, by splintering and proliferation of the elastic fibers. Figure 2.8. shows such splintering and increase of the elastic fibers ($\rightarrow$ 1) together with an old thrombus. The lumen of the artery is partly filled with collagenous connective tissue containing a few blood vessels (cicatrized granulation tissue, $\rightarrow$ 2). The yellow homogeneous mass ($\rightarrow$ 3) is the residue of the old thrombus. In the old scar tissue in the muscle of the media can be seen a few blood vessels ($\rightarrow$ 4) that have arisen in the adventitia and grown into the thrombus.

Macroscopic: Lipidosis: Yellow, flat deposits. *Sclerosis and atheroma:* lumen narrowed by grayish yellow or yellow plaques which are frequently focal. *New thrombus:* reduction or complete closing of the lumen by gray-red masses. *Old thrombus:* grayish brown to grayish white deposits on the vessel wall, often in a form resembling a rope ladder. Preferred localization of coronary arteriosclerosis: usually 1 cm. below the origin of the descending branch of the left coronary artery.

Blood Vessels

Non-inflammatory Diseases of Blood Vessels

Medial calcification

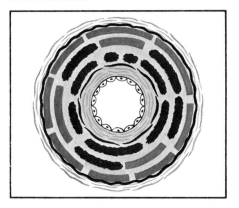

Aortic medial necrosis

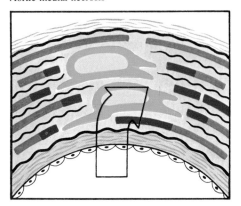

Fibromuscular arterial dysplasia

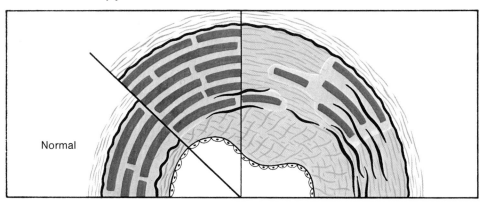

Radiation vasculopathy

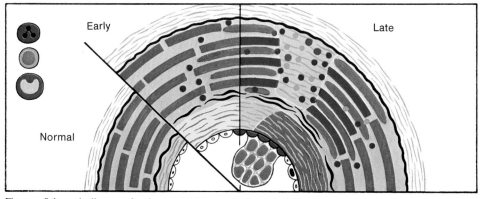

Fig. 2.9. Schematic diagram of various non-inflammatory diseases of blood vessels.

Non-inflammatory Vascular Diseases (Fig. 2.9)

Mönckeberg's Sclerosis or Medial Calcification

Affects chiefly arteries of the extremities. The calcification starts in the middle and luminal side of the media where focal deposits of calcium (calcium apatite) are laid down on the collagen and elastic fibers of the media resulting in a pipe-stem appearance of the vessels (detected by palpation). A metabolic disturbance (e.g. diabetes mellitus) which injures the myocytes in the walls of the blood vessels precedes the calcification. In part the resulting cellular detritus serves as the nidus for deposition of calcium and in part the fibrillary ground substance is so altered both qualitatively and quantitatively that calcification takes place (dystrophic calcification described by Virchow). Bony lamellae frequently form in the larger foci of medial calcium.

Aortic Medionecrosis—Idiopathic Cystic Medial Necrosis

In this condition focal areas of necrosis of myocytes and cysts filled with mucopolysaccharides (so-called mucoid lakes) develop between the elastic lamellae. The elastic framework of the media is broken here. Degenerating and necrotic medial myocytes lie at the margins of the mucoid-filled cysts, which may coalesce and cause local weakening of the wall of the aorta which can lead to rupture of the intima and portions of the media and result in a dissecting aneurysm. Such an aneurysm may rupture, typically 1–2 cm above the aortic valve; the blood stream may then dissect the media and a retrograde perforation occur in the abdominal aorta. The cause of aortic medial necrosis is probably some metabolic disturbance of mesenchymal tissues. It occurs in Marfan's syndrome in which the patients have spindly fingers and a malformed vascular system. Similar changes also occur in the pulmonary vessels in fibrocystic disease of the pancreas.

Fibromuscular Dysplasia of Arteries

This lesion occurs mostly in the large renal arteries and causes thickening of media or both media and intima resulting in stenosis of the involved artery and circulatory insufficiency. Fibrosis of the intima develops and the internal elastic lamina splits. In contrast segments of the media are thickened by collagen fibers and/or abnormal elastic fibrous tissue. There is no calcification. The disease occurs most frequently in persons between 40 and 50 years of age. The cause is thought to be a local functional disturbance of medial myocytes. It may result in renal hypertension.

Radiation Vasculopathy

The earliest lesion following x-ray radiation is injury and swelling of endothelial cells leading to seepage of plasma protein into the intima which becomes edematous. Later the media and adventitia of the vessel wall become hyperplastic.

In the late stages of radiation injury of blood vessels there is widely distributed necrosis of medial myocytes. The internal elastic lamina splinters and breaks. Fibrin from the blood stream is forced into the media. Thrombi may form on the damaged endothelium and in combination with the intimal fibrosis may occlude the vessel. Inflammatory leucocytes are seen in the areas of the necrotic medial myocytes.

Vascular Inflammation

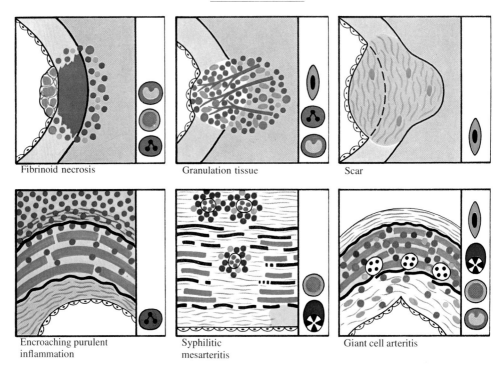

Periarteritis Nodosa

Fibrinoid necrosis   Granulation tissue   Scar

Encroaching purulent inflammation   Syphilitic mesarteritis   Giant cell arteritis

Thromboangiitis Obliterans

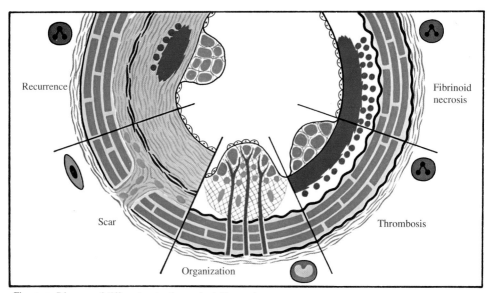

Recurrence

Fibrinoid necrosis

Scar

Thrombosis

Organization

Fig. 2.10. Diagram of different sorts of vascular inflammations.

Inflammations of Blood Vessels

Figure 2.10 on the opposite page shows the chief sorts of primary arteritis. The changes occurring in **periarteritis nodosa** (KUSSMAUL and MAIER, 1866) will serve as an example of their pathogenesis. The earliest change, or first stage, is *fibrinoid necrosis and leukocytic infiltration involving a segment of the intima and media of arterioles* (see Fig. 2.11). In the *second stage,* the fibrinoid material is reabsorbed and replaced by *granulation tissue* (see Fig. 2.12), with the result that discrete nodules form in the adventitia (periarteritis nodosa; in reality, a panarteritis). The *granulation tissue becomes cicatrized (third stage),* with consequent narrowing of the lumen, which may be marked (see Fig. 2.13). As a consequence of the inflammation and scarring, circulatory obstruction and infarction may develop (e.g., anemic infarcts in the kidney and spleen).

Giant cell arteritis (granulomatous giant cell mesarteritis) manifests itself by *fibrinoid degeneration* and a *granulomatous reaction at the intimal-medial boundary* (see Fig. 2.14). The internal elastic membrane is destroyed by the inflammatory process and the fragments of the elastic fibers elicit a foreign-body response (foreign body giant cells). Chiefly affects the temporal artery.

Note: Fibrinoid degeneration is always followed by granulation tissue and scarring (examples: verrucous endocarditis, rheumatic fever, periarteritis nodosa, thromboangiitis obliterans, giant cell arteritis, etc.).

Thromboangiitis obliterans, also called **endarteritis obliterans** (Winiwarter-Buerger's disease), shows essentially the same inflammatory process that occurs in periarteritis nodosa. The disease process is initiated by fibrinoid necrosis and leakage of blood plasma into the intima. Organization is brought about by mobilization of histiocytes and granulation tissue. The disease affects chiefly the arteries of the lower extremities *(juvenile gangrene of the extremities).* Occasionally, the cerebral, mesenteric or coronary arteries are involved.

The *earliest changes* in the disease consist of *fibrinoid degeneration (necrosis) of the intima,* with a sparse leukocytic reaction extending as far as the internal elastic membrane. *Thrombi* may or may not form on the injured intima. This is followed either by granulation tissue growing from the adventitia into the site of injury *(organization)* or by mobilization from the local connective tissue of fibrocytes and histiocytes which reabsorb the fibrinoid and thrombotic material. The *final residue is* an *intimal* or *intimal-medial scar* (see p. 71). Arteriosclerosis may develop secondarily. Recurrences localize in a previous scar.

Syphilitic Aortitis begins with *inflammation around the vasa vasorum in the adventitia* and only *secondarily involves the media and destroys the elastica.* Shrinkage of the resulting scars leads to contracture of the intima over the scar sites (p. 71).

The vascular changes of **Raynaud's disease** (Raynaud's gangrene) do not properly belong in the group of inflammatory vascular diseases. The disease is seen chiefly in women and is a progressive disease of the arterioles of the fingers, knees and ear lobes and runs a chronic course. There is hypertrophy of the medial musculature and slight fibrosis of the intima. The malady is thought to be an angioneuropathy.

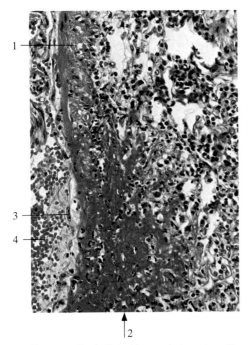

Fig. 2.10. Fresh fibrinoid necrosis in periarteritis nodosa;
H & E, 220×.

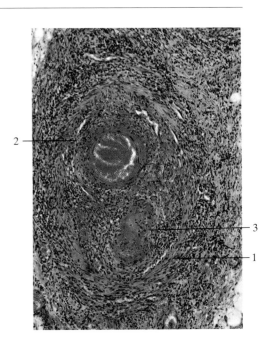

Fig. 2.11. Recurrent periarteritis nodosa;
H & E, 95×.

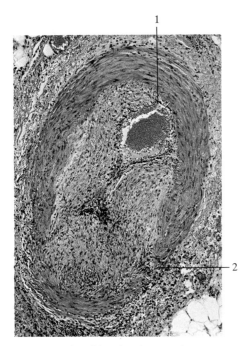

Fig. 2.12. Periarteritis nodosa (scar stage);
H & E, 74×.

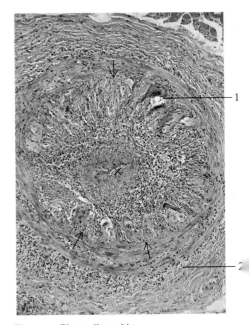

Fig. 2.13. Giant cell arteritis;
H & E, 100×.

Periarteritis Nodosa (Panarteritis)

The *earliest stage* is shown in Figure 2.11 (**fresh fibrinoid necrosis in periarteritis nodosa**). *Fresh fibrinoid necrosis* (homogeneous, strongly eosinophilic) has developed in segments of the intima and media (→ 2). In the surrounding tissues there are leukocytes and a beginning granulomatous reaction. At → 1, slightly edematous but otherwise unaffected vascular media can still be seen. The intima is lifted off the area of fibrinoid necrosis (→ 3: endothelial cells) and a loose network of fibrin and erythrocytes lies on the intimal endothelium (→ 4).

Under very low magnification, it is seen that vascular changes are nodular, being formed of red or bluish red, focal areas of exudate in the arterial wall. The appearance of a *fully developed lesion with superimposed subacute inflammation* is shown in Figure 2.12 (**recurrent periarteritis nodosa**). The lumen of the artery, with the exception of a small channel, is almost completely closed by granulation tissue which extends into a portion of the media, the adventitia lumen. The granulation tissue consists of proliferated capillaries, fibroblasts, histiocytes and lymphocytes (infrequently plasma cells and eosinophils). The media is preserved in large part (→ 1). A new vascular space with a muscularis and containing erythrocytes has developed in the granulation tissue filling the original lumen (→ 2). Fresh fibrinoid necrosis (exacerbation?) is seen at → 3, the homogeneous eosinophilic material of which is invaded by histiocytes.

The **scar stage** (Fig. 2.13) resembles the appearances seen in Figure 2.12. Fibroblasts and young cellular scar tissue have reduced the lumen to a small channel (→ 1). The place where the artery has been breached by granulation tissue arising from the adventitia can be clearly seen (→ 2), as well as the collagenous scar tissue and occasional lymphocytes.

Macroscopic: Bead-like nodules 1–2 mm. in diameter especially well seen in the heart (beneath the epicardium) or mesenteric arteries.
NOTE: Clinically the diagnosis of panarteritis may be difficult because of the great variation in symptoms.

The consequences of the vascular occlusions are multiple infarcts of the kidney and spleen, red infarcts of the liver and necrosis in the gastrointestinal tract with ulceration.

Practically any organ can be affected. Neuromuscular symptoms follow involvement of the arteries of the peripheral nerves and muscles. A biopsy of the skin or muscle may confirm the clinical diagnosis. The disease particularly attacks men 20–40 years old. The course is mostly subacute (1 year) and death results from uremia, myocardial necrosis, intestinal infarction or rupture of a blood vessel.

Giant cell arteritis (Fig. 2.14). This relatively benign form of periarteritis nodosa was once thought to affect chiefly the temporal artery of older women. However, more recent statistics indicate men and women are equally affected. Next to the temporal artery in incidence comes involvement of the ophthalmic artery (blindness), brain, heart, liver, spleen, etc. Fibrinoid necrosis develops locally in the region of the intima, with destruction of the internal elastica. As Figure 2.14 shows, the involvement is preponderantly in the intima and media. In this particular vessel, the intima shows both inflammatory exudate and granulation tissue and only a small lumen remains (→ ×). The boundary between intima and media is marked by the arrow. The internal elastica is broken into fragments that are surrounded by giant cells (→ 1). The media is diffusely infiltrated with lymphocytes and histiocytes. The exudate involves the adventitia only slightly (→ 2: adventitia).

Macroscopically and clinically, the temporal arteries are thick (pulseless) and the overlying skin is red; migraine-like headaches.

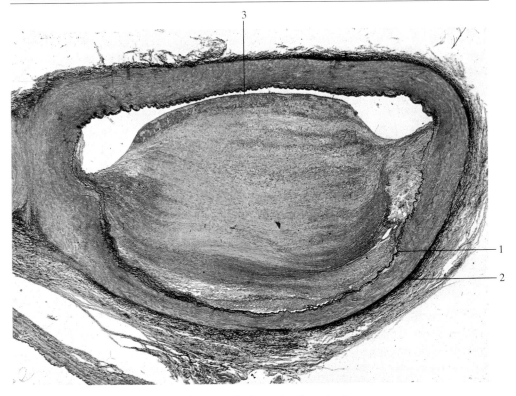

Fig. 2.15. Thromboangiitis obliterans in a leg artery; elastica-nuclear fast red stain, 19×.

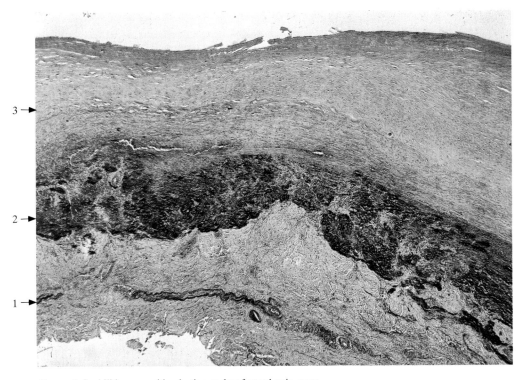

Fig. 2.16. Syphilitic mesaortitis; elastica-nuclear fast red stain, 32×.

Thromboangiitis obliterans. Figure 2.15 is a very low magnification of a cross-section of an artery of the leg stained for elastica. The lumen is almost completely filled by poorly cellular fibrous tissue. The internal elastica (→ 1) and the external elastica (→ 2) show as black bands. The media appears as a red, homogeneous layer. The internal elastica is slightly split in several places. Proliferation of intimal connective tissue has almost completely filled the lumen of the artery. Fresh fibrinoid necrosis (exacerbation, → 3) can be seen in the upper portion in the form of red, band-like streaks.

Thromboangiitis obliterans may have various morphological appearances. The *earliest stage,* which is often fleeting, consists of *fibrinoid degeneration* and is seldom seen. The most frequently seen stage is of a *recurrent thrombus* showing organization and a *sclerotic base.* The final stage can often scarcely be differentiated from arteriosclerosis, especially if a secondary thrombus has formed on a sclerotic plaque (see p. 67).

The disease process attacks the arteries of the legs (65%), is decidedly focal with cushion-like intimal thickening, fresh thrombosis and corresponding reduction in vessel lumen. Distal to the obstruction, the artery shows intimal proliferation, which may act as a sort of plug. The disease runs a course with many exacerbations and affects mostly a single lower extremity, particularly of young men (juvenile gangrene of the leg with intermittent claudication). Endarteritis of small arteries shows the same histological picture and attacks in particular the arteries of the brain (32%) and the renal (86%), mesenteric (60%) and coronary arteries (myocardial infarct! 96%) or aorta (90%).

Syphilitic Mesaortitis (Fig. 2.16). *This in an inflammation of the adventitia and media of the aorta developing in tertiary syphilis.* Figure 2.16, taken at low magnification, shows the typical "motheaten" pattern of the destruction of the medial elastica. The adventitia (→ 1) shows an increase in collagenous fibrous tissue (scar formation). The greater part of the media (→ 2) is irregularly replaced by nodular, sparsely cellular scar tissue. The intima (→ 3) is greatly thickened by secondary arteriosclerosis. In the right hand side of the figure hyalinization of the intima has occurred. The disease process begins with a lympho-histiocytic and plasma cell inflammation around the vasa vasorum of the adventitia and creeps along the vessels into the media. The small medial arteries then show an endarteritis which results in medial ischemia (necrosis), formation of granulation tissue, destruction of elastica and replacement of the lost tissue by a scar. Since the scar tissue shrinks, the intima is pulled inward over the scar.

From this result the characteristic *macroscopic* ridges (wrinkles) or tree-bark appearance of the intima, especially prominent in the thoracic portion. In addition, the wall of the aorta is thin and the vessel dilated (ectasia). Frequently, the inflammation also encroaches upon the cusps of the aortic valve, causing widening of the commissures and formation of a channel between them. In addition, the cusps contract so that aortic insufficiency develops. Furthermore, the coronary ostia can become obstructed by intimal proliferation, so that death is not infrequently due to a myocardial infarct.

Medium and small sized arteries, in particular those at the base of the brain, can also be affected in tertiary syphilis, chiefly in the form of an endarteritis with intimal proliferation.

Thrombosis – Thrombophlebitis – Organization

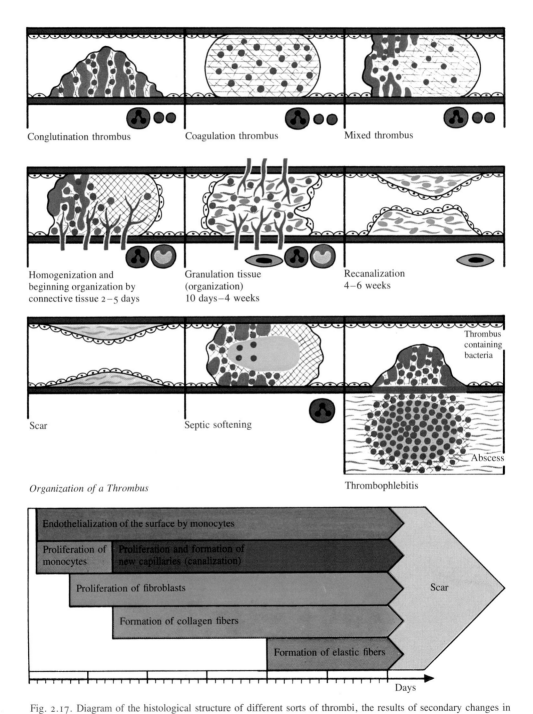

Fig. 2.17. Diagram of the histological structure of different sorts of thrombi, the results of secondary changes in a thrombus and the process of organization. Thrombophlebitis.

Thrombosis—Thrombophlebitis

Thrombosis is the intravascular coagulation of blood during life. Figure 2.17 illustrates in diagrammatic fashion the histological structure and fate of the different sorts of thrombi and the temporal events in the course of organization.

1. A **conglutination** or **agglutination thrombus,** shown adhering to the vessel wall (a mural or parietal thrombus) has a typical form. Conglutinated blood platelets are built up into a coral-like laminated scaffold. Fibrin surrounds and also lies between the columns of platelets, giving an appearance like that of a reinforced steel building. Leukocytes are enmeshed in the fibrin and accumulate like mantles around the blood platelets. Between the fibrin columns lie masses of erythrocytes (see p. 74).
Macroscopic: Rib-like projections of platelets are seen on the surface of the thrombus, giving it a rippled appearance crosswise to the direction of blood flow like the pattern of a wind-swept sand dune. Grayish red in color and friable.

2. A **coagulation thrombus** completely fills the vessel lumen and histologically consists of fibrin lamellae arranged parallel to the vessel wall. Between the lamellae stretches a delicate, irregularly constructed framework of fibrin in the meshes of which erythrocytes have become trapped. Platelets cannot be seen with the light microscope. There is a scanty sprinkling of leukocytes.
Macroscopic: A red, structureless column of coagulated blood.

3. A **mixed thrombus** consists of a headpiece, which has the structure of a *conglutination thrombus,* and a tailpiece, which has the structure of a *coagulation thrombus.* In the femoral vein, both conglutination and coagulation thrombi are frequently intermingled.
Macroscopic: Intermixed red and gray parts. *Postmortem clots,* in contrast to thrombi, have an elastic consistency (clots formed slowly are gray due to the buffy coat; clots formed quickly are red) and show no stratification or other signs of a structure.

4. In **septic thrombophlebitis**[1] there is a purulent inflammation of the vessel wall of bacterial origin. A thrombus containing bacteria forms at the site of the inflammation and histologically shows irregularly arranged masses of platelets and fibrin and bacterial colonies. If thrombotic material comes loose, then pyemic abscesses develop in the lung or elsewhere (see p. 88). Thrombophlebitic liver abscess in appendicitis!
Macroscopic: Gray to grayish white, cheesy coating of the walls of veins.

5. **Hyalin thrombi** have a red homogeneous appearance in H & E sections and are composed of platelets and fibrin. They are found in capillaries and venules particularly in shock (see pp. 84, 167).

Fate of Thrombi

1. *Emboli:* parts of a thrombus, or even the whole thrombus, may become detached and circulate with the blood. The danger of embolism is reduced when the thrombus has become organized (10 days). 2. *Alterations in the structure of the thrombus (homogenization):* In the course of disintegration, the contained erythrocytes, granulocytes and platelets fuse with the fibrin and cell fragments and form a homogeneous mass. This process of homogenization begins in the center of the thrombus as early as the second day and proceeds continuously. The fibrin may be dissolved over a long time (years) as the results of streptokinase therapy in chronic obstruction of the leg arteries demonstrate. 3. *Dissolution of the thrombus:* a) *by granulocytes* (putrid softening). When the proteolytic enzymes of the granulocytes are released they dissolve the fibrin, erythrocytes and platelets, especially in the center of the thrombus. A pus-like fluid results that is flushed away by the blood stream. b) *by the fibrinolytic system* (thrombolysis): By the conversion of plasminogen to plasmin, the fibrin in the thrombus can be dissolved by proteolysis (plasmin has a high specificity for fibrin, but does not lyse platelet masses). Plasminogen is present in flowing blood and is absorbed by the fibrin fibers in the thrombus. The fibrinolytic system can be activated therapeutically by bacterial products (streptokinase). c) *by granulation tissue* (organization). Early as one day after it starts to form monocytes cover the surface of the thrombus and grow into it (transformed to histiocytes and fibroblasts). Sprouts of vascular endothelial cells or subendothelial cells (myelocytes?) grow into the base of the thrombus (vascular endothelial cells have fibrinolytic activity).

---

[1] Note: in clinical use "thrombophlebitis" means "bland," i.e., non-infective venous thrombosis associated with the external signs of inflammation (rubor, tumor, dolor, calor).

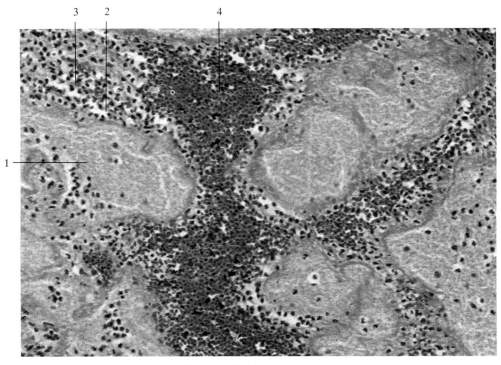

Fig. 2.18. Conglutination (agglutination) thrombus; H & E, 246×.

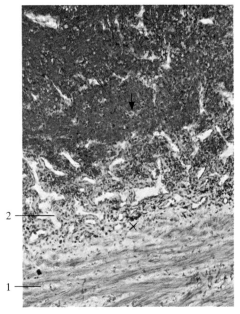

Fig. 2.19. Organizing thrombus; H & E. 101×.

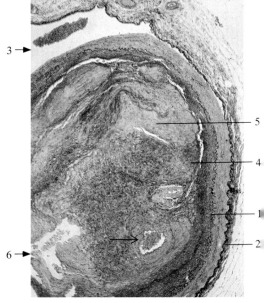

Fig. 2.20. Recanalized arterial thrombus; elastica-van Gieson stain, 40×.

Capillaries develop from these endothelial cells and grow into the thrombus (about 10 days). About day 5 fibroblasts invade the base of the thrombus. About day 10 they form collagen fibers and later a lesser number of elastic fibers. Thus the cellular response of the vessel wall is formation of granulation tissue. Such granulation tissue, by virtue of its contained proteolytic enzymes, has the ability to dissolve a thrombus including the homogenized portions and replace it with connective tissue. In this way a scar may be formed after 4–6 weeks. The new capillaries bring about recanalization of the formerly thrombosed blood vessel.

Special Sorts of Organization: The newly formed connective tissue may become calcified or ossified (phleboliths). The new blood channels in the thrombus can be especially large and numerous (cavernous.) Involvement of the valves of the veins in the process of organization of thrombi in the leg veins may be very important in the development of post-thrombotic syndromes (e.g. varicosities, stasis ulcers). 4. *Propagation or "growth" of thrombi:* Simultaneously with the processes of dissolution, a thrombus can also increase in size through the addition of a new thrombus. Such propagation of a thrombus occurs–particularly in the veins of the lower extremities (calf veins–femoral, iliac) and always carries a high risk of embolization.

Conglutination (agglutination) thrombus. When a section of such a thrombus is examined under very low magnification, the vessel wall is seen to be covered with a thrombus having a rough, undulating surface. Projecting columns of platelets fill the spaces between erythrocytes. Under medium magnification (Fig. 2.18), the coral-like structure of the platelet masses ($\rightarrow$ 1) is easily recognized. Under high magnification, the platelets appear as finely granular material. Fibrin appears as homogeneous bands ($\rightarrow$ 2) which envelop the platelets. Outside the bands of fibrin is a zone of leukocytes ($\rightarrow$ 3). In the spaces between the platelet columns there are thickly massed erythrocytes ($\rightarrow$ 4) and a loose fibrin network. In old thrombi it may be difficult to distinguish between platelets and fibrin. Azan stains are helpful, since platelets stain blue, whereas fibrin stains red.

Organizing thrombus (Fig. 2.19). The early stages of resorption and organization begin from the vessel wall and lumen (monocytes!) and are already under way at two to four days after the onset of thrombosis. Very low magnification shows red material completely filling the lumen. The wall of the vein ($\rightarrow$ 1) appears as a light red band. Low-power magnification discloses a brighter red, sparsely cellular zone in the vessel wall near the thrombus. Medium magnification (Fig. 2.19) shows granulation tissue developing in this zone of the vessel wall where markedly dilated capillaries ($\rightarrow$ 2) and erythrocytes are clearly visible. In between lie fibroblasts and histiocytes, and formation of new connective tissue fibers has already started. Vessels are still sparse in the interior of the thrombus. Isolated histiocytes (precursors of granulation tissue) are present, lying in part around empty spaces ($\rightarrow$ 2) (compare the organization of a myocardial infarct and pericarditis, pp. 42, 54). The brownish black granules ($\times$) in the organizing tissue are intracellularly situated products of hemoglobin-hemosiderin.

Macroscopic: Firmly attached, grayish red to brown layer. Fresh coagulation thrombi are only loosely attached to the vessel wall.

Recanalization of an arterial thrombus (Fig. 2.20). The microscopic appearance depends on the age and mass of the thrombus and the degree of recanalization. In Figure 2.20, the internal elastic lamina ($\rightarrow$ 1) and external elastic lamina ($\rightarrow$ 2) are present. The former is partly split and fragmented. At $\rightarrow$ 3, the external elastic lamina is lifted off the media and blood fills the breach (artifact of preparation). The true lumen of the blood vessel is obstructed by connective tissue of different ages (richly cellular young granulation tissue $\rightarrow$ 4: older fibrous connective tissue $\rightarrow$ 5). In the midst of the connective tissue there are spaces lined by endothelium and containing erythrocytes ($\rightarrow$ 6 and arrow). These dilated blood vessels pass through the organized thrombus and have terminations in the main lumen of the artery, both before and behind the thrombus.

Macroscopic: Depending upon the stage of organization and recanalization, any of the following may be seen: a mural scar, web-like adhesions (particularly in thrombi of leg veins) and sinusoidal transformation of blood vessels (e.g., thrombosis of the portal vein). Usually, the surrounding tissues are stained brownish (hemosiderin). A less frequent consequence of the organization of a thrombus is the formation of phleboliths or of a so-called myxoma (organization of thrombi in the heart) considered by many authors a primary tumor.

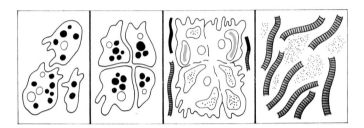

Fig. 2.21. Schematic representation of the pathogenesis of thrombosis (after RODMAN et al., 1963).

Thrombus formation starts with agglutination of thrombocytes, which is associated with loss of granulation (so-called *viscous metamorphosis*). Later, fibrin accumulates. The results of studies with the electron microscope show that this viscous metamorphosis takes place in four stages (Fig. 2.21). Normal thrombocytes (Fig. 2.21a) consist of a *clear* portion (ground substance) and a *granular* portion containing the cellular organelles. In the *first stage* of agglutination (preagglutination), the thrombocytes *swell* (membrane injury?), form *pseudopods* and stick together (Fig. 2.21b). The existing ATP begins to disintegrate (because of ATPase activity). The integrity of the outer membranes of the thrombocytes is probably preserved through the mediation of ADP and calcium. In the *second stage* of agglutination, the outer membrane of individual thrombocytes is still largely intact (Figs. 2.21b, 2.22). The granular ground substance disappears from the center of the platelets (Fig. 2.22). During the *third stage (thrombocytic rhexis),* the outer membranes of the thrombocytes disintegrate (Fig. 2.21c,d). In the center, the various constituents of the granular ground substance deteriorate. At the outer margin, protrusions are formed. Now, for the first time, fibrin is visible at the margins of the aggregates (Fig. 2.21c). In the last stage, that of *thrombocytolysis* (Fig. 2.21d), the thrombocytes disintegrate completely into granular material and membrane fragments. A large amount of fibrin is intermingled with this remaining wreckage. During this stage of viscous metamorphosis, the thrombocytes give up the following substances: 1. those effecting plasma coagulation (factor 3 = thromboplastin (thrombokinase) and factor 4 = calcium); 2. those affecting fibrinolysis–platelet proactivator antiplasmin; 3. those with an effect on the blood vessel wall–adrenalin, noradrenalin, serotonin.

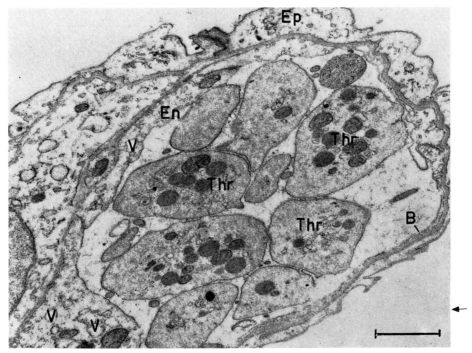

Fig. 2.22. Lung capillary with agglutinated thrombocytes (Thr) in the lumen (histamin shock, rabbit). The platelets are heaped on one another, the granular ground substance has concentrated in the center. The endothelium (En) shows numerous vesicles (V), as does the alveolar epithelium (Ep) (accumulation of fluid in vacuoles). B = basement membrane, → alveolar clearing. 20,000× (Nikulin et al., 1965).

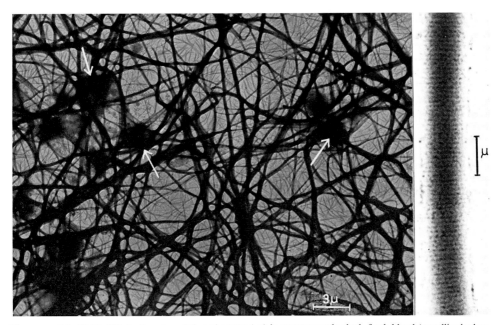

Fig. 2.23.a) Scaffold of fibrin threads and thrombocytes (→) in spontaneously shed, fresh blood (metallic shadowing). Fibrin fibers have formed in both thick bundles and a fine network. b) shows a single fibrin fiber with distinct cross-bands (periodicity of 230 Å). Magnifications, a) 3,000×, b) 100,000× (see Köppel, 1962).

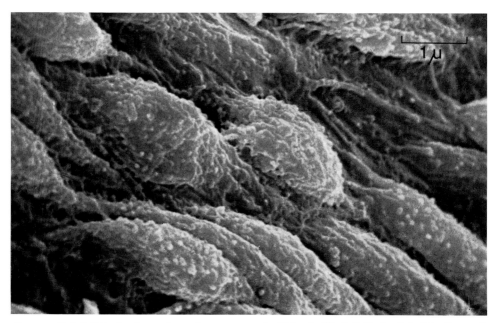

Fig. 2.24. Endothelial cells of normal aorta from a one-month-old female. The individual endothelial cells are spindle shaped and have a bed-like arrangement. The cells have numerous processes and numerous small, villous-like outpouchings on the surfaces of the cellular membranes. Scanning electron microscope, 1800×.

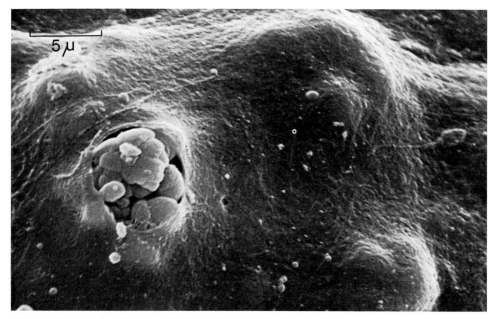

Fig. 2.25. Rupture of an atheromatous lesion in the arteriosclerotic aorta of a 67-year-old-man. At this particular location in the artery the vascular endothelium is covered by a thick film of fibrin. Scanning electron microscope, 4500×.

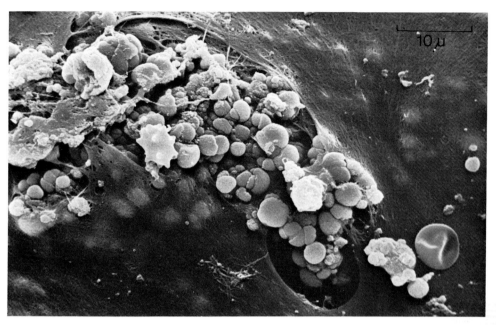

Fig. 2.26. Intimal break in the arteriosclerotic aorta of a 67-year-old man, showing globular particles (lipids) discharged from an atheromatous mass that has broken through a layer of fibrin (scanning electron microscope) 2500×.

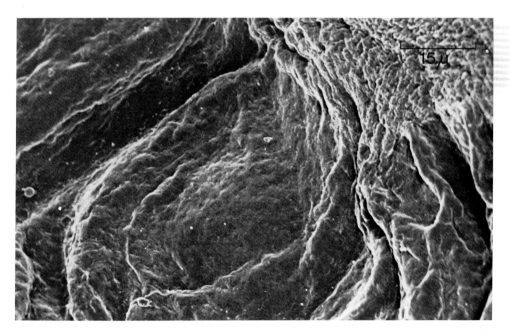

Fig. 2.27. Intimal surface of the aorta of a 76-year-old woman with syphilitic mesaortitis showing circumscribed elevation of endothelium subsequent to injury of elastica with resulting scarring, scanning electron microscope, 2000×.

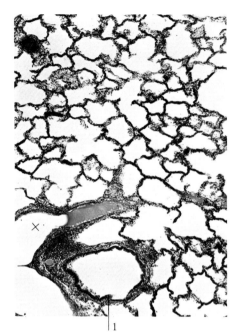

Fig. 3.1. Normal lung;
H & E, 53×.

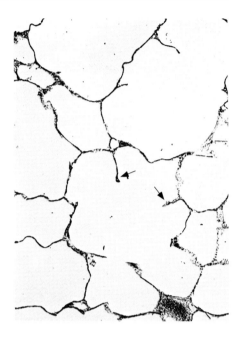

Fig. 3.2. Emphysema;
H & E, 53×.

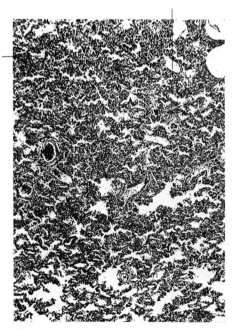

Fig. 3.3. Atelectasis;
H & E, 53×.

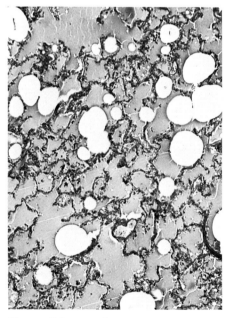

Fig. 3.4. Pulmonary edema;
H & E, 53×.

3. Lung

Histological evaluation of lung sections is often difficult for the beginner, particularly so when the disease has altered the normal architectural pattern of the lung. Frequently, in inflammatory processes, the alveolar spaces can no longer be recognized as empty sacs. Therefore, in order to identify the organ it is necessary to search for the bronchi (→ 1 in Fig. 3.1, normal lung) with their characteristic tall cylindrical epithelium, annular muscular wall and bronchial cartilage, and to look as well for the branches of the pulmonary arteries which lie adjacent to bronchi (x in Fig. 3.1; an artery partly filled with blood plasma). Caution: in the newborn the bronchi are not fully developed and this can lead one to an incorrect diagnosis!

The answers to the following questions will provide *clues* to the pathological diagnosis: Is the lung affected focally or diffusely? Does the lesion involve the alveolar or bronchial spaces, or their walls? Are the alveolar or bronchial spaces distended or not? Is the lung tissue preserved or destroyed? When such questions are properly answered, then a correct interpretation will be reached.

Chronic vesicular emphysema (Fig. 3.2). *The pulmonary alveoli are enlarged because of atrophy and destruction of the alveolar septa.* In comparison to normal lung tissue (see Fig. 3.1), there are large, optically empty spaces bounded by thin, ruptured alveolar septa. The stump-like remnants of the septa (→), which project into the alveolar spaces, are noteworthy. In contrast to acute insufflation of the lung, emphysema shows actual destruction of the septa. Examination under high magnification of tissue stained for elastica demonstrates degenerative changes in the elastic fibers such as thinning, fusion, increased staining, etc. Types: emphysema of the aged, obstructive emphysema, cicatricial emphysema.

Macroscopic: Small, medium or large vesicles. Bullous emphysema is particularly noticeable just beneath the pleura. Frequently: obstructive chronic bronchitis. Infrequently: A genetic defect (α-antitrypsin, Laurell & Eriksson). Proteases are not eliminated → destruction of lung tissue.
Complications: Rupture of vesicles and spontaneous pneumothorax; hypertrophy of the right ventricle of the heart.

Pulmonary atelectasis (Fig. 3.3). *This consists of alveolar collapse with diminished pulmonary air capacity and is usually coextensive with the territory supplied by a bronchus (e.g., reabsorption atelectasis).* Microscopic examination shows alveoli with such closely placed walls that the cellular content of the lung tissue appears to be increased. The arrow in Figure 3.3 indicates the slit-like alveolar spaces. The capillaries are mostly dilated.

Histologically, the various **forms** of atelectasis [compression atelectasis (e.g., in pneumothorax, or pleural effusion), obstructive or reabsorption atelectasis (e.g., with bronchial tumors)] all have the same appearance. In fetal atelectasis, the development and differentiation of the lung is defective.

Macroscopic: The entire lung may be dark bluish red or there may be sharply delimited, depressed zones of firm, rubbery consistency. The tissue does not float in water.

Pulmonary edema (Fig. 3.4). *Fluid exudate has escaped from the blood stream into the alveoli (intra-alveolar edema)[1].* Microscopically, the alveoli are seen to be filled with homogeneous, eosinophilic, cell-free fluid. A few solitary exfoliated alveolar epithelial cells are present. The capillaries are congested. In some places, the alveolar fluid has been lost during preparation of the section, so that empty spaces have resulted (artifacts).

Macroscopic: Heavy lungs, the cut surfaces of which exude frothy fluid.
The *pathogenesis* is concerned with an increase in pressure in the pulmonary circulation accompanied by altered permeability of the terminal vascular channels (due to toxins or oxygen lack).

---

[1] Intra-alveolar-edema = frothy fluid may be pressed from the lungs. Interstitial pulmonary edema = heavy, dusky red lungs without frothy fluid. Occurs chiefly in shock.

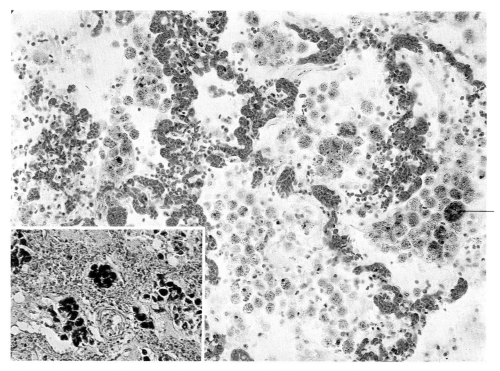

Fig. 3.5. Congestion of the lung (passive hyperemia, stasis); H & E, 240× – the inset in the lower left corner shows the Berlin-blue reaction, 132×.

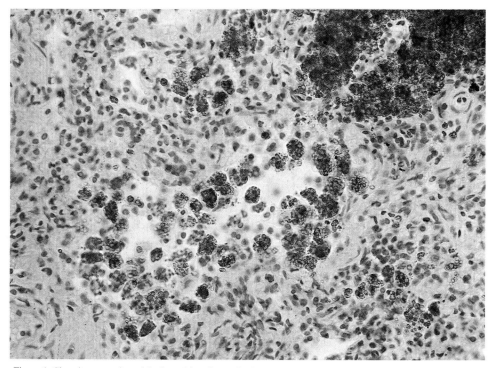

Fig. 3.6. Chronic congestion of the lung (chronic passive hyperemia or stasis); Nuclear fast red stain, 330×.

Congestion of the Lungs

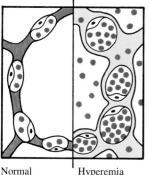 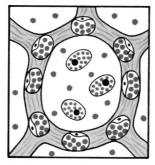 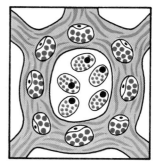

Normal	Hyperemia	Beginning induration	Chronic congestion
Alveolus	Acute	Subacute	(Stasis)

Fig.3.7. Different stages of congestion of the lung.

Passive congestion of the lungs *results from obstruction to the flow of blood from the left side of the heart (e.g., in mitral stenosis). The condition is therefore one of passive hyperemia with morphological alterations corresponding to the severity of the congestion or stasis.* In the **acute stage** (Fig. 3.7), there is simple hyperemia, the dilated capillaries projecting into the alveolar spaces in knob-like fashion. The capillaries are filled with thickly packed erythrocytes.

Macroscopic: Large, heavy, often bright red lungs, so-called red induration. Pulmonary edema.

Passive congestion of longer duration (subacute to subchronic) (Figs. 3.5, 3.7) leads to increased extravasation into the alveoli of erythrocytes which are phagocytosed by alveolar epithelium) and the hemoglobin converted into *hemosiderin* (heart failure cells laden with brown intracytoplasmic pigment). An increase in connective tissue and the basement membrane thickens the alveolar walls.

Chronic passive congestion (brown induration) (Figs. 3.6, 3.7) is manifest by greatly thickened alveolar septa (collagenous fibrosis), thickening of the basement membrane, and heavy loading of the alveolar epithelium with hemosiderin (heart-failure cells may appear in the sputum). Iron is liberated and may be deposited along with calcium in both the connective and elastic tissue (iron-calcium incrustations).

Macroscopic: Heavy, cinnamon-brown or brick-red lungs.

Congestion of the lung. Figure 3.5 shows a subacute stage with marked hyperemia of the capillaries so that they project into the alveolar spaces. The alveolar walls are not fibrotic or thickened. The alveolar spaces contain exfoliated alveolar epithelial cells (→), the cytoplasm of which contains finely granular, brown, refractile hemosiderin pigment. The Berlin-blue reaction (inset in the lower left-hand corner) shows that the pigment is an iron-containing product of hemoglobin breakdown.

Chronic passive congestion of lung (Fig. 3.6). Inspection under very low magnification shows a thicker lung framework than normal. Alveolar spaces appear narrow because of great thickening of the walls by collagenous tissue. Van Gieson stain demonstrates an intensely red staining network of fibers. The cell content, however, is not substantially increased (compare with interstitial pneumonia, p. 94). Numerous heart-failure cells, with clearly visible brown pigment, are found in the alveolar spaces. In many cases there is also an increase in smooth muscle.

Shock Lung (**electron microscopy,** Fig. 3.9)

The alveolar walls are lined with Type I(1) and Type II(2) alveolar cells. Type I alveolar cells make up most of the alveolar epithelium and are amitotic. Type II alveolar cells are intermitotic and produce surfactant factors which reduces the surface tension of the alveoli thus counteracting the natural tendency of alveoli to collapse. The membrane for gaseous exchange normally consists of narrow cytoplasmic processes of Type I alveolar cells, the epithelial basement membrane, a narrow gap in the interstitium, the endothelial basement membrane and endothelial cytoplasmic processes (4). The interstitium contains fibroblasts (5) which produce the collagen, elastin and proteoglycides of the supporting septal framework.

During the *acute stage of shock* the capillary endothelium is injured—later the alveolar walls also—and this injury may progress to necrosis. As a result epithelial and especially endothelial cell contacts are loosened (6). Leucocytic exudate appears in the interstitium. Platelet and fibrin thrombi form on the injured vessel walls (7). Fibrin masses appear in the interstitium (8) and alveoli and form hyaline membranes (9). The resultant interstitial edema of the acute stage may go into a *late stage of shock*. Endothelial cells and particularly Type II alveolar cells proliferate and block exchange of blood gasses (10). Some unknown factor in the edema fluid stimulates synthesis and proliferation of interstitial fibroblasts thus causing further fibrotic thickening of the alveolar septa which are already thickened by epithelial proliferation. This is the morphologic basis for respiratory insufficiency (diffusion defect of shock). Cellular microthrombi (7) obstruct pulmonary capillaries with resulting pulmonary hypertension and development of arteriovenous shunts. The result is reduced oxygen saturation of the blood (perfusion defect of shock).

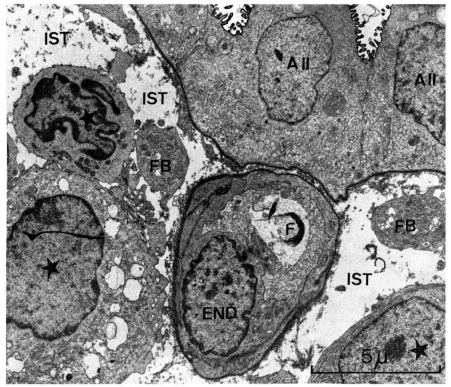

Fig. 3.8. Shock lung (male, 18 days of septic hemorrhagic shock). A II = Type II alveolar cells, IST = interstitium, END = capillary endothelium, F = fibrin, FB = fibroblasts,* = histiocytes, 7500×.

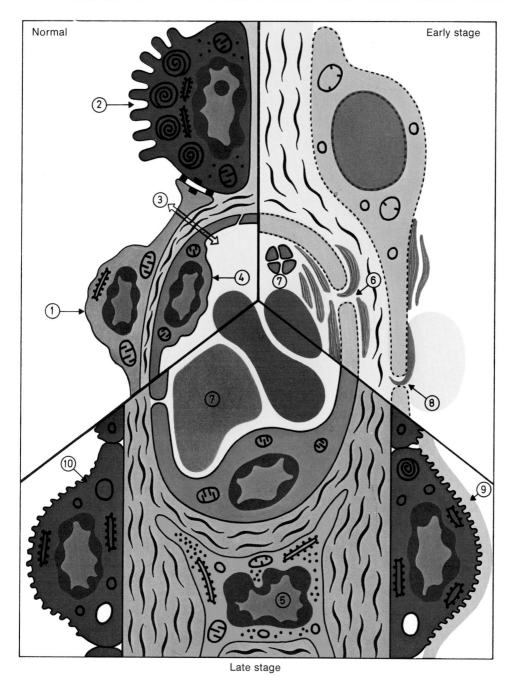

Normal

Early stage

Late stage

Fig. 3.9. Shock lung. Diagram of ultrastructural changes.

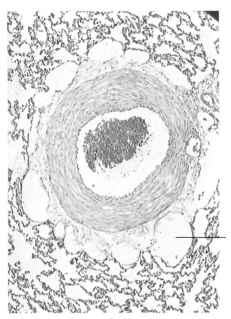

Fig. 3.10. Dilated perivascular lymph spaces in shock lung; H & E, 60×.

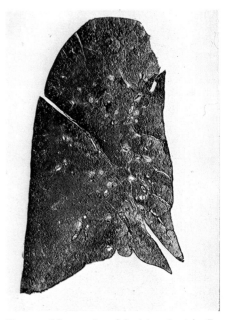

Fig. 3.11. Macrosection of shock lung (unstained).

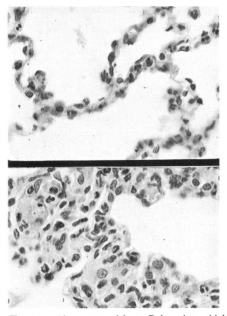

Fig. 3.12. Above: normal lung. Below: interstitial edema in shock lung; H & E, 300×.

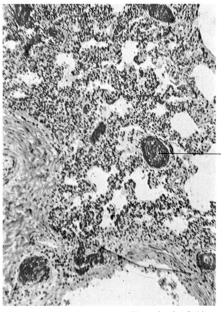

Fig. 3.13. Microthrombosis of lung in shock (Azan stain. Fibrin red), 30×.

Shock Lung

Shock describes a general failure of peripheral circulation with tissue damage resulting from decreased perfusion of blood. Central to its clinical manifestations are anuria and a decrease of the circulating mass of blood platelets (platelet failure – consumption coagulopathy – disseminated intravascular coagulation, see Sandritter and Lasch, 1966). The anuric phase of shock can be controlled by peritoneal dialysis or the artificial kidney. The respiratory insufficiency of shock patients has been given more attention in the past five years. Clinically the patients have hypoxia due to short circuiting of blood through arteriovenous anastomoses (up to 67% of the cardiac output), diminished O_2 uptake and increased blood CO_2 tension. Morphologically and roentgenologically during the first hours of shock there is spindle-shaped widening of the blood vessels (Fig. 3.14 – first hour) due to perivascular edema. Fig. 3.10 shows the greatly **dilated perivascular lymph spaces** that are almost cystic in size ($\rightarrow$). Pulmonary lymph flow through these lymph channels is reduced. In the following days (3 – 5 days, Stage II in Fig. 3.14) the perivascular edema intensifies and progresses to interstitial edema. X-rays of the lung now show a cloudy, milk-glass appearance (Fig. 3.14). Grossly the lung is dusky red and has a spongy, leather-like quality. Fig. 3.11 is a **macrosection of such a lung** that shows hyperemia and alveolar lumens that have been reduced in size by edema of the alveolar walls. These changes are shown more clearly in Fig. 3.12 where the normal lung tissue in the upper portion is contrasted in the lower portion with the **broad edematous septa** containing an increased number of cells (histiocytes, granulocytes, fibroblasts). Simultaneously (1 – 2 days) **microthrombi** appear in the lungs. Fig. 3.13 shows **red thrombi** (fibrin stains red with azan) in the small and medium sized vessels ($\rightarrow$). In the third stage of shock fibroblasts proliferate in alveolar septa, so that roentgenologically there is **reticular striation** (irreversible, progresses to pulmonary fibrosis, Ostendorf et al, 1975).

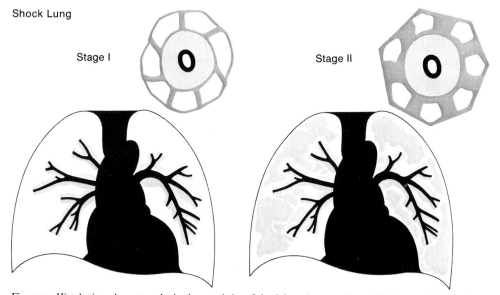

Fig. 3.14. Histologic and roentgenologic characteristics of shock lung (gray = edema, black = vessels and alveolar walls).

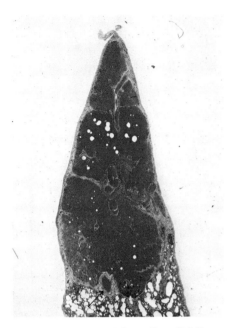

Fig. 3.15. Hemorrhagic infarct of lung; H & E, 5×.

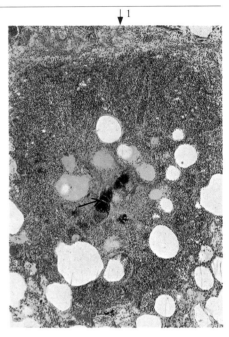

Fig. 3.16. Pyemic lung abscess; H & E, 42×.

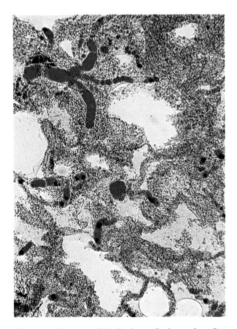

Fig. 3.17. Fat emboli in the lung; Sudan stain, 58×.

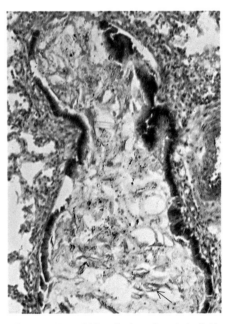

Fig. 3.18. Bronchial aspiration of amniotic fluid; H & E, 162×.

Hemorrhagic infarct of lung (Fig. 3.15). *This denotes focal necrosis and hemorrhage of lung tissue following embolic occlusion of a branch of the pulmonary artery in the presence of passive hyperemia of the bronchial circulation.* Naked eye inspection of a section usually shows a wedge-shaped, red, homogeneous lesion. The tissue in Figure 3.15 is from the lingula of the lung so that the wedge shape of the infarct is fortuitous. The embolic occlusion (→) of the nutrient branch of the pulmonary artery can be easily seen. Medium and high magnification disclose a monotonous picture: the alveolar spaces are filled with densely packed erythrocytes. In older infarcts, these show only as shadowy forms or are disintegrated into crumbled, eosinophilic, homogeneous, dingy, reddish brown masses. The alveolar septa can scarcely be distinguished from the contents of the alveoli. Septal nuclei have disappeared (evidence of *necrosis*).

Infarcts must be *differentiated from aspirated blood*, in which necrosis is lacking as well as from an embolus.
Macroscopic: Subpleural, wedge-shaped, firm, dark red masses which project above the surface of the lung and show fibrinous pleurisy.
Outcome: Leukocytic demarcation, organization and scar formation. Eventually, sequestration, abscess or gangrene may develop.

Pyemic lung abscess (Fig. 3.16). *This occurs if a branch of a pulmonary artery is obstructed not by a bland embolus but by a bacteria-containing embolus arising from a purulent thrombophlebitis (pyemia). A subpleural abscess then develops in the tissue supplied by the obstructed artery.* Low-power magnification again shows a wedge-shaped, compact mass (→ 1: pleura) that has a blue-stained appearance because of its high cellular content. Medium magnification shows that the alveoli are crowded with leukocytes. The nutrient branch of the pulmonary artery is filled with an embolus containing large, bluish black bacterial colonies (→) and many leukocytes. At the center of the lesion, the alveolar septa are necrotic and there is beginning dissolution of lung tissue (*abscess* formation) (compare with purulent thrombophlebitis, pp. 73, 95).

Macroscopic: In the early stages there is no tissue softening: instead, there are grayish yellow raised, firm subpleural masses with overlying fibrinous pleuritis and pleural necrosis (pleura is white). After *softening:* abscesses from which grayish yellow material discharges. Secondary empyema.

Fat embolism (Fig. 3.17). *Release of fluid fat from bone marrow (also from subcutaneous fat tissue or a fatty liver) after trauma (e.g., burn injury) may cause obstruction of the pulmonary capillaries and eventually escape into the arterial circulation.* In part the fat may also come from non-traumatized fat tissue (adrenalin caused lipolysis, so-called fat mobilization syndrome). Low magnification reveals small red flecks in the lung parenchyma. Medium magnification shows sudan-positive material in the capillaries, which have a stag-horn or small round disk shape (cross section). There is usually hyperemia and pulmonary edema also. NOTE: Fat embolism is a form of shock. Hyaline thrombi are always present.

Fat embolism must be *differentiated from hyperlipemia* (diabetes, a fat-rich meal), which is much more common.

Aspiration of amniotic fluid (Fig. 3.18) *This occurs during premature, intrauterine respiration.* Microscopically, the signs of aspiration consist of golden brown or greenish amniotic fluid and meconium in small bronchi and in occasional alveoli. Figure 3.18 shows a small bronchus, the lumen of which contains abundant squames (→). These consist of cross-sectioned desquamated squamous epithelium of the vernix caseosa. The masses stained golden brown (bilirubin) consist of meconium. The small round bodies are known as meconium bodies (probably desquamated colonic cells of the fetus). Secondary aspiration pneumonia may develop (infected amniotic fluid) in which maternal leukocytes participate. Aspiration of amniotic fluid occurs chiefly in premature births.

Bronchitis

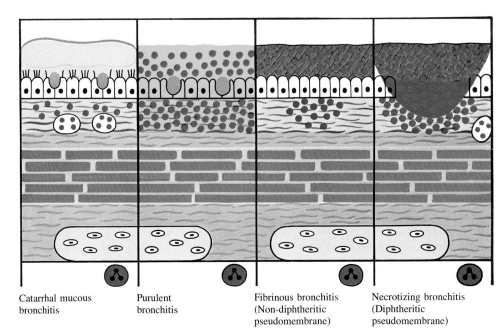

Catarrhal mucous
bronchitis

Purulent
bronchitis

Fibrinous bronchitis
(Non-diphtheritic
pseudomembrane)

Necrotizing bronchitis
(Diphtheritic
pseudomembrane)

Characteristics of Different Degrees
of Inflammation and Necrosis

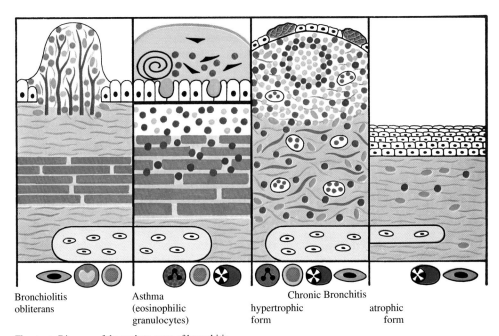

Bronchiolitis
obliterans

Asthma
(eosinophilic
granulocytes)

Chronic Bronchitis

hypertrophic
form

atrophic
form

Fig. 3.19. Diagram of the various sorts of bronchitis.

Bronchitis—Tracheitis

Figure 3.19 shows the different forms of bronchitis in diagrammatic form. Acute **sero-mucous catarrh** shows edema and hyperemia of the tunica propria as well as a layer of mucus containing a few leukocytes. The exudate contains mucus mixed with protein material, occasional leukocytes and shed epithelium. **Purulent catarrh** is recognized by its richly cellular exudate. Erythrocytes appear in **hemorrhagic inflammation.** In **fibrinous inflammation,** grayish white, cohesive, detachable membranes *(pseudo-membrane, croup[1], non-diphtheritic inflammation)* develop which often extend widely (bronchial casts may be formed, e.g., in *diphtheria*), whereas **pseudomembranous necrotizing inflammation** (diphtheritic) is distinguished by a patchy, tightly adherent, putty-like layer. In the first case, the fibrin is superficial, lying on top of the epithelium, and the connective tissue is unchanged. In the second case, the fibrin infiltrates both the epithelium and the underlying necrotic connective tissue (deeply penetrating fibrinous necrosis). Necrotizing fibrinous inflammation is always followed by proliferation of granulation tissue. When bronchioles are affected in this way, the result is **bronchiolitis obliterans.** In **chronic bronchitis,** all coats are infiltrated by cells and the goblet cells are increased in number. Metaplasia of the epithelium often becomes prominent (see also p. 93).

Fibrinous tracheitis in diphtheria (Fig. 3.20). A cross-section of the trachea viewed under low magnification shows the cartilaginous rings which stain blue. Medium magnification (Fig. 3.20) shows the hyperemia and edema of the tunica propria (→ 1). The ciliated epithelium is lacking. The basement membrane (→ 2) is overlaid with densely packed bundles of fibrin fibers (→ 3) (see p. 96).

Necrotizing tracheitis in influenza (Fig. 3.21). In contrast to diphtheria, the fibrin layer is scaly and less marked. The basement membrane is no longer recognizable (→ 1). Homogeneous material (fibrin and necrotic tissue) extends into the outer layers of the tunica propria (deeply penetrating diphtheritic pseudomembrane or false membrane, × in the picture). Bacterial colonies are seen in the necrotic material (→ 2). The cellular reaction (leukocytes, lymphocytes) is more marked than in diphtheria. Accumulated secretion in the excretory duct of a mucus gland is shown at → 3 (→ 4 is cartilage). (NOTE: Non-diphtheritic pseudomembrane shows a fibrinous layer and only the surface epithelium is affected: diphtheritic pseudomembrane shows fibrinous exudate plus necrosis of connective tissue (diphtheria, scarlet fever, ulcerative colitis).

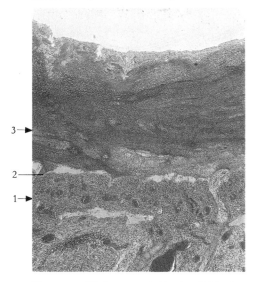

Fig. 3.20. Fibrinous tracheitis in diphtheria; H & E, 42×.

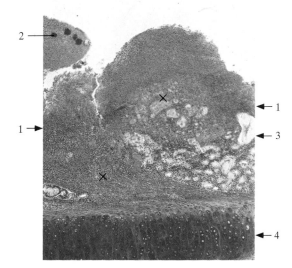

Fig. 3.21. Necrotizing tracheitis in influenza; H & E, 42×.

---

[1]Croup (acute obstructive laryngitis): condition characterized by stridor, dyspnea, high pitched cough—measles, influenza, etc.).

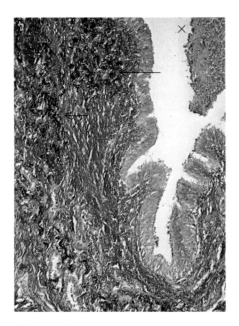

Fig. 3.22. Chronic bronchitis; elastica-
van Gieson stain, 100×.

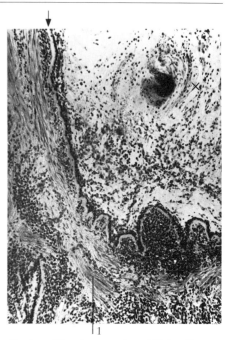

Fig. 3.23. Chronic mucous bronchitis in asthma;
H & E, 120×.

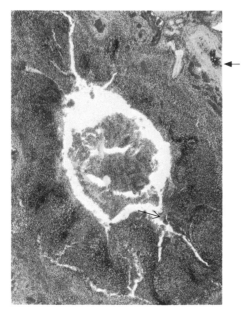

Fig. 3.24. Severe chronic proliferative bronchitis;
H & E, 32×.

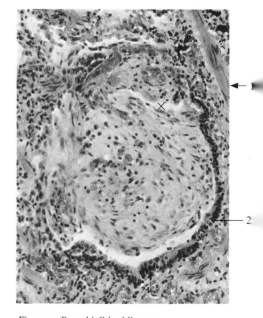

Fig.3.25. Bronchiolitis obliterans;
H & E, 195×.

Chronic bronchitis (Fig. 3.22). Histologically, there is moderate infiltration of the bronchial wall by lymphocytes, plasma cells and polymorphonuclear leukocytes. In the figure, the ciliated epithelium is intact and slightly hypertrophic. The lumen of the bronchus contains numerous polymorphonuclear leukocytes and mucus (×). The excessive production of mucus is due to an increased number of goblet cells in the mucosa as well as enhanced secretion by the seromucous glands. Elastic stains show an increase in elastic fibers (black in the photograph), which, moreover, show splitting (→) and degenerative granular fragmentation. In addition, there is a decrease in the number of collagen fibers. The muscle may show hypertrophy (see Figs. 3.19, 3.23). If the elastic membranes and muscle are destroyed, the bronchial lumen will dilate *(bronchiectasis)*.

Macroscopic: The mucous membrane is red, thickened and velvety with longitudinal and cross ripples, especially in *hypertrophic bronchitis* (increase in connective tissue, elastica and muscle fibers, see p. 90). In *atrophic bronchitis*, which is essentially the end-stage of chronic hypertrophic bronchitis, the mucosa is grayish white and smooth (atrophy of the supporting elements of the bronchial wall, see p. 90). *Complications:* cor pulmonale, pulmonary emphysema, bronchiectasis and brain abscess, amyloidosis, recurrent pneumonias. In 50% of the deaths in England.

Chronic mucous bronchitis in asthma (Fig. 3.23). *This is an allergic bronchitis, which is accompanied during the attacks by increased secretion of tenacious, highly viscous mucus.* Figure 3.23 shows the bronchial lumen filled by mucus which has formed a whirling spiral with a dark blue center *(Cushman's spiral, ×)*. Both the mucus and the bronchial wall are infiltrated with eosinophils. In addition, there is a lymphocytic infiltrate in the wall. The basement membrane (→) is thickened and the bronchial muscle hypertrophied (→ 1). Frequently, lance-shaped eosinophilic crystals are found in the mucus and these arise from the destruction of leukocytes *(Charcot-Leyden crystals)*.

Macroscopic: Stringy, glistening mucus that can be pulled from the opened bronchi.

Severe chronic proliferative bronchitis (Fig. 3.24). Under low magnification, the thickened bronchial wall appears blue (increased cell content) and the breadth of the peribronchial connective tissue is greater than normal. A bronchial cartilage is shown at →. The tunica propria of the bronchus is greatly widened and partially projects into the lumen. The thickening of the bronchial wall is due to granulation tissue which has completely destroyed the muscle and mucous glands. The granulation tissue is particularly well developed in the inner layers of the wall and is heavily infiltrated with granulocytes, lymphocytes and plasma cells. The bronchial epithelium is largely lacking, being replaced by flat ulcers covered with fibrin (→). Mucus and leukocyte-rich exudate fill the lumen.

Macroscopic: Thickened bronchial walls; narrowed lumens; secondary bronchial stenosis.

Bronchiolitis obliterans (Fig. 3.25). *In pseudomembranous, necrotizing bronchiolitis, the necrotic tissue and fibrin are replaced secondarily by granulation tissue. In this way, a web of tissue is formed which can completely fill the bronchi and bronchioles. Such a plug of granulation tissue can also form in proliferative bronchiolitis.* Under low magnification, single bronchioles are seen to be filled with cellular granulation tissue. Medium magnification shows that the ciliated epithelium (×) is partly denuded. The lumen is filled with a plug of granulation tissue (fibroblasts, fibrous tissue, capillaries and lymphocytes). The wall of the bronchus shows a chronic inflammatory infiltrate. At →1 can be seen the smooth muscle of the bronchial wall (→ 2: ciliated epithelium).

Macroscopic: The cut surfaces of the lung show a very fine, white stippling.

Inflammation of the Lung

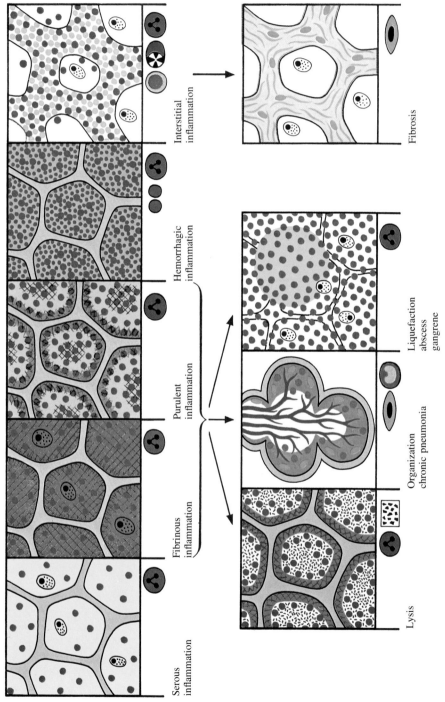

Lobar Pneumonia – Interstitial Pneumonia

Serous inflammation

Fibrinous inflammation

Purulent inflammation

Hemorrhagic inflammation

Interstitial inflammation

Lysis

Organization chronic pneumonia

Liquefaction abscess gangrene

Fibrosis

Fig. 3.26. Summary of the various sorts of inflammation of the lung, the results of healing and the complications that may develop.

Inflammation of the Lung (Pneumonia, Pneumonitis)

Two large groups of inflammations of the lung can be distinguished (Fig. 3.26):

1. **Pneumonias characterized by an intra-alveolar exudate.**

2. **Pneumonias characterized by interstitial inflammation** (alveolar or connective tissue septa).

1. **Pneumonias characterized by an intra-alveolar exudate** are commonly *focal;* called *broncho-pneumonia* or *lobular pneumonia*, since the inflammation arises within the bronchi (see Figs. 3.27, 3.28). *Peribronchial lobular pneumonia* is characterized by a zone of peribronchial exudate (see Figs. 3.27, 3.29).
When a *whole lobe of a lung* is affected, it is called *lobar pneumonia*. Lobar pneumonia (see p. 98) in-volves all the alveoli of a lobe of the lung. The exudate is of uniform appearance, at first serous, then fibrinous and finally purulent. In *bronchopneumonia,* by comparison, the inflammatory foci are in dif-ferent stages of development (serous, purulent or fibrino-purulent). Moreover, fibrinous or purulent exudate is often found in the central portion, whereas at the periphery the exudate is serous. The charac-ter of the alveolar exudate varies (Fig. 3.26). A *serous exudate* may be present (inflammatory edema = blood serum and a small amount of fibrin with a few leukocytes; for example, the stage of congestion in lobar pneumonia which must be distinguished from pulmonary edema). Or, again, there may be a *fibri-nous exudate* with large amounts of fibrin in the alveoli, usually intermixed with a few leukocytes and alveolar epithelial cells (e.g., uremic pneumonia), or *purulent exudate* (with little fibrin) or *hemor-rhagic exudate* (e.g., in influenza).

2. **Interstitial pneumonia** (Fig. 3.26 and pp. 102, 318) shows accumulations of lymphocytes, plasma cells or histiocytes in the alveolar walls.

Results of pulmonary inflammations. a) **Usual result:** lysis of the exudate by leukocytic proteolytic enzymes. Complete restitution of the lung to normal. b) **Organization by granulation tissue** (chronic pneumonia, carnification). c) **Liquefaction** (abscess or gangrene, finally sequestration). d) **Interstitial fibrosis** following incomplete healing of an interstitial pneumonia (p. 102).

Various Forms of Focal (Patchy) Pneumonia

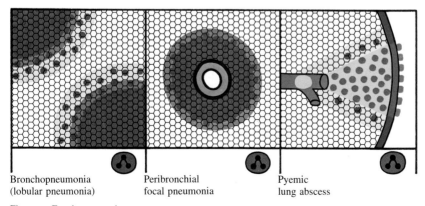

| Bronchopneumonia (lobular pneumonia) | Peribronchial focal pneumonia | Pyemic lung abscess |

Fig.3.27. Focal pneumonias.

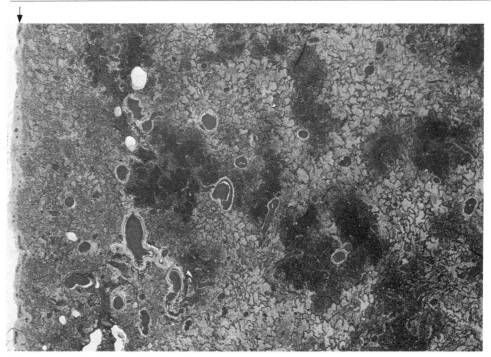

Fig. 3.28. Bronchopneumonia; H & E, 12.5×.

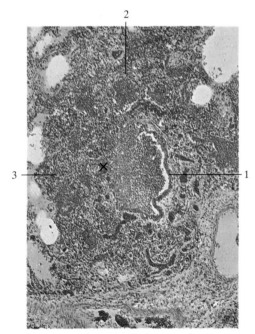

Fig.3.29. Peribronchial focal pneumonia;
H & E, 64×.

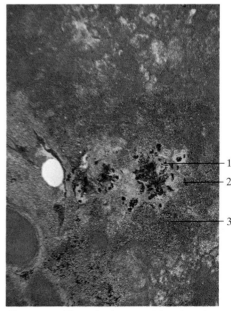

Fig. 3.30. Hemorrhagic necrotizing bronchopneumonia; H & E, 36×.

Focal (Patchy, Lobular) Pneumonia

Focal pneumonias may have a variety of causes and their pathogenesis may be different (endobronchial, peribronchial, hematogenous). Common to all forms is the spread from multiple small foci to the rest of the lung tissue.

Bronchopneumonia (Figs. 3.27, 3.28). *There is patchy inflammation of lung tissue with involvement of single groups of alveoli and not sharply limited to the anatomical units (lobules).* With low magnification, irregular, poorly defined, blue staining foci are seen in the lung (→ pleura). The alveoli between these foci contain palely stained red exudate. If the center of one of the nodules is examined with higher magnification, the alveoli will be seen to be thickly packed with polymorphonuclear cells. Alveolar walls are preserved and the capillaries are hyperemic. The further one looks toward the periphery the fewer the number of leukocytes and fibrin threads that can now be seen. Adjacent alveoli are filled with inflammatory edema, shed alveolar epithelium and a few polymorphonuclear leukocytes *(focal inflammatory edema)*. The bronchi contain purulent exudate and shed ciliated epithelial cells.

Macroscopic: The cut surface shows grayish red to gray, slightly raised nodules with a firm consistency, which can often be better felt than seen. The lung tissue is easily torn. If the nodules have fused with one another, a confluent pneumonia arises. Staphylococci, pneumococci, streptococci and gram-negative organisms are common causes.

Peribronchial focal pneumonia (Figs. 3.27, 3.29). In *this type, the inflammation extends from the bronchial wall into adjacent lung tissue so that mantle-like peribronchial lesions develop.* Low-power magnification shows blue-stained lesions, in the center of which lies a small bronchus. With medium magnification, the bronchus can be recognized by its ciliated epithelium (→ 1), which is missing in one place (×) in the illustration. Reddish fibrinous membranes can be seen in the bronchi (pseudomembranous inflammation). During the healing process, such an area may develop into bronchiolitis obliterans (see Fig. 3.25). The lumen of the bronchus is filled with leukocytes and the wall is densely infiltrated with them. The blood vessels are hyperemic. The adjacent alveoli contain fibrin (→ 2) and leukocytes (→ 3). More distant alveoli are filled with inflammatory edema fluid.

Macroscopic: Small gray nodules with centrally situated small bronchi[1]. It occurs in measles, scarlet fever, diphtheria and influenza, chiefly because of superimposed streptococcal or staphylococcal infection.

Hemorrhagic necrotizing bronchopneumonia (Fig. 3.30). *Lobular or focal peribronchial pneumonia with hemorrhagic exudate occurs chiefly in infectious diseases (e.g., in influenza) caused by a mixture of etiologic agents (a virus plus influenza bacilli or various cocci).* The microscopic picture is variegated. Low magnification shows large, irregularly shaped, red and blue focal lesions. Bacterial colonies (→ 1) are seen in the center of the lesion. The surrounding lung tissue is necrotic (→ 2). Outside of this lies a zone of leukocytes (→ 3) mixed with exuded erythrocytes. Farther toward the periphery, the exudate is entirely hemorrhagic.

In very acute and toxic cases of influenza there is only hemorrhagic edema with hemorrhagic infarction and hyalin vascular thrombi (shock).

Macroscopic: An extremely variegated bronchopneumonia with nodular foci of red, gray and grayish yellow color. Necrosis may develop, particularly in mixed streptococcal infections.

---

[1]These bronchi lack cartilage rings.

Lobar Pneumonia

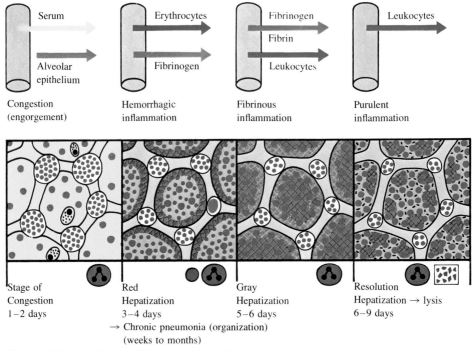

Fig. 3.31. Schematic diagram of the course and the character of the exudate of lobar pneumonia.

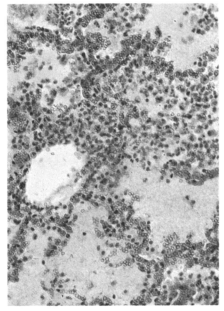

Fig. 3.32. Lobar pneumonia: stage of congestion; H & E, 190×.

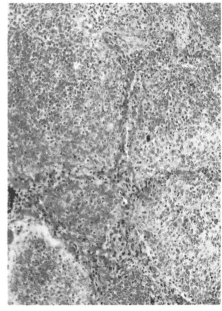

Fig. 3.33. Lobar pneumonia: stage of red hepatization; H & E, 148×.

Lobar Pneumonia

This acute inflammation of a whole lobe of a lung is initiated by pneumococci and both clinically and pathologically follows a progressive course with definite stages. In contrast to focal pneumonia, an entire lobe of a lung (occasionally only a part of a lobe) suddenly becomes inflamed. This occurs in such a way that the different stages of the inflammation do not occur together, but rather follow one another in orderly succession. It is generally supposed that an allergic host reaction plays a part in the development of lobar pneumonia whereby a previous, banal pneumococcal infection acts as a sensitizing agent (Lauche).

Figure 3.31 shows the different stages of the disease in diagrammatic form. In the **stage of congestion or engorgement** (Fig. 3.32) the alveoli are filled with a *serous exudate*. The capillaries are hyperemic. The exudate contains shed alveolar epithelium and occasional leukocytes. Next follows the stage of **red hepatization** (Fig. 3.33), in which the hyperemia increases further and erythrocytes and fibrin appear in the alveoli. **Gray hepatization** (Fig. 3.34) is marked by the appearance of fibrinous exudate. Leukocytes are especially increased in number and dominate the picture. Later, they undergo fatty degeneration and are destroyed (**resolution,** yellow hepatization, Fig. 3.35). At the same time, proteolytic enzymes are liberated which digest the fibrin (**lysis,** 9–28 days). If the fibrin is not digested, organization by granulation tissue occurs (**chronic pneumonia,** Fig. 3.36). All forms of pneumonia may be accompanied by pleuritis (**pleurisy**).

This strict division into stages naturally is not valid in every case, since estimates of the time intervals of the various stages are uncertain and different authors have differing opinions about them. Congestion and red hepatization often fuse into a single stage; there are also various opinions about the sequence of red and gray hepatization and resolution (yellow hepatization). Understandably, there are also transitional forms such as red-gray hepatization and gray-yellow hepatization.

Lobar pneumonia: Stage of engorgement (Fig. 3.32). This very early stage is seldom seen at autopsy, since death usually occurs during red or gray hepatization. Microscopic examination shows alveoli filled with an inflammatory exudate, similar to the focal edema we have already seen in bronchopneumonia (p. 97). There is a finely granular or homogeneous protein precipitate in the alveoli as well as abundant shed alveolar epithelium, but only a few leukocytes and erythrocytes. The capillary hyperemia is striking, and many of the capillaries project into the alveolar lumen in nodular fashion.

Macroscopic: Red, bloody, moist cut surfaces from which reddish, frothy fluid can be scraped off (prune-juice sputum, rusty sputum).

Lobar pneumonia: Stage of red hepatization (Fig. 3.33). In this stage, the most prominent feature under low magnification is the red color caused by extravasated erythrocytes. The firm consistency (like liver = hepatization) is caused by the fibrin. Both medium and high-power magnification show great numbers of erythrocytes, between which lie clusters of numerous leukocytes and alveolar epithelium. In the H & E stain, the thick network of fibrin fibers can be seen only when the condensor diaphragm is closed as much as possible. In the illustration, the hyperemia of the alveolar septa has already disappeared (compressed by the intra-alveolar fibrin). Fibrin thrombi may develop in the capillaries (shock!).

Macroscopic: The cut surfaces are red, firm, friable. As the exudation of fibrin increases, the lungs lose their red color and become gray.

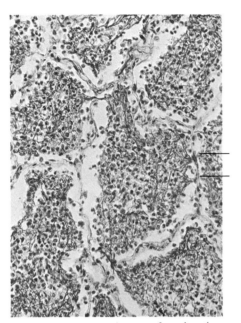

Fig.3.34. Lobar pneumonia: stage of gray hepatization;
Stained by WEIGERT's method (fibrin), 263×.

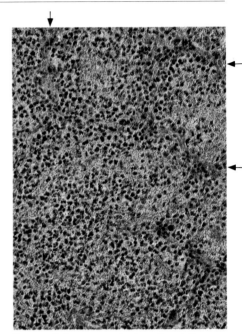

Fig.3.35. Lobar pneumonia:stage of resolution: van Gieson stain, 255×.

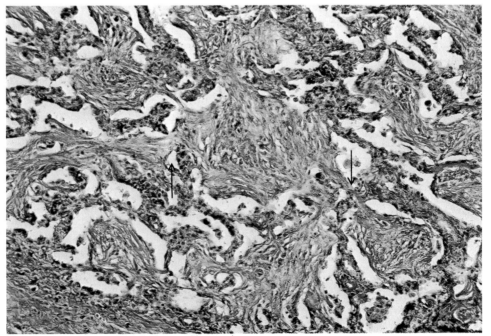

Fig. 3.36. Chronic pneumonia; elastica-van Gieson stain, 152×.

Lobar pneumonia: Stage of gray hepatization (Fig. 3.34). This stage begins after about 5–6 days and is recognized by the intense exudation of fibrinogen which polymerizes to fibrin in the alveoli. Microscopically, under low power and with H & E stains, the alveoli are seen to be filled by a network of red-stained fibers. With Weigert's method for demonstrating fibrin, they stain blue. Medium and high magnification show delicate, interlacing threads and bundles of threads which almost completely fill the alveoli. In several places, the plugs of fibrin are detached from the alveolar walls as a result of fixation. It should be noted that the fibrin threads extend through the pores of Kohn (KOHN, 1893) in the alveolar wall and fuse with those in neighboring alveoli. (Both the lines in Fig. 3.35 lie beside such a fibrin bridge so as not to obscure it.) Counterstaining with nuclear-fast red permits recognition of the numerous granulocytes. The capillaries are nearly empty, the erythrocytes present in the stage of red hepatization have been dissolved.

Macroscopic: The consistency of the lungs is increased. The cut surfaces are friable, dry and finely granular (due to fibrin plugs projecting from the alveoli). The gray color comes from the scattering of light by the fibrin (Tyndall effect).

Lobar pneumonia: Stage of resolution, yellow hepatization (Fig. 3.35). Inspection under low magnification shows a homogeneous appearance. In H & E sections, all the alveoli are filled with blue-stained material. Figure 132 shows a section stained by van Gieson's method. The alveolar septa are clearly seen (→) which indicates that destruction of lung tissue (abscess) has not occurred. The septa surrounded by cellular exudate can be seen also in H & E stains. The figure likewise shows the great numbers of granulocytes and the yellow-stained fibrin bundles.

Macroscopic: Soft, yellow cut surfaces. The more extensive the lysis from digestion of the fibrinous exudate by proteolytic leukocytic enzymes, the more intense the yellow color of the lung tissue and the greater the amount of creamy, yellowish red fluid that can be scraped from the cut surfaces (turbid, mucopurulent expectoration). The lung tissue is easily torn.

A *fibrinous pleurisy* is found in all stages of lobar pneumonia and the regional lymph nodes are swollen (*nonspecific lymphadenitis*). There is usually an accompanying infectious *splenomegaly* and frequently toxic *cloudy swelling* of the kidneys and liver (may result in hepatocellular jaundice). *Pericarditis, enteritis* and *pneumococcal meningitis* are less common complications. In addition, thrombotic occlusion of vessels can lead to complications such as *aseptic ischemic necrosis* with *sequestration* of a pulmonary segment, *lung abscess* (following secondary infection with streptococci or staphylococci) or *gangrene*.

Clinically, lobar pneumonia begins suddenly with shaking chills. With lysis (dissolution of the exudate), profuse sweating occurs and the fever falls (crisis). Simultaneously, there is increased excretion of uric acid (from destruction of leukocytes).

Chronic pneumonia (Fig. 3.36). If a crisis fails to develop, the fibrinous exudate becomes organized by granulation tissue. This arises from the respiratory bronchioles and invades the alveoli. Histologically, the changes can best be seen with van Gieson's stain, which clearly shows the red or reddish yellow plugs that fill the alveoli. Higher magnification shows the young (yellow-stained) and older (red-stained) collagenous fibers and, lying between them, angioblasts, newly formed capillaries, fibroblasts and histiocytes. The granulation tissue replaces the fibrin bridges *(pores of Kohn)*, thus connecting the plugs of granulation tissue in neighboring alveoli (→). The alveolar septa are infiltrated with lymphocytes and histiocytes. The gaps next to the alveolar wall are due to cicatricial contraction of the granulation tissue. The clefts so produced can be secondarily covered with alveolar cuboidal epithelium forming pseudoglandular spaces. An increase in smooth muscle can also be seen *(muscular cirrhosis)*.

Macroscopic: The lungs have a fleshy consistency (carnification). At first, the lungs are red and later grayish-white and shrunken.

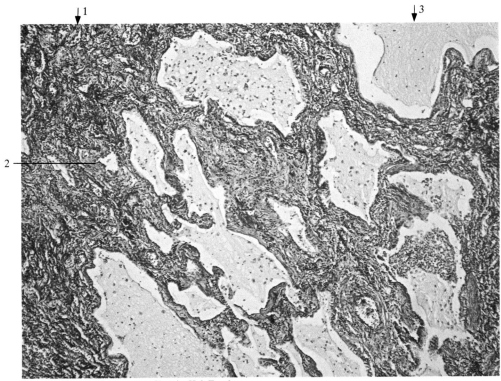

Fig.3.37. Interstitial pulmonary fibrosis; H & E, 560×.

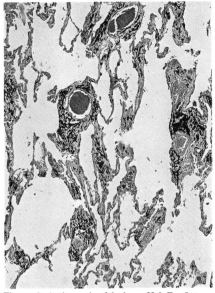

Fig. 3.38. Anthracosis of the lung; H & E, 48×.

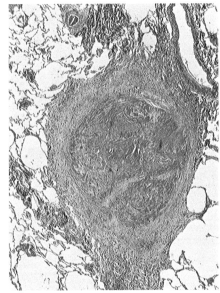

Fig. 3.39. Silicosis of the lung; H & E, 15×.

Interstitial pulmonary fibrosis (Hamman-Rich) (Fig. 3.37). *This is a non-specific inflammation of the lung of unknown etiology, which runs its course in the interalveolar septa and leads to diffuse fibrosis of the lung.* The disease begins with serous inflammation of alveolar septa. Later, the septa become preponderantly infiltrated with lymphocytes and plasma cells. This is followed by proliferation of connective tissue (chiefly fibroblasts, lymphocytes and plasma cells) and leads to disturbance of pulmonary gas exchange.

Figure 3.37 shows this later stage. There is proliferation of richly cellular granulation tissue (→ 1) which has arisen from the alveolar septa. The alveoli are thereby considerably narrowed. Only remnants of the alveolar spaces remain and these are lined with cubical epithelium (→2). Granulation tissue gradually replaces the normal lung tissue so that, eventually, only collagenous fibrous tissue is visible. In isolated places, compensatory overdistention (→3) of the less-affected alveoli has occurred (emphysema). These distended alveoli are filled with protein-containing material (edema).

Causes: antigens such as bird excrement (pigeon handler's disease), mouldy dust (farmer's lung, virus infections, irradiation, busulfan and other cytostatic drugs. Unknown (Hamman-Rich). Auto-aggression? Also seen in shock!

Anthracosis of the lung (Fig. 3.38). *In this condition, coal pigment is deposited in the interstitial tissues.* Coal dust reaching the alveoli is phagocytosed by alveolar epithelium (pneumocytes 1). Since the coal dust is insoluble, it enters the lymphatics and accumulates there. The host reaction consists of slight fibrosis of the perilymphatic connective tissue. Figure 3.38 shows the black pigment (the differential diagnosis of various pigments is given on p. 9) and the slight perivascular fibrosis and lack of cellular infiltration. Occasionally, the deposits fuse into nodules.

Macroscopic: There are fine black cords and small nodules, particularly well seen beneath the pleura.

Silicosis of the lung (Fig. 3.39). Particles of quartz dust ($1-5$ μ in size) entering the lung are phagocytosed and deposited in the lymphatics. The liberated silicates induce histiocyte formation and proliferation of reticular fibers, which later hyalinize, resulting in acellular fibrous nodules. In Figure 3.39 can be seen several large, concentrically arranged, fibrous nodules which are raised above the surface of the lung (→: pleura). Histiocytes containing coal pigment can also be seen at the periphery of the silicotic nodule. Because of their high refractive index, the quartz particles can be detected readily in histological preparations mounted in water and examined with polarized light. Emphysema is present in the areas adjacent to the silicotic nodules. Similar changes are observed in the hilar lymph nodes of the lungs.

Macroscopic: Firm, gray, dry, round nodules.
Pulmonary emphysema, chronic bronchitis and cor pulmonale are the common *complications. Tuberculosis* commonly accompanies silicosis (30–60% of cases). Silicosis and silico-tuberculosis are recognized as compensatory diseases under Workmen's Compensation Laws. Most studies indicate no association with bronchial carcinoma.

Asbestosis of the lung (Fig. 3.40). Asbestos acts as a nidus for the formation of silicate spicules composed of magnesium, silica and iron. The asbestos dust elicits diffuse pulmonary fibrosis, in which are seen dumbbell- or club-shaped asbestosis needles encrusted with protein and iron (brown color). In Figure 3.40, typical asbestos bodies are seen in poorly cellular scar tissue.

Macroscopic: Diffuse fibrosis of the lung. Rather commonly, there is also secondarily a bronchogenic carcinoma. Asbestos which occurs in street dust (automobile tires, brake linings), may also cause pleural mesothelioma. In animal experiments glass fibers are also carcinogenic.

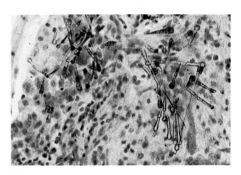

Fig.3.40. Asbestosis; H & E, 255×.

Tuberculosis

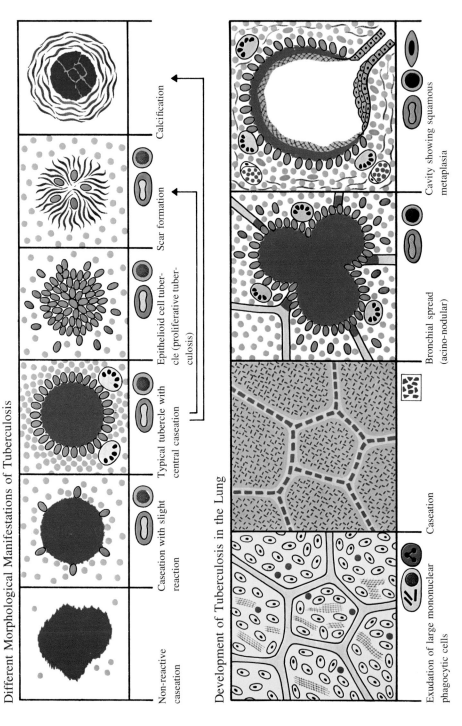

Different Morphological Manifestations of Tuberculosis

Non-reactive caseation — Caseation with slight reaction — Typical tubercle with central caseation — Epithelioid cell tubercle (proliferative tuberculosis) — Scar formation — Calcification

Development of Tuberculosis in the Lung

Exudation of large mononuclear phagocytic cells — Caseation — Bronchial spread (acino-nodular) — Cavity showing squamous metaplasia

Fig. 3.41. Various histological manifestations of the tubercle. Development of pulmonary tuberculosis.

Tuberculosis

Figure 3.41 illustrates the **various histological appearances of a tubercle.** The *"typical"* tubercle consists of a *necrotic center (caseation),* a zone of *epithelioid cells* (modified histiocytes) *Langhans giant cells* and *granulation tissue,* and a more or less well-marked outer margin of *lymphocytes.* In lymph nodes and in certain diseases *(Boeck's sarcoid)*[1], the principal manifestation of tuberculosis may be proliferative, i.e., the formation of a *tubercle composed of epithelioid cells* and showing no central caseation. Occasionally Langhans giant cells are present as well as slight secondary caseation (see pp. 28, 30, 106).

All the manifestations of the tubercle shown to the *right* in the diagram (Fig. 3.41) indicate a *defense reaction* by the host (productive tuberculosis). Epithelioid cell-tubercles as well as caseous tubercles heal by removal of the necrotic material and increased production of collagen fibers and scar formation (e.g., hyalin scars in lymph nodes, indurated slate-colored nodules in the lung). The caseous material may calcify secondarily *(calcified nodules).*

The manifestations to the *left* in Figure 3.41 arise when there is reduced host resistance (exudative tuberculosis). In these cases, the caseation is progressive. Epithelioid cells are always scanty and the chief host reaction is necrosis. Finally, acute bacteremia and sepsis develop with non-reactive necrosis (fulminant tuberculous sepsis).

In the **development of tuberculosis in the lung** (Fig. 3.41), there is an exudative preliminary stage consisting of an acute serous inflammatory exudate containing many large mononuclear phagocytic cells (Fig. 3.42). Alveolar epithelial cells with ingested tubercle bacilli fill the alveoli. Necrosis then ensues very rapidly *(caseation).* *Cavities* develop as a consequence of the tissue destruction (i.e., softening of the caseous necrosis) and may lead to bronchial spread with development of *acino-nodular tuberculosis* characterized by cockade-shaped areas of necrosis and typical tuberculous granulation tissue.

---

[1] NOTE: Epithelioid cell tubercles are a special sort of tissue reaction which occurs in several conditions—Boeck's sarcoid, regional enteritis, etc.

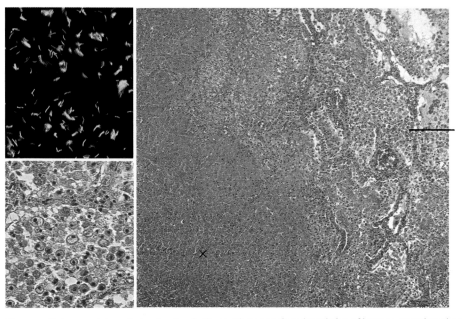

Fig. 3.42. Pulmonary tuberculosis, showing fresh caseation necrosis and exudation of large mononuclear phagocytic cells. H & E, 82×. Upper left: tubercle bacilli in alveolar epithelial cells. Auramin stain (fluorescence microscopy), 1,000×. Lower left: exudate with numerous mononuclear macrophages. H & E, 195× (see description on p. 107.

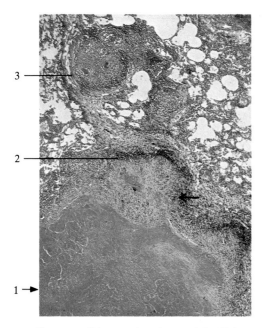

Fig. 3.43. Primary tuberculous nodule (Gohn tubercle) with lymphatic spread;
H & E, 32×.

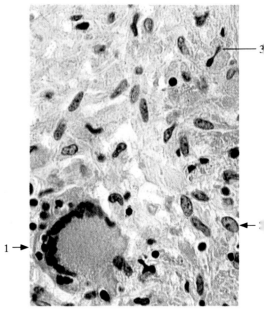

Fig. 3.44. Langhans giant cell and epithelioid cells;
H & E, 576×.

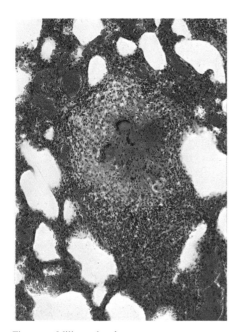

Fig. 3.45. Miliary tubercle;
H & E, 99×.

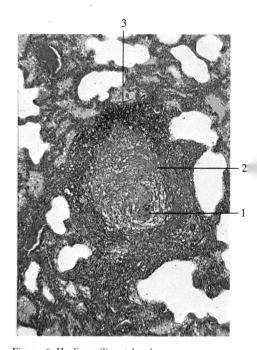

Fig. 3.46. Healing miliary tubercle;
elastica-van Gieson stain, 56×
(see description on p. 109).

Pulmonary tuberculosis, showing fresh caseation necrosis and exudation of large mononuclear phagocytic cells (p. 105). Examination with very low magnification shows a large, irregularly bordered, blue to bluish red area and an adjacent red zone. Medium and high magnification reveal that the blue area consists of crumbled, finely granular, bluish red material (×: necrotic tissue and nuclear fragments). The alveolar walls cannot be seen, but the elastic fibers can still be distinguished with elastica stains. There is a gradual transition without cellular demarcation from the necrosis to the zone containing the exudate of macrophages. In this area, the alveoli are completely filled with alveolar epithelial cells (→). Nearby there is seen a granular, proteinaceous exudate with fibrin and leukocytes. The inset in the upper left corner of Figure 3.42 shows *tubercle bacilli* (bright yellow rods with fluorescence microscopy) which have been phagocytosed by alveolar epithelial cells. In the lower left corner of the picture, the *macrophages of the exudate* are seen under high magnification. The alveolar epithelial cells are spherical and have abundant cytoplasm and round, eccentrically placed nuclei. The cytoplasm in many cells is finely granular and vacuolated.

Macroscopic: Grayish yellow, gelatinous lesions.

Primary tuberculous nodule with lymphatic spread (Fig. 3.43). *At the time of the first infection with tubercle bacilli, a primary nodule develops at the site of entry. In the lung, the primary nodule is beneath the pleura. In extrapulmonary primary tuberculosis, for example in the intestine, the primary nodule is in the intestinal mucosa (see p. 126). Extension from the primary nodule occurs by way of a tuberculous lymphangiitis to the nearest draining lymph node (hilus of the lung, mesenteric lymph node). The lung tubercle and tuberculous lymph node together constitute the primary tuberculous complex.*

Air-borne bacilli lodge in the lung and are taken up by alveolar epithelial cells (Fig. 3.42). Liberation of toxins may then evoke a serous inflammatory reaction *(macrocytic exudation, desquamative macrocytic pneumonia)*. The resulting caseous necrosis becomes walled off by tuberculous granulation tissue. Histologically, at low magnification, round, red, anuclear lesions (blue if calcified) can be seen in the lung with small satellite lesions nearby. Medium magnification (Fig. 3.43) shows the tuberculous necrosis (→ 1), bounded by partially cicatrized granulation tissue (→ 2) containing many Langhans giant cells (→). Air-containing alveoli and a small satellite tubercle can be recognized in the neighboring portions of the lung (→ 3: a nodule arising from lymphatic spread and showing central necrosis and a broad capsule of granulation tissue and lymphocytes). Examination of the margin of the necrotic zone under high magnification (Fig. 3.44) discloses *epithelioid cells* and typical *Langhans giant cells* (→ 1 in Fig. 3.44, see also p. 30). The nuclei of the giant cells are arranged in the shape of a crescent with the opening of the crescent facing the necrosis. The cytoplasm is finely granular. The giant cells arise chiefly by coalescence of epithelioid cells. *The epithelioid cells present two morphological forms:* plump epithelioid cells (→ 2) with poorly defined cytoplasm, oval nuclei and small nucleoli; or as shrunken cells with nuclei resembling a cat's tongue (slipper shaped → 3).

Macroscopic: Yellowish, map-like, subpleural nodules about 1 cm. in diameter, frequently with neighboring miliary tubercles.

Miliary tubercle (Fig. 3.45). *These are millet seed sized tubercles of lymphogenous or hematogenous (miliary tuberculosis) origin.* In miliary tuberculosis, low magnification shows numerous small, richly cellular nodules scattered throughout the lung tissue. Higher magnification shows a small central zone of necrosis surrounded by epithelioid cells and lymphocytes. In the illustration, many Langhans giant cells can be seen at the edge of the necrotic zone.

Macroscopic: Firm, gray, glassy nodules of pinhead size are present in both lungs.

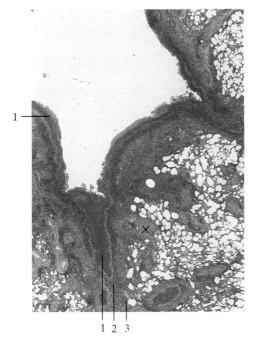

Fig. 3.47. Tuberculous cavity;
H & E, 8×.

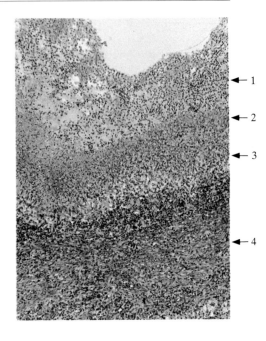

Fig. 3.48. Tuberculous cavity (detail);
van Gieson stain, 82×.

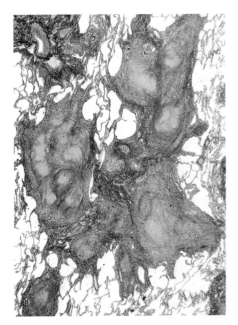

Fig. 3.49. Bronchial spread (acino-nodular)
in pulmonary tuberculosis;
van Gieson stain, 21×.

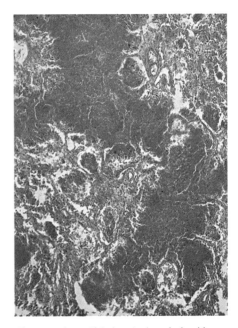

Fig. 3.50. Acute (fulminant) tuberculosis with
extensive caseous necrosis;
H & E, 66×.

Healing miliary tubercle (Fig.3.46, p. 106). Under the influence of tuberculostatic drugs (e.g., streptomycin), miliary tuberculosis can heal fairly quickly. In such a situation, small nodules of epithelioid cells are seen, in the center of which remnants of caseation still persist (yellow in van Gieson's stain → 1) walled off by a broad zone of red fibrous tissue (→ 2). The epithelioid cells have been transformed into histiocytes and fibrocytes and have formed mature reticular and collagenous fibers. In the illustration, there is an increase of elastic fibers at the margin of the tubercle (→ 3). Adjacent lung tissue shows slight emphysema.

Macroscopic: Completely healed tubercles are small white stellate scars.

Tuberculous cavity (Figs. 3.47, 3.48). *As a result of enzymatic digestion of the caseous material (leukocytic enzymes) and removal of the liquefied material by way of a draining bronchus, a cavity may develop in the wall of which three layers can be recognized histologically* (Fig. 3.47). The innermost layer (→ 1) consists of a narrow band of homogeneous, eosinophilic, *necrotic tissue* (yellow in van Gieson's stain), next comes a dark blue layer in which *cellular granulation tissue* and epithelioid cells (→ 2) can be seen under high magnification. Finally, the third and outside layer consists of *cicatrized granulation tissue* (→ 3) infiltrated with nodular collections of lymphocytes. Notice that the blood vessels in the region of the cavity (×) are nearly completely obstructed by intimal proliferation. At a distance from the cavity there are small and large caseous nodules.

Still **higher magnification** (Fig. 3.48) shows the **cavity wall in more detail.** Fibrin is present in the innermost zone (→ 1). Then comes a necrotic zone (→ 2), infiltrated and bordered by epithelioid cells (→ 3). A layer of granulation tissue exhibits numerous vessels and lymphocytes. In the outer portions there is cicatrized granulation tissue (→ 4), with red-staining connective tissue fibers (van Gieson's stain).

Macroscopic: 1. *Fresh cavities:* irregular, grayish white, shaggy wall. 2. *Old cavities:* shiny, grayish yellow or grayish white wall, often showing squamous metaplasia. Scarred, strand-like vessels and bronchi may traverse the cavity.

Bronchial spread in pulmonary tuberculosis (acino-nodular tuberculosis) (Fig. 3.49). *The lesions give a characteristic appearance as they cluster around the bronchial passages.* The tubercle bacilli either lodge in the territory served by a terminal bronchus (pulmonary acinus) or cause peribronchial inflammation, a focal peribronchial pneumonia. As a result, many closely grouped caseous nodules are found, some of which have fused, while others are completely enveloped by fibrous tissue. Higher magnification shows all the typical features of a tubercle (necrosis, a collar of epithelioid cells, Langhans giant cells, and granulation tissue). Figure 3.49, which is stained with van Gieson's method, shows the yellow, central area of necrosis, surrounded by red collagenous connective tissue and peripheral lymphocytes. Numerous giant cells are seen. Notice the emphysema next to the nodules.

Macroscopic: Yellow nodular lesions arranged in grape-like clusters, decreasing in size and extent from the apex to the base of the lung.

Acute (fulminant) tuberculosis with extensive caseous necrosis (Fig. 3.50). *Acute tuberculosis results from marked reduction of host resistance (or increased virulence of the infectious agent). It is sometimes seen as a terminal stage in the treatment of tumors with cytotoxic drugs or in advanced cachexia.* Histologically, there are eosinophilic, map-like areas of necrosis without significant cellular reaction. The illustration shows necrotic pulmonary lesions with serofibrinous exudate and occasional lymphocytes. The alveolar septa are destroyed or indistinct.

Macroscopic: Miliary and larger than miliary-sized, gray, poorly defined, map-like lesions.

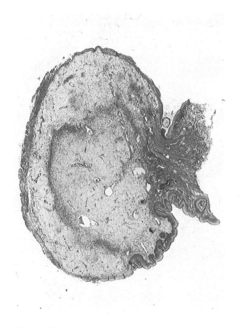

Fig. 4.1. Hemangiomatous epulis (granuloma pyogenicum);
H & E, 20×.

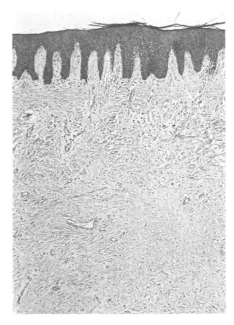

Fig. 4.2. Fibroma;
H & E, 60×.

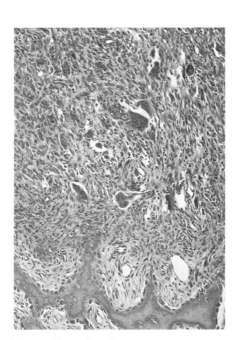

Fig. 4.3. Giant cell epulis;
H & E, 60×.

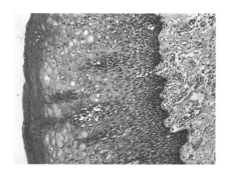

Fig. 4.4. Pachydermia;
H & E, 40×.

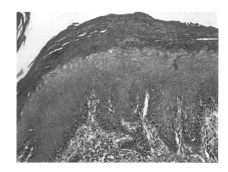

Fig. 4.5. Leukoplakia;
H & E, 40×.

4. Oral Cavity—Gastrointestinal Tract—Pancreas

From ancient times the **oral cavity** has been considered a *mirror of disease*, since many diseases manifest themselves there (e.g., leukemia, agranulocytosis, infectious diseases, etc.). Only a few examples have been selected for consideration here, chiefly because they occur frequently or have special diagnostic or therapeutic significance.

Hemangiomatous epulis ("granuloma pyogenicum"). Fig. 4.1. This is a rather common condition of the lower lip or tongue. Macroscopically there are bright red nodules about 0.5 cm in size partly covered with squamous epithelium (Fig. 4.1). On the right-hand side of the figure the oral mucous membrane is unaltered. The spongy structure of the lesion is clearly shown in the illustration. Proliferation of capillaries occurs just as it does in a capillary hemangioma (see p. 308). In addition there is a sparse infiltration of granulocytes. The lesion usually results from trauma, infrequently it is a true tumor. Women are preferentially affected.

Fibroma (Fig. 4.2) is the most frequent "tumor" of the oral cavity. This *true fibroma* is rich in fibrocytes (occurs especially in the cheeks near the line of closure of the teeth) and is different from a fibroma due to irritation which is a fibrous hyperplasia resulting from chronic pressure, e.g., a prosthesis or tooth crown. Fig. 4.2 shows a fibroma due to irritation that is covered with non-cornified squamous epithelium and composed of broad tongues and bands of collagen fibers and a few fibroblasts.

A **giant cell epulis** (Fig. 4.3) occurs on the gingiva or alveolar process as a nodular bluish or gray tumor (chiefly near front teeth, the mandible; in young women). It always shows a relation to periodontal tissue. Histologically there is a rich proliferation of capillaries and foreign body type giant cells derived from vascular endothelium. Frequently microhemorrhages occur with hemosiderin laden macrophages. Later plasma cells may appear *(granulomatous epulis)* and even bony deposits (osteoplastic epulis). A giant cell epulis is a reactive granulomatous lesion caused by minor trauma for example in reconstructive processes in the periodontium (see also osteoclastoma, p. 267).

Pachydermia (Fig. 4.4). White flecks on the mucous membranes of the cheeks or lips (chiefly in men) that cannot be distinguished grossly from leukoplakia. Histologically there is orderly hyperplasia of the squamous epithelium with hyperkeratosis (rarely parakeratosis). Transition to leukoplakia?

Fig. 4.5 shows harmless changes in the neighborhood of **leukoplakia** which itself is regarded as a precancerous lesion and frequently develops on the alveolar process of the lower jaw or on the mucous folds of the cheeks. Histologically there is *hyperkeratosis, parakeratosis* (nuclei are present in the horny layer), *acanthosis* and *dysplasia* (mitosis present in all layers, loss of polarity in the epithelial layer, hyperchromasia of nuclei) *as well as dyskeratosis* (cornification of single cells). Additionally the submucous is infiltrated by *inflammatory cells*. Transition to carcinoma is 5–10% within 5–10 years. Men are chiefly affected. Causes: tobacco abuse. Either carcinoma in situ or frank carcinoma may hide beneath a lesion that grossly appears to be leukoplakia.

Ameloblastoma (adamantinoma, Fig. 4.6). A benign, cystic tumor arising in the region of the molar teeth of the lower jaw. Histologically there are islands of teeth corresponding to the ameloblasts of developing teeth. The cells have a palisade arrangement and are surrounded by reticulum-like cells (→). Hollow spaces lined with pavement epithelium that sometimes has a horny layer may develop.

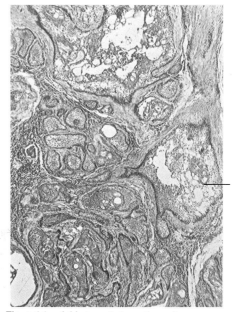

Fig. 4.6 Ameloblastoma (adamantinoma); H & E, 60×.

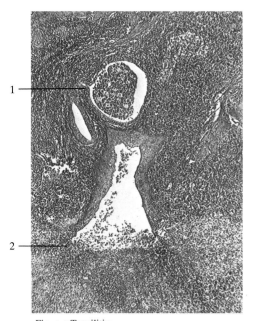

Fig. 4.7 Tonsilitis;
H & E; 100×.

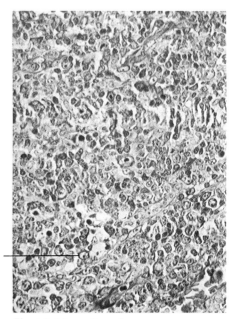

Fig. 4.8. Monocytic angina;
Giemsa stain; 380×.

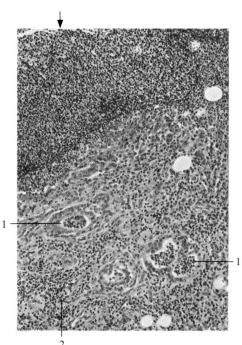

Fig. 4.9. Purulent sialadenitis with abscess;
H & E, 120×.

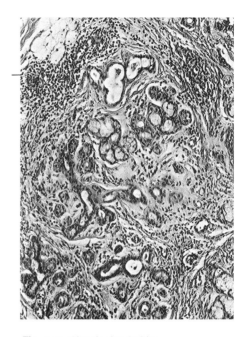

Fig. 4.10. Chronic sialadenitis;
H & E, 100×.

Tonsils and Salivary Glands

Tonsilitis (Fig. 4.7). *Chiefly due to streptococcal infection of the faucial tonsils*. The term *angina* is used when all the lymphoid tissues of the mouth are affected. The tonsilar crypts may be filled with plugs of pus (→ diagonal section of a crypt filled with leukocytes). An abscess has ruptured into the longer portion of the crypt → 2 (necrotic tissue and leukocytes). In the upper part of the figure there is scar tissue indicating previous inflammation.

Necrotizing tonsilitis occurs in scarlet fever (hemolytic streptococci), diphtheria and Vincent's angina (fusiform bacteria and spirochetes). In chronic recurrent tonsilitis the crypts contain cellular detritus, fibrin, leukocytes, fungal and bacterial remnants.

Angina of infectious mononucleosis (glandular fever), Fig. 4.8. In this condition there may be a superficial necrotizing tonsilitis as an expression of generalized infection with Epstein-Barr virus (EBV of the herpes group), accompanied by enlargement of liver, spleen and lymph nodes. Smears of peripheral blood contain up to 90% lymphoid cells (normal lymphocytes plus abnormal lymphocytes or glandular fever cells) which are derived from lymphatic tissue. Lymph nodes and tonsils contain many of these abnormal basophilic lymphocytes (immunoblasts →), lymphoblasts and plasma cells so that the normal structure of the nodes is erased. The reaction centers of secondary lymphoid follicles may be preserved.

Age: 15–25 years, chiefly males. Diagnosis: heterophil agglutination (Paul-Bunnell) test.
Epstein-Barr virus is also thought to be the cause of *Burkitt lymphoma* (see p. 288), *nasopharyngeal carcinoma*, occurring in the south Chinese and perhaps other malignant lymphomas (lymphogranuloma?).

Inflammation of salivary glands may be caused by bacteria, viruses, fungi, irradiation or an immunologic agent. Virus infections like mumps (epidemic parotitis) cause bilateral swelling of the parotic glands (interstitial serous inflammation with lymphocytic infiltrate). Testes, pancreas and meninges may also be affected (viremia). *Cytomegalic inclusion* disease is seen in newborn infants or adults (see p. 29) with lowered resistance or undergoing cytostatic therapy. Typical findings include large, round, DNA-rich nuclear inclusions in the epithelium of parotid ducts. All organs may be affected. *Sjögren's syndrome* is an autoimmune disease (antibodies against parotid duct extract) which affects postmenopausal women and leads to atrophy of the parotid and tear glands (sicca syndrome: xerostomia, keratoconjunctivitis sicca) and sometimes may be associated with chronic rheumatoid arthritis.

Purulent sialadenitis with abscess (Fig. 4.9), usually bilateral, occurs in debilitated patients with poor resistance, frequently following an operation. Calculi may form in ascending infection, mostly in the submandibular gland and chiefly in men. Histologically, dilated excretory ducts and their branches contain granulocytes (→1). The gland itself is edematous and packed with polymorphonuclear leukocytes and lymphocytes (→ 2). Often there is tissue destruction and abscess formation (→).

Chronic sialadenitis of the submandibular gland (Fig. 4.10) presents as a hard, tumor-like lesion. Cause: duct calculi. Men are mostly affected. Histologically there is scanty infiltration of lymphocytes (→) and collagenous connective tissue surrounding excretory ducts. The glandular acini are distorted by chronic inflammation. The result is sclerotic scarring of the gland similar to that seen in cirrhosis of the liver.

Granulomatous inflammation with many epithelioid cells may occur in sarcoidosis (see p. 236). The parotid glands are involved most frequently (6%), but the submandibular and lacrimal glands may also be affected (Mikulicz syndrome).

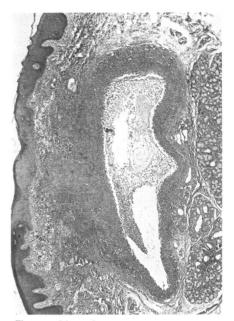

Fig. 4.11. Mucocele;
H & E, 20×.

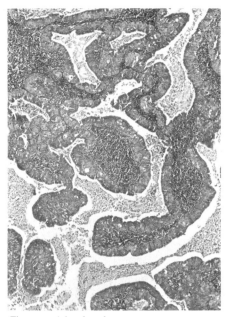

Fig. 4.12. Adenolymphoma;
H & E, 60×.

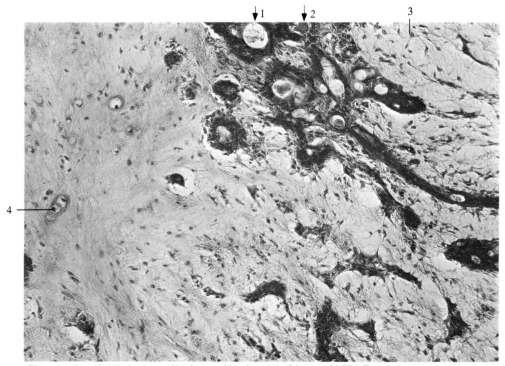

Fig. 4.13. So-called "mixed tumor" (pleomorphic adenoma) of the parotid; H & E, 130×.

Salivary Gland Tumors

Mucocele (retention cyst of salivary gland, salivary gland granuloma, Fig. 4.11). Occurs chiefly in the lower lip as a result of injury of the salivary excretory duct from biting. They are pseudocysts without epithelial lining (true cysts have an epithelial lining). Mucous secretion accumulates in the tissues as a result of the trauma (or of chronic inflammation) leading to a granulomatous tissue reaction which walls off the mucous. On the left hand side of the illustration, there is surface epithelium; on the right, salivary gland. A large true cyst is called a *ranula* (submaxillary or sublingual gland).

Adenolymphoma (Warthin tumor, Fig. 4.12.) A benign tumor, almost exclusively of the parotid glands, mostly unilateral, virtually restricted to elderly men. Macroscopically the cut surface is finely cystic. Histologically there are cystic spaces lined by a double layer of epithelium with red staining (H & E) cytoplasm. Characteristically lymphoid tissue lies between the cysts.

Mixed tumor of the parotid (pleomorphic adenoma Fig. 4.13). Mixed tumors may arise in any of the salivary glands of the oral cavity but are most frequent in the parotid gland. The current opinion is that the tumor is a *true adenoma* showing pseudomesenchymal differentiation. Foci of mucous, hyalin and cartilage are thought to be derived either from cells of the glands or from myoepithelium. Examination of the tumor with a scanning lens reveals foci of several different sorts of tissue: solid strands of cuboidal and cylindrical epithelium forming glands ($\rightarrow$ 1). Masses of homogeneous hyaline fill the lumens of the glands ($\rightarrow$ 2). The solid strands border homogenous tissue containing abundant blue staining ground substance and branched cells having stellate processes (mucoid portion $\rightarrow$ 3) or cells with halos that resemble cartilage cells ($\rightarrow$ 4). The epithelial formations are derived from salivary gland ducts.

Macroscopic: Well defined grayish white tumors often with a gelatinous cut surface. Prone to recur. In elderly men about 5% show malignancy (adeno- or squamous carcinomas).

Adenoidcystic carcinoma (Cylindroma Fig. 4.14). This is a locally malignant epithelial tumor, which grows by local infiltration, frequently recurs after removal, but metastasizes only rarely (lungs). It shows a Swiss cheese pattern histologically, with adenoid cellular structures having both small and large cystic spaces filled with mucous. The cysts are formed from the mucous secreted by epithelial cells that are embedded in hyaline stroma. Typically there is a PAS positive basement membrane.

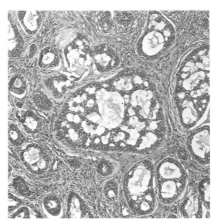

Fig. 4.14. Adenoidcystic carcinoma; H & E, 60×.

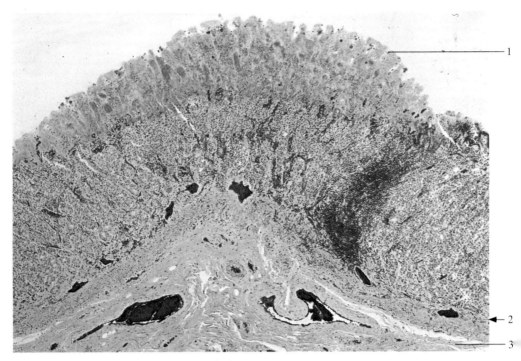

Fig. 4.15. Corrosive injury of gastric mucosa; H & E, 50×.

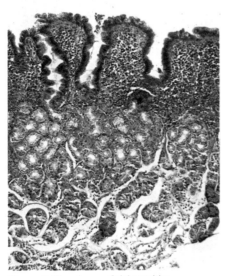

Fig. 4.16. Chronic superficial gastritis;
H & E, 90×.

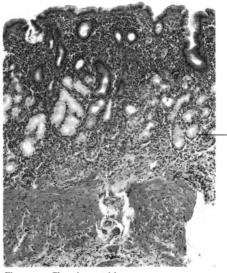

Fig. 4.17. Chronic gastritis
with early mucosal
atrophy; H & E, 90×.

Gastrointestinal Tract

A knowledge of the normal architecture of the gastrointestinal tract is helpful in interpreting histopathological appearances (mucosa: squamous epithelium-cylindrical epithelium-glands; character of the villi; tunica propria, muscularis mucosae, submucosa, muscularis propria and subserosa). It is important to note the cellular constituents of the individual coats and any defects in the mucosa or atypical proliferation of the glands.

Corrosive injury of the gastric mucosa (Fig. 4.15). Corrosive acids cause coagulation necrosis of the gastric mucosa, while lye causes liquefaction necrosis. Figure 4.15 shows an area of fresh corrosion of the gastric mucosa due to HCl. The necrosis (coagulation necrosis $\rightarrow$ 1) can be seen on the surface. The cytoplasm of the necrotic cells in the glands is stained more strongly with eosin than the cells that lie deeper. The cells in the necrotic area lack nuclei. The necrotic zone is bordered by a narrow rim of granulocytes, scant numbers of which are also present in the submucosal stroma. With the passage of time, the necrotic mucosa sloughs off and an ulcer results. $\rightarrow$ 2 muscularis mucosae, $\rightarrow$ 3 submucosa.

Macroscopic: In the early stage of scab formation, there are different colors, depending upon the kind of corrosive: sublimate (HgCl$_2$)-grayish white, HNO$_3$-yellowish, H$_2$SO$_4$ and HCl-dark brown. The following sequelae may develop: perforation, cicatricial stricture (e.g., in the esophagus).

Gastritis

Gastritis. Normally there is slight inflammation of the entire gastrointestinal tract with infiltration of small numbers of granulocytes ("physiological" inflammation). For the diagnosis of gastritis histologically there should be necrosis of epithelium with a tissue defect and a more marked inflammatory reaction. Histological gastritis may not have a clinical counterpart.

1. **Acute gastritis:** Catarrhal inflammation, edema and a small epithelial defect. Recovery in a few days (alcohol abuse!).

2. **Chronic superficial gastritis** (Fig. 4.16): Chiefly confined to the antrum but also encroaching on other regions of the stomach. Fig. 4.16 shows the alterations in mucous glands in the antrum. The tips of the villi are widened by inflammatory exudate (lymphocytes, plasma cells, granulocytes) and appear plump. Small defects in the superficial epithelium are visible. Epithelium with dark nuclei and basophilic cytoplasm has replaced the normal mucus-secreting superficial epithelium.

3. **Chronic gastritis with early atrophy of mucosa** (Fig. 4.17). The diagram on p. 119 illustrates the loss of mucosa compared to normal and the extension of inflammatory exudate to the mucosa muscularis. The inflammatory process extends from the surface to involve the entire mucosa. In contrast to superficial gastritis the mucosa is reduced in width and has bulky borders and flat foveolae. The inflammatory exudate consists of granulocytes, plasma cells and many lymphocytes. Typical lymph follicles may be present. Both chief cells (pepsinogen production) and parietal cells (HCl production) are reduced in number. Likewise the mucous glands ($\rightarrow$) in the antrum are decreased.

4. **Chronic atrophic gastritis** (Fig. 4.18). The mucosa is markedly atrophied (Figs. 4.18, 4.22). Both chief cells and parietal cells have vanished as have antral mucous glands. The entire mucosa consists only of the surface epithelial layer and broad gastric pits with elongated marginal tips. Frequently the lymphoid tissue is hyperplastic (lymph follicles). Clinically: achlorhydria, achylia gastrica.

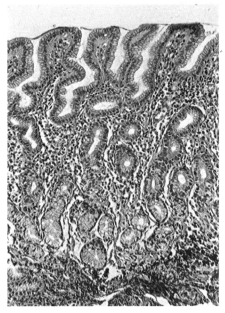

Fig. 4.18. Chronic atrophic gastritis;
H & E, 100×.

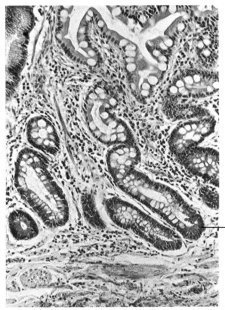

Fig. 4.19. Atrophy and intestinal metaplasia of
gastric mucosa;
H & E, 200×.

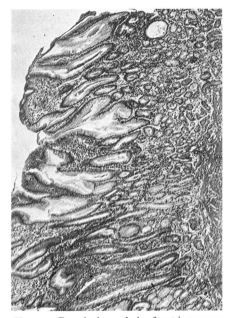

Fig. 4.20. Foveolar hyperplasia of gastric mucosa;
H & E, 100×.

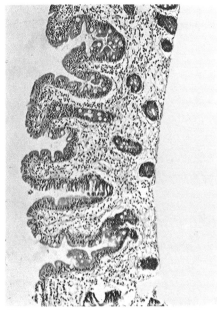

Fig. 4.21. Celiac disease (non-tropical sprue);
H & E, 100×.

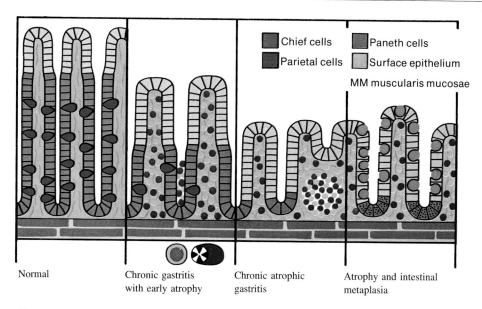

Normal   Chronic gastritis   Chronic atrophic   Atrophy and intestinal
with early atrophy   gastritis   metaplasia

Fig. 4.22. Diagram of different sorts of chronic gastritis (redrawn from Oehlert).

5. **Atrophy of gastric mucosa with intestinal metaplasia** (Fig. 4.19). The mucosa is atrophied just as in chronic atrophic gastritis. The foveolae extend to the muscularis mucosae and resemble the crypts of the jejunal mucosa. Goblet cells are abundant and there are granular Paneth cells ($\rightarrow$). For the most part the epithelium is basophilic (dark red cytoplasm, no pale secreting epithelium). Occurs in the end-stage of chronic atrophic gastritis, pernicious anemia, senile atrophy and in the margins of chronic gastric ulcers. It is regarded as a precancerous lesion and may result in early cancer (see p. 301).

6. **Atrophy of gastric mucosa.** Occurs in the aged, in chronic atrophic gastritis and in pernicious anemia. Normally extrinsic factor (vitamin B_{12}) is bound to intrinsic factor of the parietal cells and thus protected from destruction. Loss of parietal cells (atrophy, chronic gastritis, after gastrectomy) may lead to a deficiency of B_{12}. A genetic defect may also operate.

Causes of gastritis: chronic alcohol abuse, age-determined disturbance of regenerative capacity (after 60 years 50–80% of persons have superficial chronic atrophic gastritis, Simala et al, 1968), autoaggression.

Hyperplasia of gastric mucosa (Fig. 4.20, 4.22). In the *Zollinger-Ellison syndrome* there is glandular hyperplasia of the mucosa that is markedly mammilated macroscopically. The mucosa is thickened because of hyperplasia of the glands and of both chief cells and parietal cells. The usual cause is a gastrin producing tumor of the pancreas. *Result:* multiple gastric and duodenal ulcers. *Giant hypertrophic gastropathy.* Gigantic mucosal folds and increase in thickness of mucosal epithelium. Increased mucous production $\rightarrow$ protein loss $\rightarrow$ hypoproteinemia.
Foveolar hyperplasia in chronic gastritis (Fig. 4.20). Mucosal epithelium is widened with loss of chief and parietal cells.

Celiac disease (non-tropical sprue, gluten enteropathy) Fig. 4.21. The malabsorption syndrome occurs after resection of the small intestine, in Whipple's disease (see p. 124), exudative enteropathy and sprue. In **non-tropical sprue** (Fig. 4.21) there is sensitivity to gluten-enzyme defect. There is villous atrophy (flattening and broadening with increase of parietal cells) and a lymphoplasmacytic infiltrate. *Clinical:* large, fatty stools.

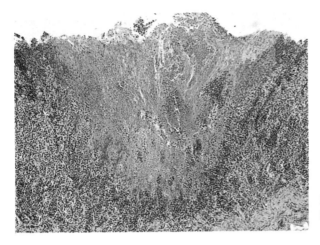

Fig. 4.23. Hemorrhagic infarct of the gastric mucosa; H & E, 72×.

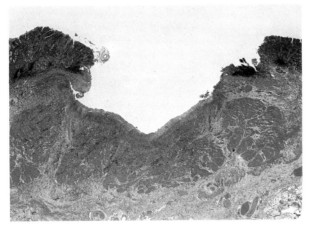

Fig. 4.24. Fresh gastric ulcer, H & E, 14×.

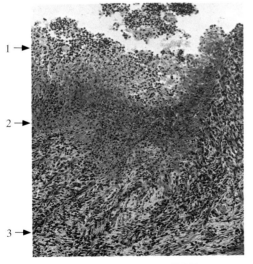

Fig. 4.25. Base of a gastric ulcer; H & E, 102×.

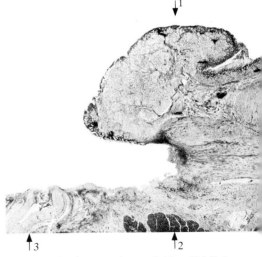

Fig. 4.26. Chronic penetrating gastric ulcer; H & E, 6×.

Gastric Ulcer

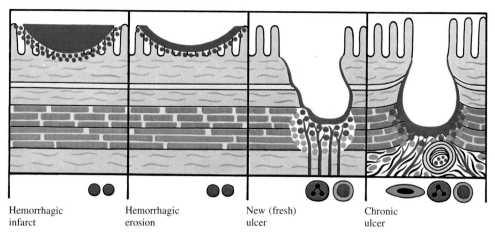

| Hemorrhagic infarct | Hemorrhagic erosion | New (fresh) ulcer | Chronic ulcer |

Fig. 4.27. Probable pathogenesis of a gastric ulcer.

First stage: *hemorrhagic infarction of the mucosa* (see Fig. 4.23). The necrotic material is being excavated into the lumen (*hemorrhagic erosion*). The erosion can either heal or progress to ulceration. A *new ulcer* (Fig. 4.24) frequently is step-like on the oral edge, while on the aboral edge it rises steeply. A *chronic ulcer* (Fig. 4.26), in contrast, is flask shaped with a margin of dense scar tissue.
NOTE: Erosion: defect limited to mucosa. Ulcer: defect involves stomach wall.

Hemorrhagic infarct (Fig. 4.23). A wedge-shaped area lacking stained nuclei is seen in the mucosa. Medium magnification shows erythrocytes lying in anuclear necrotic tissue, the greater part of which stains only faintly. The villi of the surface mucosa have disappeared (slight erosion).

Macroscopic: Irregularly shaped black foci with shallow mucosal defects.

Fresh gastric ulcer (Fig. 4.24). Under low magnification, the defect in the wall can be seen extending to the muscularis and showing the usual mucosal overhang (on the aboral edge to the left of the illustration). In the base of the ulcer, there is a pale grayish red zone (fibrin) and a darker zone (necrosis and granulation tissue). Under higher magnification, it is easier to analyze these layers. **Base of a gastric ulcer** (Fig. 4.25). At the top, there is a loose layer of fibrin and polymorphonuclear leukocytes (→ 1) lying on an intensely eosinophilic band-like zone of fibrinoid necrosis (→ 2): necrotic material composed of fibrin and nuclear fragments. Granulation tissue (→ 3) surrounds the necrotic layer and invades it. The capillaries in the granulation tissue run perpendicularly to the surface. Fibroblasts, lymphocytes, histiocytes and mature connective tissue make up the lower third of this zone.

Macroscopic: A step-like or flat, round or oval defect in the wall. The base is gray.

Chronic penetrating ulcer (Fig. 4.26). In this figure, the mucous membrane has been elevated (→ 1) and contains hyperplastic pyloric glands. In the neighborhood of the ulcer, there is an increased amount of connective tissue. The defect in this instance extends to the pancreas (→ 2). The necrosis has eroded a large artery →3 (clinically: fatal hemorrhage).

Macroscopic: A round defect with firm margins and a smooth base. Pancreatic lobules can often be seen in the base of the ulcer.

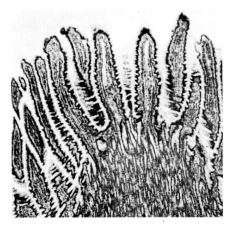

Fig. 4.28. Normal jejunum (dog); H & E, 40×.

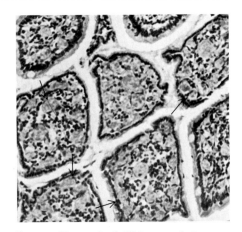

Fig. 4.29. Hyperemia of villi (cross section); H & E, 170×.

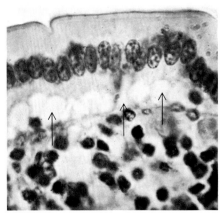

Fig. 4.30. Serous exudation with elevation of surface cells; H & E, 700×.

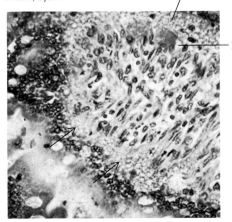

Fig. 4.31. Marked protein exudation in the subepithelial space; H & E, 400×.

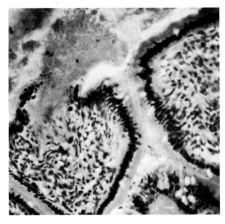

Fig. 4.32. Beginning necrosis of the tip of a villus; H & E, 180×.

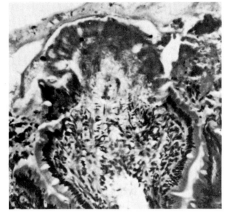

Fig. 4.33. Complete necrosis of the tip of villus; H & E, 190×.

Enterocolitis

All the infectious agents or their toxins, as well as noninfectious toxic agents (e. g., allergy, uremia) cause a similar series of tissue reactions in the intestinal mucosa, which succeed one another in an orderly progression and have as a common basis changes in the terminal vascular system. The early stages cannot be as well seen in humans as in experimental animals because of the rapid onset of autolysis. The photographs on page 122 illustrate such a series of experiments in dogs given dysentery toxin intravenously (Croneberg and Sandritter, 1952).

The dysentery toxin first causes shock, with a fall in blood pressure, then an increase in peripheral resistance due to contraction of the arterioles. Following this, a disturbance of the microcirculation develops, resulting in aggregation of erythrocytes (sludge phenomenon) and of platelets (see p. 77) which cause reduced venous return to the heart. In the terminal phase, hyalin thrombi form in the arterioles and venules and cause necrosis and hemorrhage. The central feature of this sort of shock is an alteration of blood coagulation in which consumption of coagulation factors and blockade of the reticuloendothelial system (see p. 18) play an essential part (for *consumption of coagulation factors,* see Lasch, 1963, 1964; for morphology, see Sandritter and Lasch, 1966). In the dog, the intestine must be regarded as a shock organ. The alteration in the microcirculation first becomes apparent as hyperemia (Fig. 4.29 → hyperemic capillaries) of the villi of the small intestine (compare them with the slender villi of normal *jejunum* in Fig. 4.28). Simultaneously with the hyperemia, there is exudation into the stroma of the villi.

The exudate lifts the epithelium. The result is the formation of a *subepithelial space* (→ in Fig. 4.30). With increasing capillary circulatory disturbance (hyalin thrombi), more fluid accumulates in the subepithelial space (→ in Fig. 4.31), so that the entire epithelium is elevated. Figure 4.31 shows the **granular protein masses** (formed from the fluid during fixation) under the epithelium (→). The stasis has led to circumscribed *necrosis of the tips of the villi* (Fig. 4.32), characterized by a homogeneous mass of epithelium, villus stroma and fibrin. Finally, the entire upper third of the villi becomes necrotic (**complete necrosis of the tips of the villi,** Fig. 4.33). In the end stage, one sees a broad necrotic zone with nuclear fragmentation, exudate and leukocytes.

The experimental observations just described can serve as a model for the development of the morphological consequences of shock (e. g., renal cortical necrosis, hemorrhagic necrosis of the adrenal or Waterhouse-Friderichsen syndrome, etc.) and for enteritis in man. In the subacute and chronic stages, the necrotic material is cleared away (by mechanical means or leukocytic ingestion). Ulcers develop which may extend deeply and so lay bare the muscularis (*ulcerative colitis,* p. 125). In chronic cases, secondary proliferation of the mucosa occurs at the edges of the ulcers (so-called pseudopolyposis, p. 125).

In many cases, a fibrinous exudate predominates, with more or less marked necrosis of the tips of the villi (pseudomembranous colitis, e.g., in uremia).[1] Figure 4.34 (**superficial fibrinous and necrotizing colitis**) shows such an inflammation with a broad layer of fibrin and leukocytes (→ 1) and beginning necrosis of the tips of villi. The mucosa is markedly hyperemic and the submucosa is thickened by edema (→ 2: muscularis mucosae).

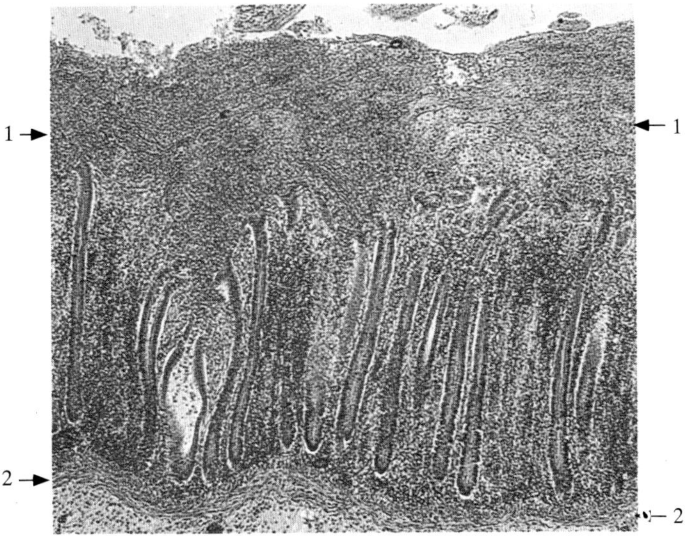

[1] Pseudomembranous colitis occurs chiefly after antibiotic therapy as a result of overgrowth of staphylococci.

Fig. 4.34. Superficial fibrinous and necrotizing colitis; H & E, 46×.

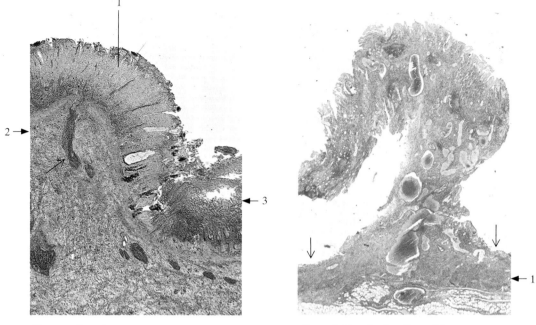

Fig. 4.35. Dysentery;
H & E, 28×.

Fig. 4.36. Chronic ulcerative colitis;
H & E, 11×.

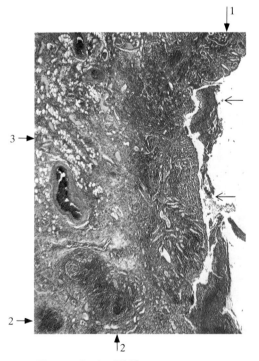

Fig. 4.37. Regional ileitis;
H & E, 20×.

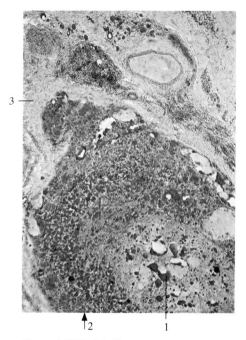

Fig. 4.38. Whipple's disease:
Sudan-hematoxylin, 64×.

Dysentery (Fig. 4.35). *Intestinal infestation by Shigella organisms or amebae. The colon is most frequently affected, and less frequently the distal ileum. In the early stages, there is edema and hyperemia of the mucosa, which is followed by hemorrhagic inflammation, necrosis, and a fibrinous exudate on the surface of the mucosa (pseudomembranous, necrotizing inflammation). The terminal stages show ulceration.* (Amoebic dysentery is discussed on p. 328.) Figure 4.35 shows an area of expanding necrosis of the colonic mucosa ($\rightarrow$ 1) and considerable edematous loosening of the submucosa ($\rightarrow$ 2). The blood vessels are widely dilated and partly filled with erythrocytes and fibrin thrombi ($\rightarrow$). There is a longitudinal pseudomembranous layer of fibrin ($\rightarrow$ 3). For electron microscopy see Takeuchi et al., 1965.

Macroscopic: Redness and edema of the intestinal wall. Mucosal necrosis is forming a dirty yellowish brown, clay-like covering. Sharply circumscribed ulcers with undermined margins. The colon contains blood mucus.

Chronic ulcerative colitis (Fig. 4.36). *This is a chronic relapsing, noninfectious inflammation of the mucosa of the colon (an autoimmune disease with mucosal ulceration and granulomatous inflammation $\rightarrow$ clinical bleeding, scarring, polypoid mucosal regeneration and in about 7% of cases carcinoma; normally 0.3%. Seen chiefly in neurotic young persons, but may occur at any age).* In the fully developed disease, there are extensive ulcers ($\rightarrow$) extending to the muscularis propria ($\rightarrow$ 1), together with islands of preserved colonic mucosa. These islands of colonic mucosa are polypoid and have stalks containing connective tissue (the elevation of the mucosa to the left in the illustration is an artifact).

Macroscopic: Extensive, irregular, longitudinal mucosal defects with polypoid overgrowth of mucosal islands. The wall is stiff and the lumen narrowed. The muscularis shows cross rippling.

Regional ileitis (terminal ileitis, regional enteritis, Crohn's disease, Fig. 4.37). *This is a chronic, recurring disease of the intestine or colon involving all intestinal coats. Etiology is unknown. Age: 15–35 years. Frequently familial.* After the edema, hyperemia and hemorrhage of the acute stage, the chronic stage is characterized by extensive ulceration ($\rightarrow$) with thickened mucosa ($\rightarrow$ 1) and accompanied by a chronic inflammatory infiltrate and epithelioid cell granulomas ($\rightarrow$ 2) with Langhans type giant cells (this is not tuberculosis, but rather a non-specific granuloma). In Figure 4.37, the ulcer extends to the subserosa ($\rightarrow$ 3). Beneath this, there is an increased amount of collagenous connective tissue (scarring) and hypertrophy of the muscularis.

Macroscopic: In the chronic stage, the intestinal wall is thick and rigid, the surrounding tissues are adherent and there are irregular mucosal defects.

Complications: Perforation, hemorrhage, stenosis, fistulas, extension, frequent recurrence.

NOTE: Often multiple segments are involved with frequent recurrences.

Whipple's disease (intestinal lipodystrophy, Fig. 4.38). *This is a progressive disease of the small intestine and mesenteric lymph nodes in which there is stasis of chyle, fat storage and granulomatous inflammation. It is probably caused by a bacterial infection (Corynebacteria?, Hemophilus?,* Chears and Ashworth, 1961; Kjaerheim et al., 1966). Histologically, the intestinal lymph vessels are dilated and filled with fat. The sinuses of enlarged mesenteric lymph nodes are also dilated, cystic and crammed with phagocytosed fat (partially dissolved during fixation $\rightarrow$ 1). Histiocytic granulation tissue is present throughout ($\rightarrow$ 2) with large foam cells containing lipid droplets (also glycoproteins). It is in these cells that the above-mentioned bacteria have been demonstrated. In the later stages, scarring may result from the chronic inflammation ($\rightarrow$ 3).

Macroscopic: Chylous ascites, dilated, yellow lymphatic channels in the intestinal serosa, enlarged cystic lymph nodes with yellow contents.

Pathogenesis: Bacterial infection.
Clinical: Chiefly rheumatic complaints, endocarditis, steatorrhea, anemia, cachexia. Obstruction of the thoracic duct (stasis?).

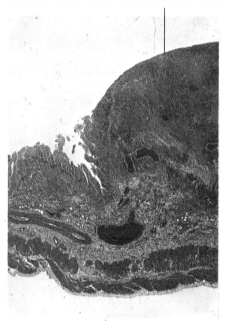

Fig. 4.39. Typhoid fever: marked inflammatory swelling; H & E, 26×.

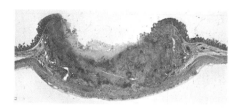

Fig. 4.40. Typhoid fever: ulceration and scab formation;
H & E, 6×.

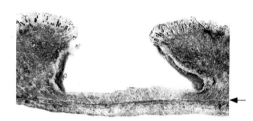

Fig. 4.41. Typhoid fever: ulcer
H & E, 8×.

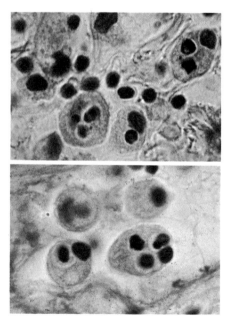

Fig. 4.42. Typhoid fever: large macrophages;
H & E, 640×.

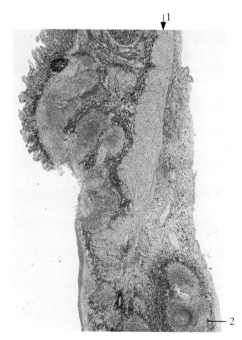

Fig. 4.43. Tuberculous ulcer of intestine;
van Gieson stain, 12×.

Typhoid Fever

The typhoid bacillis (Salmonella typhi) *causes an inflammatory disease of the lower ileum and occasionally the colon that runs a characteristic course. The inflammation starts in the region of Peyer's patches and progresses to necrosis and ulceration. Four stages are recognized, each lasting approximately one week. Both the intensity of the inflammation and the duration of the disease vary greatly.*

1st stage (1 week); **marked inflammatory swelling** (Fig. 4.39), with either diffuse or focal enlargement of the lymphoid follicles which is characterized by infiltration of swollen reticuloendothelial cells and palely stained lymphocytes (architecture erased). Figure 4.39 shows the dense cellular infiltration of a swollen follicle (bluish red), with beginning necrosis of the surface mucosa (→). **Higher magnification** (Fig. 4.42) reveals an increased number of large round macrophages with abundant cytoplasm containing pyknotic nuclei, nuclear fragments and erythrocytes within phagosomes.

Macroscopic: Pea-sized, grayish red nodules or gray plaques.

2nd stage (2 weeks); a **scab** (Fig. 4.40) can be seen in the necrotic portion of the markedly swollen and superficially ulcerated tissue (area devoid of nuclei). The necrotic area is surrounded by leukocytes.

Macroscopic: Yellowish green necrosis stained with bile.

In the third week the necrotic tissue sloughs, and this results in the *3rd stage: ulceration* (Fig. 4.41). The ulcer extends to the muscularis (→). A narrow strip of necrotic tissue can still be recognized in the edges at each side.

In the *4th stage* (4 weeks) *the ulcer is cleaned up finally* by granulation tissue, which is then converted to a *scar* and finally epithelialized from the adjacent mucosa. The scars are smooth and thin because of the absence of lymph follicles. After about four months, only a thin zone in the intestinal wall marks the previously diseased area. Typhoid scars never cause stenosis.

Clinical: temperature rises during the first week to 39–40°C and continues to week four, then falls; florid diarrhea (pea soup stools), skin rash (rose spots), splenomegaly.

Complications: Perforation with peritonitis in the ulcer stage (3 weeks), fatal intestinal hemorrhage, typhoid pneumonia, waxy hyalin, degeneration of the abdominal muscles (p. 231).

Intestinal tuberculosis (Fig. 4.43). *Tubercle bacilli may colonize the lymph follicles of Peyer's patches and cause caseous tuberculosis.* Under very low magnification, a defect is seen which extends to the muscularis (→ 1). The base is formed by a narrow zone of necrosis (caseation) containing many polymorphonuclear leukocytes (secondary infection). At the margins, there are round nodules that can be identified as typical tubercles under higher magnification. The tubercles extend through the entire wall at the base of the ulcer and into the serosa (→ 2). There is an increase in connective tissue.

Macroscopic: Flat ulcers with tattered margins, often surrounded by a circle of small white nodules on the serosa. Tuberculous lymphangiitis develops. The nearest lymph nodes draining the area are also always involved. Intestinal tuberculosis appears either as a result of ingestion of tubercle bacilli (primary intestinal tuberculosis with a primary complex) or, more frequently, as a secondary tuberculous process in association with active pulmonary tuberculosis.
Complications: Scarring of the ulcers with resultant intestinal stenosis, rarely perforation into the peritoneal cavity or into neighboring hollow organs. Bleeding may occur from a tuberculous ulcer; or generalized tuberculous peritonitis may develop.

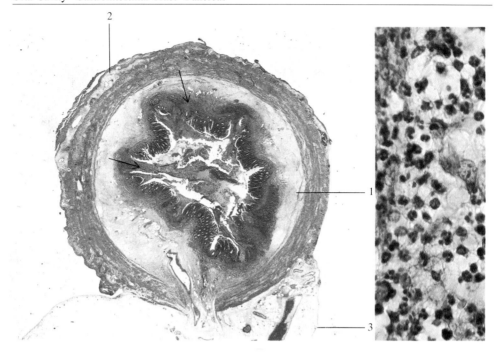

Fig. 4.44a. Phlegmonous appendicitis; H & E, 10×.

Fig. 4.44b. Higher
magnification of
the submucosa, 600×.

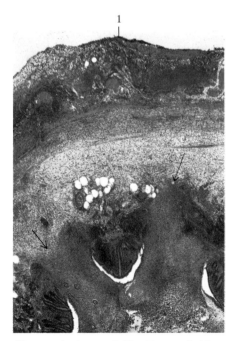

Fig. 4.45. Acute appendicitis with a so-called focus
of primary infection;
H & E, 23×.

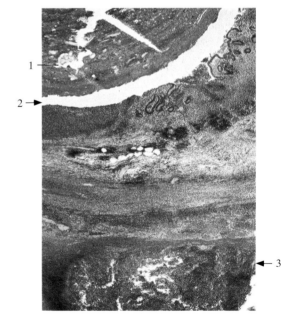

Fig. 4.46. Appendicitis with a fecalith;
H & E, 41×.

Appendicitis

Inflammation of the vermiform appendix usually has an intestinal origin (invasion of obstructed glands by intestinal bacterial flora or streptococci: or obstruction from a fecalith). Only rarely is appendicitis hematogenous, although it may follow an acute viral infection such as influenza, chickenpox or measles.

The *inflammation* starts in a small focus in the mucosa (*primary infection* of ASCHOFF, 1908) and then spreads like a *phlegmon* through all coats of the wall. Intramural abscesses, secondary ulceration, empyema, necrosis and gangrene of the wall frequently occur as a result of the development of arteritis and hemorrhagic infarction.

Figure 4.44a shows an example of **acute phlegmonous appendicitis** at very low magnification. Fibrin and leukocytes fill the lumen. Several primary sites of infection are seen with mucosal necrosis covered with fibrin and leukocytes. The markedly increased thickness of the submucosa (edema → 1) and sparsity of leukocytic infiltration are remarkable (higher magnification Fig. 4.44b). Fibrin covers the peritoneum (→ 2). The inflammation also commonly extends into the mesentery (→ 3).

In Figure 4.45, two **primary foci of infection** can be seen under higher magnification (2 arrows in the picture). The inflammation has originated in a crypt and the leukocytic exudation has involved the tunica propria. Following this, the epithelium is breached and the mucosa destroyed by focal inflammatory exudation of fibrin and leukocytes. Later the necrotic tissue may slough and an ulcer form (acute ulcerative appendicitis). In Figure 4.45, the whole wall is infiltrated with leukocytes (→ 1: peritoneum covered with fibrin and leukocytes).

Fecal stasis (Fig. 4.46) in the appendix (inadequate peristalsis?) can lead to the development of a fecalith (from deposition of calcium and magnesium). Undigested food particles (→ 1: fragment of vegetable matter) are frequently seen in fecaliths. *Mucosal ulceration* (→ 2) may develop from the trauma of the pressure of such particles and result in *phlegmonous inflammation* involving all the intestinal coats. Figure 4.46 shows also *an intramural abscess* (→ 3) in the muscularis.

Acute appendicitis is usually a rapidly progressive illness that requires prompt surgical intervention. The urgency of the intervention becomes clear when the number of serious complications of untreated appendicitis are compared with the rapidity of recovery after appendectomy.

Chronic appendicitis (Fig. 4.47) results in disappearance of the mucosa and usually obliteration of the lumen. In Figure 4.47, the lumen is closed by connective tissue containing lymphocytes and plasma cells which occurs in the acute stage if the mucosa is destroyed by necrosis. Occasional lymph follicles remain. The submucosa is greatly thickened by fibrosis (→) and contains nodules of fat tissue (→ 1). Chronic appendicitis is uncommon (2–6% of appendices examined).

Complications of appendicitis: Perforation, peritonitis, pericecal abscess (typhlitis), spreading retroperitoneal inflammation (phlegmonous), subphrenic abscess, pyelophlebitic liver abscess, chiefly in the left lobe, hydrops, mucocele.

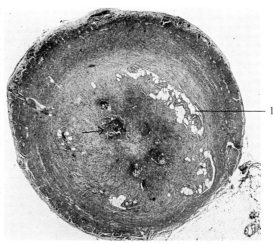

Fig. 4.47. Chronic obliterative appendicitis; H & E, 15×.

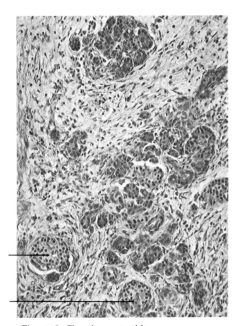

Fig. 4.48. Chronic pancreatitis
H & E, 120×.

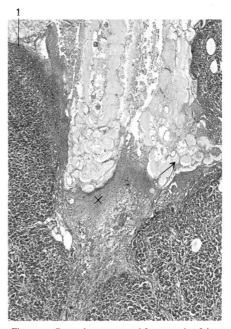

Fig. 4.49. Parenchymatous and fat necrosis of the pancreas;
H & E, 43×.

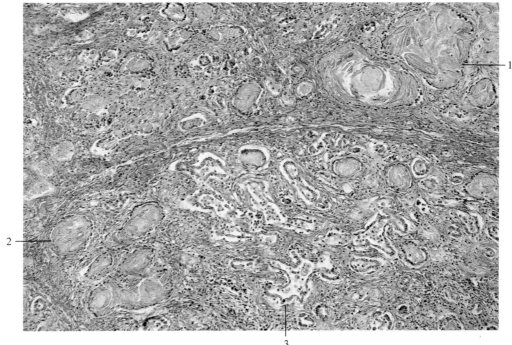

Fig. 4.50. Cystic fibrosis of the pancreas; van Gieson stain, 80×.

Pancreas

Chronic pancreatitis (Fig. 4.18). *This is a chronic, recurrent inflammation with destruction, reconstruction and replacement of the exocrine parenchyma of the pancreas by connective tissue. The etiology is varied: primary infection, metabolic (alcohol), idiopathic.*
Histologically there is marked fibrosis with foci of chronic inflammatory infiltrates rich in lymphocytes, plasma cells and histiocytes. The fibrous tissue infiltrates the acini, splitting and finally completely destroying them. Small fresh areas of pancreatic necrosis are frequently seen (enzymatic pancreatitis). Mostly the disease has a slow course, often with acute exacerbations. It is remarkable that the islets of Langerhans (→) remain intact for a considerable time. In the final stages (the burned out pancreas), however, they also are destroyed and diabetes mellitus develops. Excretory ducts may proliferate and ectasia of ducts containing pancreatic calculi may develop (X-ray!).

Clinical: pancreatic insufficiency (fatty stools, diarrhea). A past history of alcohol abuse is frequent. In 50% of cases there is latent hyperparathyroidism. Persons with pancreatic carcinoma often have had chronic pancreatitis previously.

Fat necrosis of the pancreas (Fig. 4.49). *Necrosis of the parenchyma and fat tissue of the pancreas is initiated by autodigestion (trypsin, lipase) resulting from previous disturbance of the local circulation. The pathogenesis of this very complex process is still under dispute.* Microscopically, there is necrosis of the parenchyma and islands of fat tissue in the pancreas, frequently accompanied by hemorrhage *(hemorrhagic pancreatic necrosis)*. Under low magnification, the ghost-like outlines of the fat cells can be recognized in many of the necrotic areas (→). In other areas, the fat is replaced by homogeneous, pale pink or blue material. Often, crystals of fatty acids are precipitated. Hematoidin is deposited at the edge of the area of fat necrosis (×) in Figure 4.49. The necrosis also extends into the parenchyma (→ 1), which appears eosinophilic and shows loss of nuclei. In the acute stages of the necrosis, leukocytes accumulate at the margins, while in later stages a collar of granulation tissue or mature connective tissue containing foam cells may be found. Fat necrosis developing after death lacks any evidence of tissue reaction such as exudation of leukocytes.

Macroscopic: In the initial stages, there is edema and focal parenchymatous necrosis (large, dirty-gray pancreas): in hemorrhagic necrosis, the pancreas is dark red and bloody; secondary liquefaction with cyst formation may develop. Fat necrosis appears as chalky white, freckle-sized nodules. Adipose women are especially prone and there is often alcohol abuse with fatty cirrhosis of the liver.

Cystic fibrosis of the pancreas (Fig. 4.50). *Not only is the pancreas involved in this disease but also the mucous glands of the intestine, bile ducts, lungs and salivary glands (mucoviscidosis, Anderson, 1962). It affects chiefly children who have meconium ileus. Marked inflammatory changes are present in the lungs of these children (bronchiectasis) and, finally, chronic deficiency of pancreatic enzymes leads to the development of celiac disease. The basic disease process is a "dyscholasia", that is, the development of stasis and a secretion of high viscosity.* Microscopically, the normal lobular structures are surrounded by strands of connective tissue. Both the ducts (→ 1) and acini (→ 2, 3) are widely dilated and cystic. The contents of the cysts consist of homogeneous or laminated secretions. An increased amount of interstitial tissue is distributed randomly through the lobules (red connective tissue in van Gieson stain). In addition, there is scanty infiltration of leukocytes and plasma cells. In general, the organ is reconstructed in a way similar to hepatic cirrhosis.

Macroscopic: The pancreas is firm and grayish white. In the late stages, there are numerous small cysts and the surface is granular.

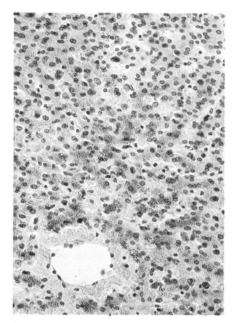

Fig. 5.1. Brown atrophy of the liver;
111×.

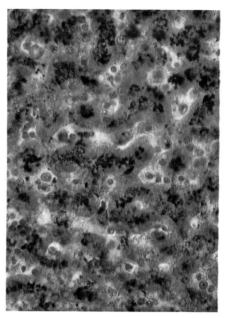

Fig. 5.2. Siderosis of the liver;
Berlin blue reaction, 456×.

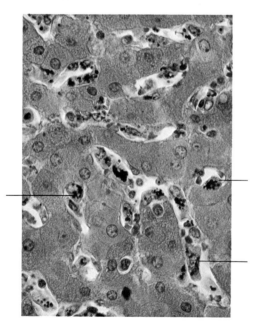

Fig. 5.3. Malarial melanin pigment;
H & E, 480×.

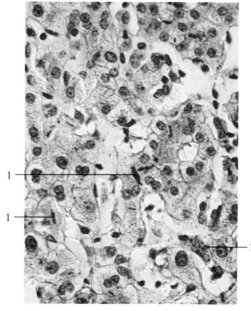

Fig. 5.4. Icterus of the liver;
H & E, 310×.

5. Liver–Gallbladder

Familiarity with the normal microscopic anatomy of the liver is an essential prerequisite for interpretation of the microscopic appearances of abnormal liver. For purposes of orientation, the *periportal field* will serve as a good starting point [Glisson's triad of bile ducts (cylindrical epithelium), artery (heavy muscular wall) and branches of the portal vein]. The periportal field is enveloped by a sheath of liver cells, known as the *limiting plate* (Popper and Schaffner). Cords of liver cells accompanied by sinusoids course toward the central vein. When trying to understand pathological changes in the liver lobules, it should be borne in mind that different parts of the liver lobule can be affected separately (e.g., either the central or peripheral zones). This depends upon peculiarities of the circulation and of the cellular complement of enzymes. Concepts about the fundamental functional unit of the liver are still not well established. For example, instead of the "classic" liver lobule centered around the central vein *(central vein unit)*, a so-called *portal vein unit* has been proposed (see Rappaport, 1954). In this scheme, the periportal zone lies at the center and the central vein marks the peripheral boundary of the liver lobule. Many pathological alterations can be well correlated with the functional findings with this concept (e.g., the pattern of stasis). *Attention should be paid to the following features in pathological material:* the cell constituents of the periportal field, the integrity of the liver cell cords, and of the liver cells themselves, particularly in the limiting plate, Kupffer cells and any deposits of pigments or other substances (e.g., fat, amyloid).

Brown atrophy of the liver (Fig. 5.1). *In brown atrophy, which may affect any internal organ and especially the heart and liver, there is an increase in lipofuscin.* The pigment is best seen in histological sections stained with hemotoxylin without a counterstain. Low magnification shows a prominent brownish cast in the region of the central portion of the lobule. Under higher magnification, brown cytoplasmic granules can be seen. Figure 5.1 shows the central vein and surrounding cords of liver cells, which contain less and less pigment the farther they are situated from the center of the lobule. In addition, the liver cells are also atrophic and have compactly arranged nuclei.

Macroscopic: Brown, shrunken organ with a wrinkled capsule.

Siderosis of the liver (Fig. 5.2). *In this condition, iron-containing pigment, usually derived from hemoglobin, is deposited in the cytoplasm of both the liver and the Kupffer cells.* In contrast to lipofuscin pigment, siderin is found chiefly in the periphery of the liver lobule, especially in the cytoplasm of cells lying next to bile ductules (see p. 9). In this way, the midline between two rows of cells becomes intensified. The pigment appears yellowish brown in sections stained with hematoxylin and eosin, but the Berlin blue reaction colors the pigment a deep blue. The stellate shaped Kupffer cells also contain deposits of iron pigment.

Macroscopic: A brown liver of normal size, often associated with siderosis of other organs (pancreas, spleen, salivary glands), especially in hemochromatosis (see p. 149).

Malarial melanin pigment (Fig. 5.3). *Brownish black pigment originating from destruction of blood cells in malaria is deposited in the reticuloendothelial cells.* Accordingly, it is found in the Kupffer cells of the liver. Figure 5.3 shows the black granules in the swollen Kupffer cells (→), and is a good demonstration of the phagocytic capacities of these lining cells of the sinusoids.

Macroscopic: Smoky gray discoloration of liver and spleen.

Icterus of the liver (Fig. 5.4). *In jaundice, granules of bile pigment appear in the cytoplasm of the liver cells and bile casts form in the ductules or larger bile ducts.* Under low magnification, greenish, sausage-shaped secretions (bile casts, incorrectly called bile thrombi → 1, see also p. 154) can be seen. Isolated, fine droplets of bile are also seen in the cytoplasm of the liver cells. In obstructive jaundice and extrahepatic jaundice, the central zone of the liver lobule is particularly affected, whereas in hepatocellular jaundice all parts of the lobule are involved.[1] The Kupffer cells may also contain bile pigment (→ 2) or phagocytosed necrotic liver cells.

Macroscopic: The liver has either a green (biliverdin) or a golden brown color (bilirubin).

---

[1] Drug induced jaundice has become very important (sex hormones, ovulation arresting drugs, psychotherapeutic drugs such as chlorpromazine).

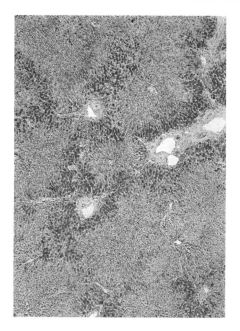

Fig. 5.5. Peripheral fatty degeneration
of the liver; Sudan stain, 22×.

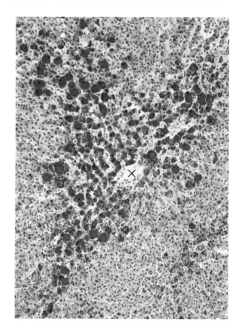

Fig. 5.6. Central fatty degeneration of the liver;
Sudan stain, 84×.

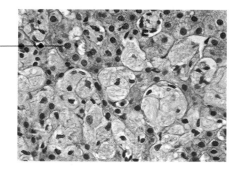

Fig. 5.7. Gaucher's disease;
H & E, 300×.

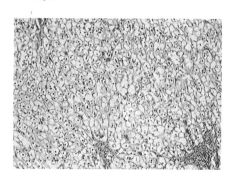

Fig. 5.8. Glycogen storage disease;
H & E, 300×.

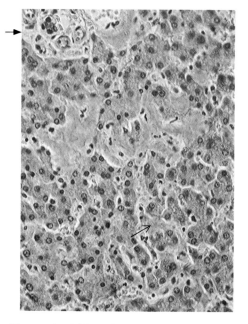

Fig. 5.9. Amyloidosis of the liver;
Congo red stain, 155×.

Fatty Degeneration of the Liver

The lipids of the liver cells are bound to the cell components and are not normally seen. When fat appears in the form of droplets in the cytoplasm of the liver cells, the condition is known as *fatty degeneration* (fatty metamorphosis). Three forms of fatty degeneration occur in the liver: *peripheral fatty degeneration* (e.g., alimentary fatty degeneration), *central fatty degeneration* (e.g., metabolic or toxic) and *diffuse fatty degeneration,* particularly in chronic alcohol abuse (see fatty liver). It occurs with excess accumulation of fats or carbohydrates in diabetes, use of antibiotics, cytostatic drugs or cortisone.

Peripheral fatty degeneration (Fig. 5.5) is manifested by the occurrence of large droplets of fat in the cytoplasm of liver cells at the periphery of the lobules. Low-power examination of preparations stained with Sudan shows a red ring surrounding the pale central zone. Higher magnification shows that the liver cells are filled with large droplets of fat; frequently, these are large round globules. The nucleus is displaced to the periphery of the cells.

Macroscopic: Yellow ring-shaped network with brownish red centers.

Central fatty degeneration (Fig. 5.6) shows the reverse picture. With the scanning lens, the central zones of the lobule appear as red areas surrounded by a blue halo. Low magnification reveals the position of the fat deposits. The central vein ($\times$) lies in the middle of the fatty area. A further point of distinction from peripheral fatty degeneration is the fact that most of the fat droplets are very fine and distributed diffusely through the cytoplasm.

Macroscopic: Small yellow point-like lesions scattered on a brown background.

Storage diseases (Figs. 5.7 and 5.8). Excessive storage of certain substances in cells is a genetic metabolic anomaly in which specific lysosomal enzymes are lacking so that degradation of these substances does not occur and they accumulate within cells. In *Gaucher's disease* cerebrosides (kerasin) accumulate because of a deficiency of glucocerebrosidase and α-galactosidase in lysosomes. The erythrocytic membranes are only partially destroyed by cells in the reticuloendothelial system and cytoplasmic accumulation of the lipids occurs in the spleen, liver and bone marrow. Figure 5.7 shows large bright red cells of the reticuloendothelial system with finely granular cytoplasm which have compressed the liver cells and even caused pressure atrophy $\rightarrow$. In **von Gierke's disease** there is a lack of the lysosomal enzyme maltase with the result that lysosomal glycogen is not metabolized. Nine different sorts of enzyme defects are known. *von Gierke's disease* involves liver and kidney, *Pompe's disease* chiefly the heart (frequency — 1:100,000 Births). Figure 5.8 shows the typical appearance of the liver with large cells having clear cytoplasm. The glycogen being water soluble dissolves out of the cells in formalin fixed tissue. In tissue fixed in alcohol, the glycogen is preserved and can be demonstrated by special stains (see p. 155).

Amyloidosis of the liver (Fig. 5.9). The amyloid, which is a pathological protein, is deposited in the space between the walls of the sinusoids and the liver cells (Dissé's space, periportal field). At first only a narrow strip of homogeneous red material (positive for Congo red) is seen next to the capillaries ($\rightarrow$ inside picture). If the deposits are marked they may cause pressure atrophy of the liver cords which may disappear completely. The lumens of the sinusoids may be greatly reduced as a consequence of the infiltration. Amyloid stains with either Congo red or methyl violet (red metachromasia, see pp. 165, 246). Amyloid stained with Congo red is doubly refractive and shows an abnormal green color when viewed with polarized light.

Macroscopic: Large, firm organ having a wooden consistency and glassy cut surfaces. Suspected cases of amyloidosis may sometimes be confirmed by either a needle biopsy of the liver or a punch biopsy of the rectum.

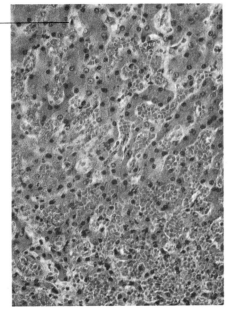

Fig. 5.10. Mild congestion (stasis) of liver; H & E, 250×.

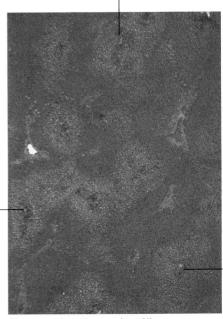

Fig. 5.11. Marked congestion of liver; H & E, 29×.

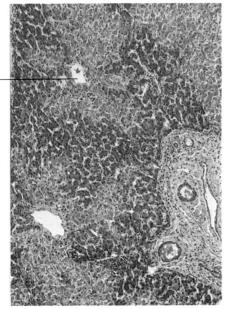

Fig. 5.12. Hypoxemic (ischemic) necrosis of liver; H & E, 60×.

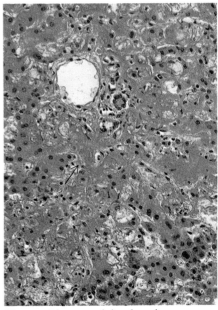

Fig. 5.13. Liver necrosis in eclampsia; H & E, 200×.

Congestion of the liver (Fig. 5.10). Stasis due to obstruction of the venous return to the right heart (right heart insufficiency) manifests itself first in the *central zone of the liver lobules*. At a later stage, lake-like vascular channels develop by fusion of the congested central zones of adjacent liver lobules. In the early stages, low-power magnification reveals red zones in the center of the lobules; higher magnification discloses the greatly dilated sinusoids. Figure 5.10 shows a section of the central zone (the central vein lies below and outside the picture), with the sinusoids greatly distended by numerous erythrocytes. If the liver cells in the uncongested upper portion of the illustration are compared with those in the congested areas, it can be clearly seen that the liver cells in the latter are atrophic because of compression by dilated sinuses. This often leads to deficient oxygenation of the cells so that they also show fatty degeneration (→: unaltered Kupffer cell).

Macroscopic: Enlarged, firm liver. The cut surfaces show dark red central areas surrounded by pale brown peripheral zones. Often, fatty degeneration is also present and imparts a yellow appearance.

Marked congestion of the liver (Fig. 5.11). When congestion has been present for a long time, it involves not only the intermediate and peripheral zones of the lobule, but also the adjacent lobule. In this manner, congested channels are formed which connect one liver lobule with another and lead to a *reversal of the normal liver pattern* so that the periportal field (→) is in the middle of a red ring of hyperemia (see notes on histology on p. 133). The red ring and the broad channels can be seen even with the scanning lens. With low-power magnification, the periportal field is seen to be at the center. Higher magnification of the congested area shows the greatly dilated sinusoids. In these areas, the liver cells have disappeared. Frequently, the walls of the sinusoids cannot be recognized. A great lake of blood has formed. Most of the intact parenchyma shows fatty degeneration.

Macroscopic: The liver is large and dark red. The cut surfaces show a dark red network on a yellow background (fatty degeneration), the so-called nutmeg liver.

Hypoxic (Ischemic) **liver necrosis** (Fig. 5.12). *Necrosis of the liver can affect either single cells (see hepatitis, p. 141) or groups of cells in either the intermediate zone of the lobules or without any particular localization.* Focal necrosis can be caused by *toxins* (e.g., diphtheria) or it may be dependent upon *acute oxygen lack.* Figure 5.12 shows geographical areas of necrosis in the centers of the liver lobules (→: central vein). The areas of necrotic liver cells are apparent from the pale red stain. Nuclei are decreased in number. Kupffer cells, for the most part, are preserved. Also seen in shock.

Liver necrosis in eclampsia (Fig. 5.13). *Eclampsia usually develops toward the end of pregnancy but before labor has occurred. The pathogenesis is now considered to be the result either of direct action of a toxin formed in the placenta on the parenchymatous cells or a secondary outcome of a disturbance of the circulation (shock?). Liver, kidney and brain are preferentially affected.* In contrast to hypoxic liver necrosis, which develops in the area of greatest oxygen deficiency, the necrosis of eclampsia is distributed at random throughout the lobule. Examination with a scanning lens discloses irregularly scattered, eosinophilic, map-like lesions. Low-power magnification shows that the liver cell cords and sinusoids in the homogeneous red areas are no longer arranged next to one another. Cell nuclei have disappeared. The cytoplasm of the liver cells has become homogeneous and structureless. The blood in the sinusoids is coagulated into solid masses (→) as a result of stasis or the formation of fibrin and platelet thrombi (hyalinethrombi → evidence of shock etiology).

Macroscopic: Gray or grayish yellow, map-like lesions.

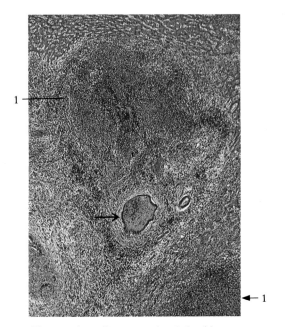

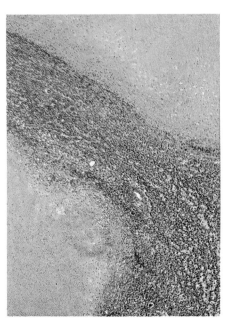

Fig. 5.14. Ascending suppurative cholangitis;
H & E, 50×.

Fig. 5.15. Gumma of the liver;
van Gieson stain, 40×.

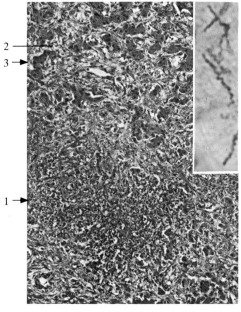

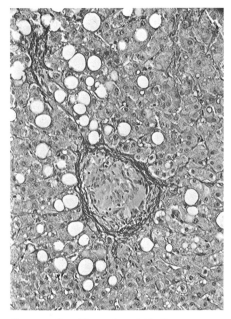

Fig. 5.16. Congenital syphilis of the liver;
H & E, 120×.
Inset: spirochetes;
Levaditi stain, 2,350×.

Fig. 5.17. Sarcoid granuloma in the liver;
H & E, 330×.

Ascending suppurative cholangitis (Fig. 5.14). *This is caused by ascending bacterial infection (most-ly* Escherichia coli) *of the bile ducts and is often associated with bile stasis (stones, tumors).* The bile ducts in the periportal spaces are dilated and contain exudate rich in polymorphonuclear leukocytes (→). The entire periportal field is infiltrated with polymorphonuclear leukocytes, which also are found in the adjacent parenchyma where there is tissue necrosis (*cholangiolytic abscess* → 1). In Figure 192 there is an increase in the periportal fibrous tissue which forms a concentric, collar-like arrangement around the bile ducts (→). This is often an indication of previous cholangitic disease (see primary cholangitis, p. 145).

Macroscopic: The liver is bile-stained, with widening and proliferation of the periportal fields and foci of greenish necrosis (abscesses).

Gumma of the liver (Fig. 5.15). *In the third stage of syphilis, granulomas (gummas) with a rubbery consistency appear in affected organs.* These are sharply demarcated, round or map-like foci of ne-crosis which, as can be easily seen with elastica and van Gieson stains, contain connective tissue or elastic fibers which arise in the surrounding tissues and penetrate the necrotic area. Figure 5.15 shows the necrotic center (yellow with van Gieson stain and lacking nuclei) surrounded by a narrow band of granulation tissue. Epithelioid cells resembling those of tuberculosis (p. 106) are seen in the granulation tissue. These, however, are present in smaller numbers than in tuberculosis. Next to this there is a layer of connective tissue vascularized with capillaries and containing fibroblasts and lymphocytes. In the outermost zone, scar tissue has formed (red in van Gieson's stain). As in tuberculosis, there are also Langhans type giant cells. However, in contrast to tuberculosis, numbers of plasma cells are present in the granulation tissue of a gumma and the neighboring blood vessels show endarteritis.

Macroscopic: Yellow, map-like areas of necrosis having a rubbery consistency.

Congenital syphilis of the liver (Fig. 5.16). Under low magnification, the normal architecture of the liver can be scarcely recognized. There are small, richly cellular, blue-staining focal lesions *(syphilomas).* The liver cords are widely separated by an interstitial cellular infiltrate, and individual groups of liver cells have been destroyed. Medium magnification reveals miliary granulomas (→ 1) showing areas of fresh necrosis, nuclear fragments, polymorphonuclear leukocytes and lymphocytes. In these areas, the liver cells are completely destroyed. In the surrounding tissue, a chronic interstitial hepatitis has developed in which the interstitial tissue is markedly distended with histiocytes (→ 2), fibroblasts, lymphocytes and fibrous tissue. Remnants of liver cords lie in between (→ 3). Numerous *spirochetes* can be demonstrated with special stains (Levaditi silver stain, inset, Fig. 5.16).

Macroscopic: The liver is of firm consistency and the cut surfaces show grayish brown flecks.

Congenital syphilis localizes principally in the skeletal system *(syphilitic osteochrondritis,* p. 260, *syphilitic saddle nose, syphilitic periosteitis),* in the skin *(syphilitic pemphigus),* lungs *(pneumonia alba)* and brain. In addition, the victims may show the so-called *Hutchinson triad* (keratitis, inner ear deafness and malformed teeth).

Sarcoid granuloma of the liver (Fig. 5.17). Sarcoidosis *(Boeck's sarcoid)* may originate in a lymph node in the lung or have a hematogenous origin and involve all organs. The liver is affected in 60% of cases and consequently a liver biopsy may be diagnostically helpful. Figure 5.17 shows an epithelioid cell granuloma with a typical collagenous ring in the outer zone (beginning scar ring). Peripheral to this zone there is fatty degeneration with large droplets of fat.

Viral Hepatitis

Massive Liver Necrosis

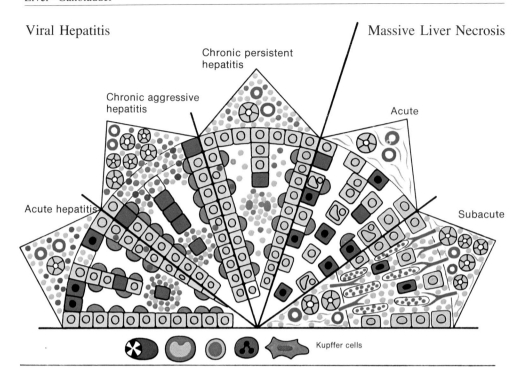

Chronic persistent
hepatitis

Chronic aggressive
hepatitis

Acute

Acute hepatitis

Subacute

Kupffer cells

Cirrhosis of the liver

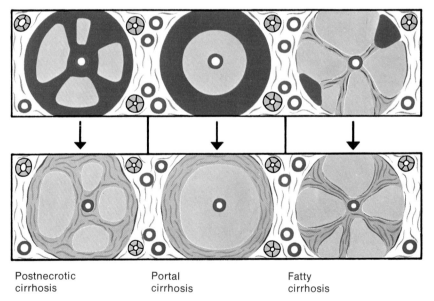

Postnecrotic
cirrhosis

Portal
cirrhosis

Fatty
cirrhosis

Fig. 5.18. Diagram of the histological changes in viral hepatitis, massive liver necrosis and cirrhosis of the liver.

Viral Hepatitis—Massive Liver Cell Necrosis—Cirrhosis

Figure 5.18 shows in schematic form the histological apppearances of these three diseases, which will be considered together because of certain similarities. *In essence, all three show destruction of liver cells (necrosis) accompanied by resorption and a secondary mesenchymal reaction that takes the form of granulation tissue. There is, in addition, reorganization of the structure of the liver and parenchymal regeneration.* In many cases of cirrhosis, *primary proliferation of granulation tissue (inflammation) with simultaneous or subsequent destruction of parenchyma* occupy a prominent place.

Viral hepatitis (see also pp. 143, 145) is initiated by *necrosis of single cells* (acidophilic necrotic cytoplasm). These are resorbed by histiocytes. The periportal zones show an infiltrate of lymphocytes and histiocytes which break through the limiting plate and extend farther into the parenchyma. *Chronic hepatitis* develops in about 5% of cases, either as *chronic aggressive hepatitis,* which shows a patchy inflammatory exudate extending from the periportal field into the parenchyma, or as *chronic persistent hepatitis* which runs a course of many years and does not show extension of the periportal inflammatory exudate into the liver parenchyma.

In massive liver cell necrosis (see also pp. 140, 147), the necrosis involves either the entire liver or a part of it. In the majority of cases, it is now thought to be a *fulminant form of viral hepatitis.* The acute stage *(massive cytolytic necrosis,* formerly *acute yellow atrophy)* is manifested by dissociation of the liver cell cords, necrosis of cells and pyknosis of nuclei. In the *subacute stages,* a large part of the parenchyma is demolished and the periportal zones collapse and are infiltrated with chronic inflammatory cells.

Cirrhosis of the liver (see also pp. 140, 149) is a disease in which there is *destruction of parenchyma* with *progressive reconstruction* of the entire liver and formation of *psuedolobules.*

Two essentially different types of cirrhosis are recognized: 1. *postnecrotic cirrhosis,* 2. *portal cirrhosis (including biliary cirrhosis).*

The diagram on the opposite page illustrates the ways in which the different sorts of cirrhosis develop (after Thaler, 1969). In **post necrotic cirrhosis** (Type 1 in Fig. 5.18) there is massive parenchymal necrosis which, as shown in the diagram, either involves isolated segments of the liver lobule or more commonly embraces several liver lobules or large areas of the parenchyma. As a result large irregular zones of fibrosis develop and surround the remaining parenchymal tissue in a disorderly fashion.

If many liver lobules are destroyed, large scars develop in which the periportal fields are packed closely. Eventually only small islands of parenchyma remain (see p. 149). *Postnecrotic cirrhosis* can also develop in fatty cirrhosis (Type III in Fig. 5.18), if there is concurrent chronic recurrent necrosis of liver lobules.

Portal cirrhosis (Type II) is due to chronic inflammation starting in the periportal field with secondary periportal necrosis resulting in the formation of large uniform islands of parenchyma bounded by a ring of fibrous tissue. The central vein may lie in the center but is often displaced to the periphery of the islands of parenchyma (see p. 149).

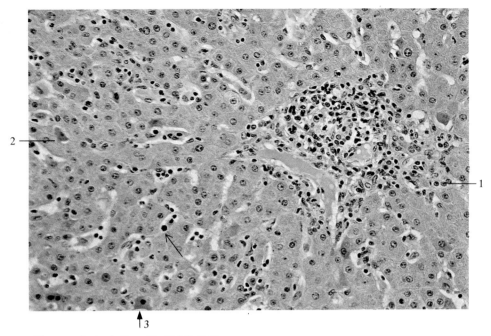

Fig. 5.19. Acute viral hepatitis; H & E, 60×.

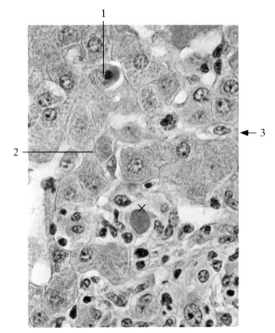

Fig. 5.20. Acute viral hepatitis, detail;
H & E, 500×.

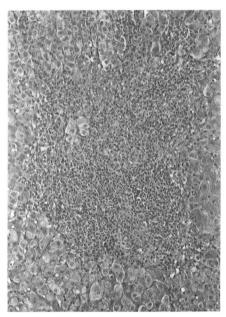

Fig. 5.21. Chronic aggressive
hepatitis; H & E, 100×.

Viral Hepatitis

Acute and chronic viral hepatitis shows a *characteristic histological picture* so that, in most cases, it is possible to diagnose the sort of hepatitis and the prognosis. Study of needle biopsy specimens has aided in unraveling the course of the disease.

Clinically **acute viral hepatitis** begins with malaise, loss of appetite, nausea and mild jaundice. SGOT is slightly elevated. The disease lasts about 6 weeks. It is transferred orally in epidemics of Virus A (infectious hepatitis). The virus has been successfully transmitted to apes (Deinhardt et al, 1967). Incubation period 15–20 days. **Serum hepatitis** (homologous serum hepatitis, Virus B) is transmitted orally or parenterally (blood transfusion, injections, "hippie" hepatitis). Incubation period 45–160 days. The viral agent can be detected in blood as a corpuscular antigen (so-called Australia antigen, hepatitis -B antigen, HB antigen). HB antigen can also be detected by immunofluorescence techniques in the cytoplasm of liver cells. With the light microscope the cytoplasm has a ground glass appearance (increase in endoplasmic reticulum). The disease is more severe and persists longer than does hepatitis A. Both forms of hepatitis have the same histological features, the necrosis of individual cells eliciting a secondary inflammatory reaction of the Kupfer cells and in the periportal fields. Since the framework of supporting fibers is preserved, it is possible for regeneration to occur without destruction of liver parenchyma. Both hepatitis A and B can progress to chronic hepatitis.

Acute viral hepatitis (Figs. 5.19, 5.20). Low magnification reveals widening and cellular infiltration of the periportal fields, but with preservation of architecture and scanty cellular infiltration of the parenchyma. Somewhat higher magnification (Fig. 5.19) shows the periportal infiltrate to consist of lymphocytes and a few polymorphonuclear leukocytes which have breached the limiting plate of the lobule and invaded the parenchyma (→ 1). Between the liver cell cords there are *swollen Kupffer cells* (stellate shaped) and round cells with a single nucleus, which appear to be immigrant blood monocytes (→ in the picture). In addition, individual liver cells are small and shrunken, with striking angular cytoplasm and pyknotic nuclei (→ 2, →3 acidophilic necrosis of single cells).

High magnification, Figure 5.20, **acute viral hepatitis detail** (see also p. 140), shows necrosis of individual cells and the reaction in the liver. At → 1, a necrotic cell with nuclear pyknosis is seen. At → 2 (also ×), there is the ghost of an anuclear cell forming a typical eosinophilic body (so-called hyalin or Councilman body, see Fig. 5.46, p. 156). These "hyalin bodies" are not specific for hepatitis, as they are also observed in other conditions. The individual necrotic cells are surrounded by lymphocytes and histiocytes with plump, oval or slightly indented nuclei (see p. 156). At → 3, there is a swollen Kupffer cell. In the acute stages there are, in addition, bile pigmentation of liver cells and bile casts in the central zones. Mitoses and multinucleated giant cells indicate the onset of liver cell regeneration.

Macroscopic: The liver is enlarged, with rounded edges and spotted, yellow, reddish brown external and cut surfaces. 90% of cases of acute hepatitis heal in 2-6 months. The others progress to chronic hepatitis.

Chronic hepatitis in 3–5% of cases develops from an acute hepatitis (chiefly hepatitis B, 15%, and less frequently hepatitis A, 1%). However, there are also cases that begin insidiously without preexisting acute hepatitis (Sherlock, 1973). Two forms are recognized:

Chronic aggressive (active) hepatitis (Fig. 5.21). This is the most severe form of chronic hepatitis and is manifest by marked inflammatory exudate in the periportal fields which invades the lamellar boundaries and sends tongue-like projections into the parenchyma (moth-eaten appearance) so that exudate bridges periportal fields, which may lead eventually to cirrhosis. Necrotic liver cells are replaced by an infiltrate of lymphocytes and histiocytes. Within 3–5 years it can develop into cirrhosis of the liver. Thirty per cent of cases show a positive reaction with Australia antigen. Lupoid hepatitis is a special form of chronic aggressive hepatitis that affects particularly young women (10–29 years). Patients show the LE phenomenon, high antibody titers (lgb, lgA) and antibodies against smooth muscle. Australia-antigen is negative. Autoaggressive disorder? The inflammatory infiltrate also contains plasma cells.

Macroscopic: finely granular surface.

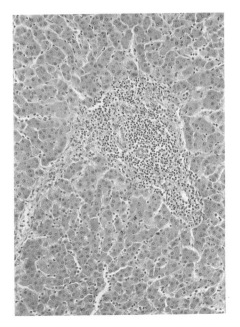

Fig. 5.22. Chronic persistent, recurrent hepatitis;
H & E, 100×.

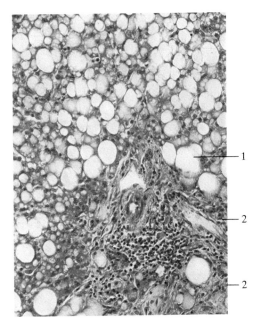

Fig. 5.23. Fatty hepatitis;
H & E, 170×.

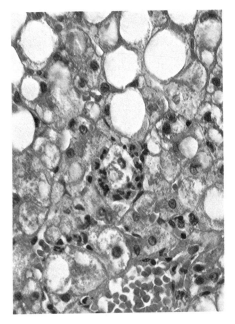

Fig. 5.24. Fatty hepatitis (detail)
H & E, 400×.

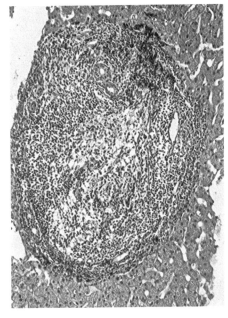

Fig. 5.25. Chronic destructive cholangitis;
H & E, 100×.

Chronic persistent hepatitis (Fig. 5.22): The periportal infiltrate consists of lymphocytes, which often form germinal centers, and does not extend into the parenchyma. The parenchyma shows a few necrotic cells and focal or generalized increase in Kupffer cells. Eighty per cent have HB antibodies. The disease may persist many years. Immunoglobulins are not elevated. It does not progress to cirrhosis.

Macroscopic: Smooth surface.

Fatty hepatitis (Figs. 5.23, 5.24). Liver injury conditioned by alcohol. In the beginning of the disease there is merely fatty change, either focal or diffuse (large or small droplets). Later single cells become necrotic as a result of fat accumulation or balloon-like swelling of liver cells (hydropic and fatty change) or the formation of fat cysts (coalescence of several fatty liver cells, → 1). Characteristically there are **Mallory bodies,** i.e., focal cytoplasmic hyalinization of liver cells (often hornshaped, Fig. 5.26). The periportal fields are widened (edema, granulocytes, proliferation of bile ducts → 2). Secondarily fibrous proliferation develops in the lobule center (so-called **network fibrosis**) so that solitary cells or a few cells are encased in fibrous tissue. Figure 5.24 shows a necrotic, fatty liver cell which has been resorbed by granulocytes. The Kupffer cells also are increased in number and granular from accumulated iron. After 10–15 years of chronic alcohol abuse either portal or postnecrotic cirrhosis may develop (see p. 149) (about 10–20% of alcoholics). The mechanism of alcohol injury is unknown: oxydation of fatty acids is decreased, NADH deficiency? Arrested protein synthesis? Increased lipolysis?

Cholangitis: An inflammation of the intrahepatic bile ducts secondary to bile stasis resulting from extrahepatic duct stenosis (gallstones, tumors, scars). Mostly there is an ascending infection with *E. coli* (see p. 138). Primary cholangitis occurs as a **chronic nondestructive, nonpurulent cholangitis** (Fig. 5.25). Histologically the bile ducts are distended by lymphocytes and plasma cells which are also found in the periportal fields (a similar picture occurs in chronic aggressive hepatitis). Bile ducts are destroyed, the inflammation extends into the parenchyma and portal biliary cirrhosis may develop.

Clinical: Chiefly women 30–60 years of age. Biliary cirrhosis develops on the average after 7 years. In 98% of cases antibodies against mitochondria can be demonstrated (autoaggression?).

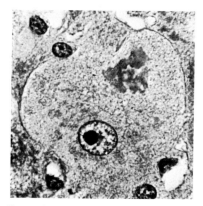

Fig. 5.26. Mallory body; H & E, 400×.

145

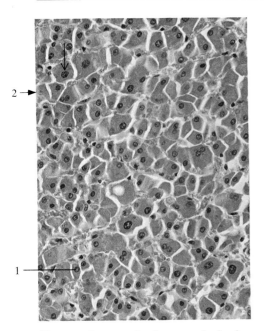

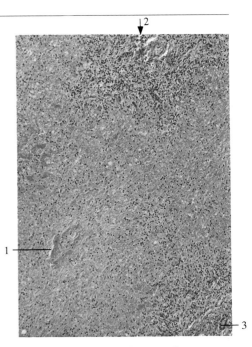

Fig. 5.27. Acute massive liver necrosis showing disorganization of the liver cell cords; H & E, 270×.

Fig. 5.28. Acute massive liver necrosis (4–6 days old); H & E, 110×.

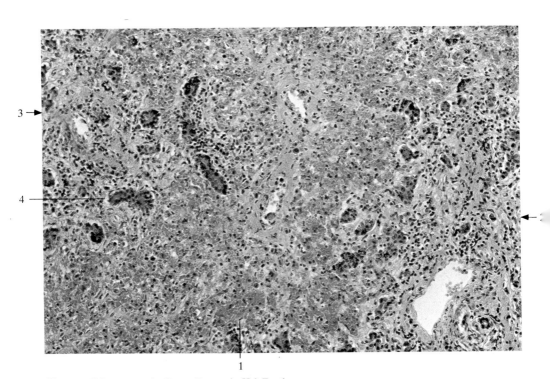

Fig. 5.29. Subacute massive liver cell necrosis; H & E, 165×.

Massive Liver Necrosis

In **acute massive liver necrosis** (Figs. 5.27, 5.28), the whole organ is necrotic. It may be caused by various etiological agents and may lead to death within a few days. Among causative agents are: 1. *Potent poisons* (e.g., phosphorus, poisonous fungi, arsenic and others: these cause so-called toxic liver necrosis). In toxic liver injury, a marked degree of fatty degeneration of liver cells is seen at the beginning of the illness. Necrosis develops secondarily and affects the peripheral zones of the lobules preferentially. 2. *Metabolic disturbances* (usually protein). 3. *Viral infection.* This causes a *fulminant* or *malignant form of viral hepatitis* and has increased greatly in incidence during the past 20 years (0.5–5% of cases of acute viral hepatitis). This is so-called acute yellow atrophy of the liver.

The microscopic picture of acute massive liver necrosis varies with the age of the illness and with the time that has elapsed between death and performance of the autopsy. In fresh cases (6–8 hours after death), there is disorganization of the liver cell cords, that is, the individual liver cells have become unattached and appear as separated cellular elements. The cells vary in size, and some are already shrunken (→ 1, Fig. 5.27). The cytoplasm is homogeneous and stains more blue than normal (decrease in glycogen content). The nuclei are small and frequently either pyknotic (→) or more faintly stained than normal (karyolysis → 2).

Figure 5.27 shows the liver of a patient who was ill of a clinically obscure "upper abdominal syndrome". At laparotomy, the liver was yellow and slightly reduced in size. An incisional biopsy was taken (see Fig. 5.27). Nineteen hours later, the patient died and at autopsy showed the typical picture of massive liver necrosis. Histologically, at autopsy the liver cells were without nuclei and the cytoplasm was faded and finely granular. There was no inflammatory infiltrate.

Acute massive liver necrosis, 4–6 days old (Fig. 5.28). If a patient with acute massive liver cell necrosis survives for a few days and then dies, almost complete dissolution of the liver cells occurs. Only homogeneous, eosinophilic material now remains. Intact individual Kupffer cells, however, are still present. The band-like areas of strongly eosinophilic material (→ 1) still contain anuclear remnants of liver cell cords. The periportal fields (→ 2) are infiltrated with inflammatory cells (lymphocytes), and show occasional proliferated bile ducts (→ 3).

Macroscopic: The liver is small and flaccid and the capsule is wrinkled. The cut surfaces are yellow, yellowish green or ocher yellow. The liver may weigh as little as 500 Gm. (normal weight is 1,500 Gm.). Frequently, crystals of leucine and tyrosine can be seen on the cut surface or on the surface of the capsule (*microscopically:* round granules or crystalline tufts).

Subacute massive liver necrosis (Fig. 5.29). When only a part of the liver is affected by the necrosis (e.g., a lobe or a part of a lobe), or if the disease runs a slow course, subacute red atrophy ensues in which cell detritus, the remnants of liver cells, can be seen between the dilated sinusoids (→ 1). Resorption of the necrotic tissue is far advanced and, as a result, the supporting hepatic framework has collapsed and the periportal spaces lie closer to one another (→ 2 and → 3 indicate respectively two portal fields). There are numerous proliferated bile ducts (→ 4) in addition to lymphocytic infiltration. Two central veins can be seen in the middle of the picture between the portal fields. At very low magnification, the increased width of the periportal fields and the proliferation of bile ducts are plainly visible.

Macroscopic: The liver is reduced in size, tough in consistency and has red and yellow, marble-like cut surfaces. The red color is due to hyperemia and pooling of blood. Islands of fatty parenchymous tissue are yellow. This is sometimes called subacute red atrophy of the liver. Duration: 3–8 weeks. Mortality: 40%.

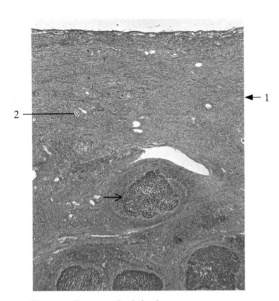

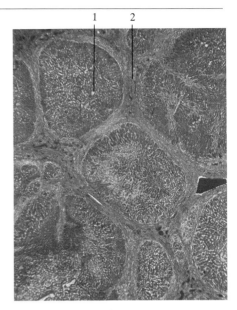

Fig. 5.30. Postnecrotic cirrhosis;
H & E, 15×.

Fig. 5.31. Portal cirrhosis;
H & E, 30×.

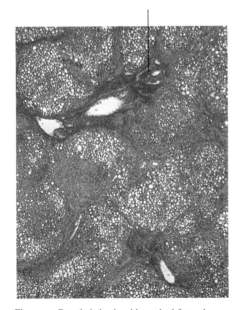

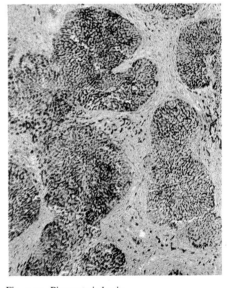

Fig. 5.32. Portal cirrhosis with marked fatty change;
van Gieson stain, 40×.

Fig. 5.33. Pigment cirrhosis;
Berlin-blue reaction, 30×.

Hepatic Cirrhosis

Postnecrotic cirrhosis (Macronodular cirrhosis, Fig. 5.30). The results of patchy parenchymatous necrosis are clearly seen in the picture. There is a large area of subcapsular tissue destruction (→ 1), the lobular pattern has disappeared and the periportal zones are collapsed and compressed on one another. This has resulted in large scars that are rich in collagenous tissue and infiltrated with chronic inflammatory cells. The periportal zones also are infiltrated with lymphocytes and, in addition, show bile duct proliferation (→ 2). Islands of remaining parenchyma (→) can still be seen in the scarred tissue. Some of these show central veins or periportal zones, but they no longer have an orderly arrangement, since the necrosis of the lobules has been irregular. The central vein, for example, may lie at the edge of the lobule or the periportal zone lie in the middle of it *(pseudolobules)*. Other masses of regenerating liver cells have formed nodules with an abnormal architectural arrangement of the liver cell cords *(regeneration adenomas)*.

Macroscopic: The liver is irregularly nodular with depressed large and small scars and coarse nodules (regenerating parenchymal remnants). This type of cirrhosis has large irregular nodules (macronodular cirrhosis): Portal cirrhosis small uniform, diffuse nodules (diffuse fibrosis). If there is no inflammatory infiltrate, it is called post necrotic scarring.

Portal or Laennec's cirrhosis (Fig. 5.31). Examination with the scanning lens discloses various sized foci of red parenchymatous tissue traversed by bluish red septa of scar tissue. With low-power magnification, the pseudolobules and connective tissue septa connecting the periportal zones can be seen more clearly. Various sized islands of liver tissue with abnormally situated central veins have been formed in this way (→ 1). The connective tissue (→ 2) is infiltrated with cells (lymphocytes, histiocytes and a few polymorphonuclear leukocytes) and contains proliferated bile ducts. The progress of the cirrhosis is indicated by the degree of involvement of the parenchyma by cellular exudate.

Macroscopic: The liver shows fine, fairly regular nodularity (so-called hobnail liver).

Portal cirrhosis with marked fatty change (Fig. 5.32). In this condition, the alteration of architecture develops in a regular fashion from the periportal zones just as in portal cirrhosis. With the scanning lens, it is scarcely possible to recognize the tissue as liver. In van Gieson preparations, red connective tissue septa can be seen, while the tissue between has a vacuolated appearance. Low magnification shows lymphocytic infiltration of the periportal fields and bile duct proliferation (→). The liver cells contain round, optically empty droplets (the fat has been dissolved out in the process of preparation). In some places, larger fat cysts have formed (from fusion of fatty cells) (see also p. 145). Fatty cirrhosis often develops from fatty hepatitis and occurs frequently in alcoholics. Mallory bodies may be present.

Macroscopic: Large, yellow, finely granular, firm liver. Sixty to seventy percent of all cases of cirrhosis result from malnutrition or toxins (alcohol abuse). Acute viral hepatitis seldom progresses to cirrhosis. There is no correlation between etiology and the kind of cirrhosis.

Pigment cirrhosis (Fig. 5.33). *This occurs mostly as a part of hemochromatosis (bronze diabetes), an illness in which siderin pigment is deposited in the pancreas, spleen, lymph nodes, salivary glands and many other organs.* Very low magnification of sections treated with Berlin blue shows irregular, blue-stained masses of parenchyma traversed by red-stained connective tissue septa of various widths. Higher magnification shows granules of blue pigment in the cytoplasm of the liver and Kupffer cells and in the lining cells of proliferated bile ducts.

Macroscopic: The liver is small, firm and brown and shows either fine or coarse granularity.

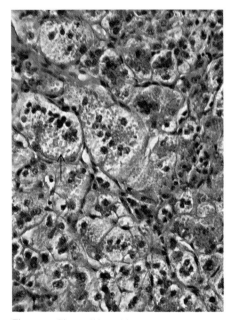

Fig. 5.34. Giant cell hepatitis;
H & E, 300×.

Fig. 5.35. Chronic myeloid leukemia of liver;
H & E, 108×.

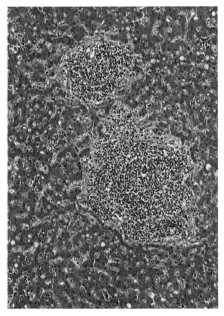

Fig. 5.36. Lymphatic leukemia involving the liver;
H & E, 108×.

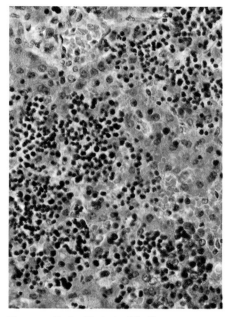

Fig. 5.37. Erythroblastosis of the liver;
H & E, 388×.

Giant cell hepatitis (Fig. 5.34).

Giant cell hepatitis of the newborn or infant is the expression of a particular reaction by the infant liver to various noxious stimuli (mainly viral hepatitis, although other causes are possible). The symptoms which are most prominent clinically are those resulting from obstructive jaundice. Microscopically (Fig. 5.34), the normal cords of liver cells are replaced by numerous, bizarre multinucleated giant cells (→). They frequently are the width of two or more liver cords. The cytoplasm of these giant cells is vacuolated and often filled with bile pigment (→ in the picture). These giant cells are an expression of faulty regeneration or fusion of cells. Proliferation of connective tissue cells (stellate cells, cells in the periportal fields) is very prominent in this phase of the disease.

Macroscopic: Enlarged liver, with a marked green discoloration.

Chronic myeloid leukemia of liver (Fig. 5.35). *In this form of leukemia, there is an unregulated increase in immature early forms of granulocytes in the bone marrow with spillover into the blood. It usually leads to infiltration of the spleen and lymph nodes and to accumulation and increase of myeloblasts, promyelocytes and myelocytes in the sinusoids of the liver* (see also p. 249). The scanning lens reveals preservation of the architecture. Low magnification shows the markedly increased cell content of the sinusoids, most of which are distended and plugged with large, nucleated blood cells (myelocytes with round, vesiculated nuclei and, when more mature, granular cytoplasm; myeloblasts with oval or bean-shaped nuclei, see p. 249). The portal fields are, for the most part, either not involved or only slightly infiltrated with leukemic cells. The liver cells may undergo pressure atrophy and show degenerative changes.

Macroscopic: The liver is enlarged, grayish red and the lobules are indistinct. In acute leukemia, the periportal zones are especially affected.

Lymphatic leukemia involving liver (Fig. 5.36, also p. 249). In contrast to myeloid leukemia, the *periportal zones* in chronic lymphatic leukemia are permeated with immature cells (lymphoblasts, lymphocytes), whereas the sinusoids contain only small numbers of nucleated cells. Under low magnification, the markedly increased, blue appearing, spherical periportal zones are at once apparent. Higher magnification shows infiltration of the periportal connective tissue by lymphatic cells, with dense or vesiculated nuclei and scanty cytoplasm.

Macroscopic: The liver is enlarged. The periportal spaces are often visible on the cut surfaces as small, white nodules.

Erythroblastosis of the liver (Fig. 5.37). *In this condition, the fetus or newborn infant develops hemolytic anemia as a result of immunization of the mother during pregnancy by the father's blood factors. (Most commonly this is Rh incompatibility and less commonly incompatibility of ABO or some other factor.) The anemia results in a marked reactive increase in blood formation in the bone marrow and other hematopoietic tissues, including the liver (this occurs normally in newborns).* Nodules of cellular infiltration are seen in the liver. Under high magnification, these can be identified as foci of intrasinusoidal hematopoiesis. The cells are chiefly erythropoietic (in particular, erythroblasts and normoblasts), with a few from the white cell series and some megakaryocytes. In addition, there is hepatocellular jaundice, since, in most cases, the liver cells are unable to produce indirect reacting bilirubin. Bile casts and siderosis may also be seen.

Macroscopic: A large, red liver. In late stages, there may be generalized edema *(congenital hydrops)*, anemia and *severe jaundice* (icterus gravis, often associated with kernicterus).

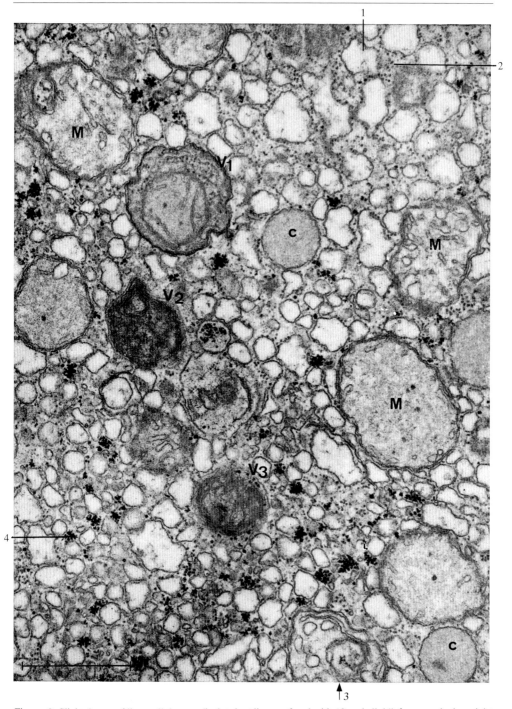

Fig. 5.38. Slight degree of liver cell damage (isolated rat liver perfused with 10 γ phalloidin[1] per gm. body weight, 30 min.). There are vacuolar dilatation of the smooth and rough ER (→ 1) and ribosomes without membranes (→ 2). There are also numbers of autolysosomes (autophagocytotic vacuoles) with accumulated mitochrondria (V$_1$; also see p. 153), and myelin figures (V$_2$ and V$_3$) which are presumably a manifestation of the digestion of membranes in these lysosomes. → 3 Golgi apparatus, M = mitochrondria, C = cytosome, → 4 glycogen. 32,000× (Miller).

[1] Amanita phalloides

Electron Microscopy of Liver Injury

The electron microscopic changes of the liver cell organelles are rather uniform and, for the most part, nonspecific. Theoretically, all the changes described on p. 16 may occur. In acute toxic injury (alcohol, carbon tetrachloride, partial hepatectomy, see Fig. 5.40, or anoxia), the mitochondria are swollen (cloudy swelling) and the endoplasmic reticulum or ground substance becomes vacuolated (hydropic degeneration). Glycogen stores disappear, the rough endoplasmic reticulum becomes disorganized and frequently loses its ribosomes (reduction of protein synthesis) and, finally, the cell membranes become fragmented, vacuolated and are destroyed (p. 152). The lysosomes contain parts of the cellular organelles (Fig. 5.39). Similar pictures are seen in acute viral hepatitis, in which hyaline bodies, also called Councilman bodies (p. 156), appear, i.e., necrotic, shrunken liver cells. Chronic liver damage entails primarily focal or diffuse proliferation of the smooth endoplasmic reticulum (intensification of the detoxification process, Jones et al, 1966). In chronic *alcoholic intoxication,* focal filamentous masses may be seen *(Mallory bodies,* alcoholic hyalin, p. 156). Terminally, the ER may be entirely disrupted. The smooth endoplasmic reticulum may also appear to form myelin-like whorls (fingerprints). Fat droplets may be seen either in acute or chronic liver damage. In chronic hepatitis, there is also proliferation of collagen fibers in the space of Dissé, and a basement membrane may form. In intrahepatic (hepatitis, toxic) and extrahepatic cholestasis the bile canaliculi are dilated, the microvilli are swollen at first, then disappear, and the pericanalicular cytoplasm has a denser appearance. Lysosomes and cytosomes (pericanalicular dense bodies), increase in number and are spread throughout the cytoplasm (activation of acid phosphatase). In addition, bile droplets can be seen in the cytoplasm (p. 154). Determination of the path of bile into the bloodstream (whether between or through hepatic cells) has not been successful even with the electron microscope. In hepatic cirrhosis, nonspecific changes again are seen (enlargement and clumping of mitochondria, myelin-like degeneration, vacuoles in the ER, proliferation of collagen fibers around the liver cells, autophagolysosomes, localized cell destruction, fat deposition, localized glycogen aggregation, pigmentation, bile tubule proliferation and hemosiderin).

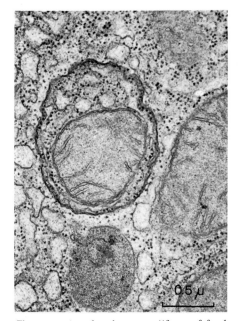

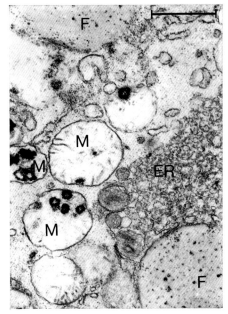

Fig. 5.39. *Autophagolysosome,* "focus of focal degradation" in a liver cell of a rat. Treatment as in Figure 5.38. Within the surrounding membrane there is a well-preserved mitochondrion and parts of rough endoplasmic reticulum (ribosomes, membranes). 45,000× (Miller).

Fig. 5.40. Acute carbon tetrachloride poisoning (after 24 hours, liver, mouse). Focal proliferation of the smooth endoplasmic reticulum (ER), fat droplets (F) as well as swollen mitochondria (matrix type) with round, black-appearing matrix aggregates (calcium deposits, Reynaulds, 1963). 35,000× (Hübner).

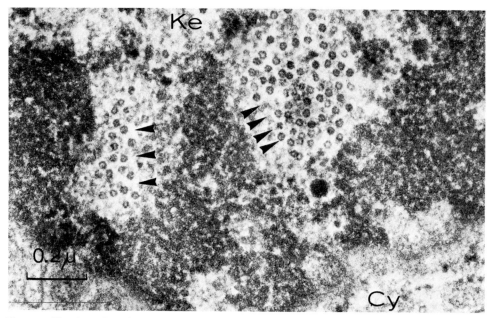

Fig. 5.41. Chronic persistent hepatitis in an 11-month-old infant. Hepatocyte nucleus (KE) with masses of virus particles (core antigen, arrows). Cytoplasm = Cy, 80,000× (Kistler).

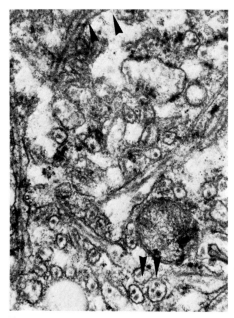

Fig. 5.42. Chronic persistent hepatitis B (SH) in a 38-year-old kidney transplant recipient. Smooth endoplasmic reticulum (arrows) of a hepatocyte with longitudinal and cross sections of SH surface antigen. 44,000× (Kistler).

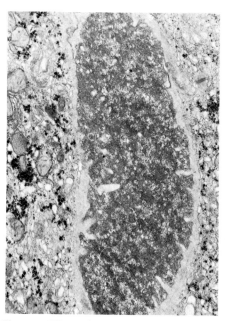

Fig. 5.43. *Bile cast* in a canaliculus (human, viral hepatitis). There are no microvilli (Fig. 11), the lumen is filled with bile pigment. 12,000× (Biava, 1964).

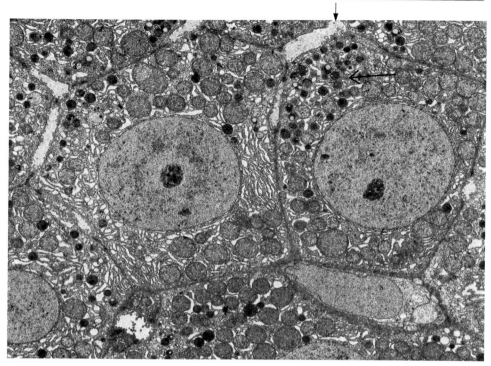

Fig. 5.44. Markedly atrophied liver cells with scanty cytoplasm, tightly packed organelles and numerous lysosomes (→) in the region of the bile capillaries (arrow above). Glycogen is absent. 5000×.

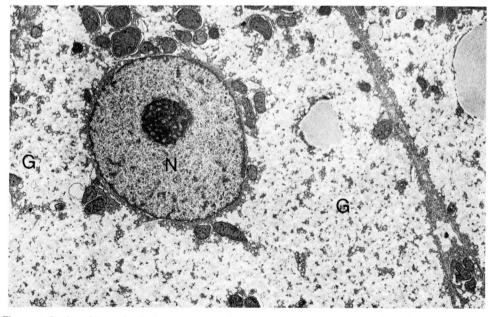

Fig. 5.45. Section of liver of a child with von Gierke's disease (glycogen storage disease Type I). In this disorder there is a deficiency of glucose-6-phosphatase, an enzyme of the endoplasmic reticulum. The cell contains practically no glycogen and only rudimentary cell organelles (N = nucleus, G = glycogen). 5500× (Spycher).

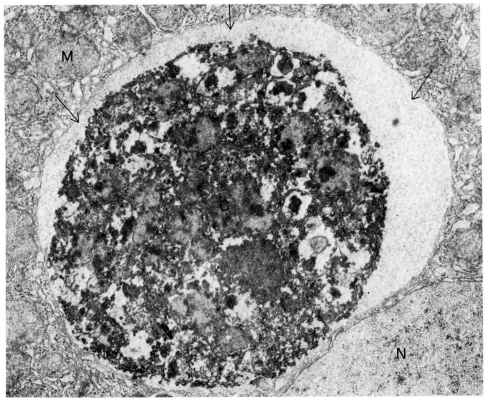

Fig. 5.46. *Hyaline (acidophile) body* in viral hepatitis, so-called *Councilman body* = C. The necrotic, rounded and shrunken liver cell containing fragments of organelles, arrow indicates the lysosomal membrane, has been phagocytosed by a liver parenchymal cell (N = nucleus, M = mitochondria of liver cell). 35000×.

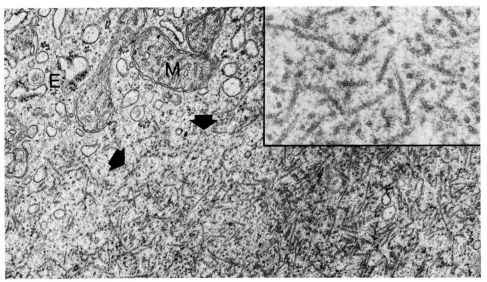

Fig. 5.47. Liver cell containing Mallory bodies, so-called alcoholic hyalin (mouse liver). Notice the nodular arrangement of the microfilaments (→ and insert above). This is probably a pathological protein (membrane). M = mitochondria, E = endoplasmic reticulum. 22000×. Inset 39000×. (Denk).

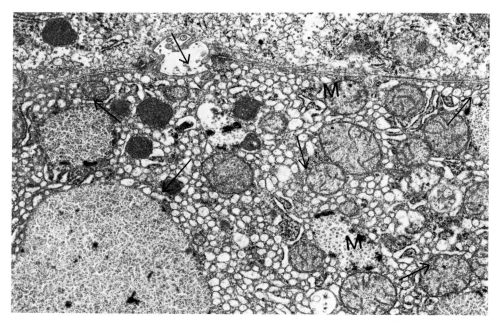

Fig. 5.48. Section of a liver cell from a child with Pompe's disease (= glycogen storage disease Type II). In this disorder there is a deficiency of the lysosomal enzyme α-1,4-glycosidase. These are gigantic storage vacuoles packed with glycogen (arrow). M = mitochondria. 1000×. (Spycher).

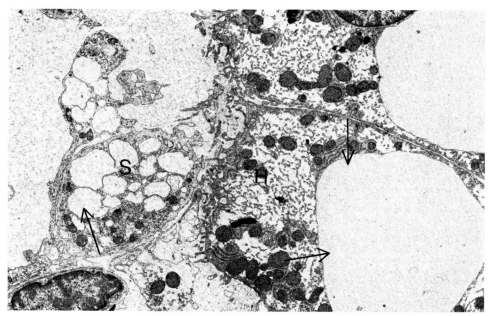

Fig. 5.49. Section of a liver cell from a child with GM-1 gangliosidosis, absence of lysosomal enzyme B-galacto-dase. Large storage vacuoles filled with GM-1 ganglioside (arrow) are present in the cytoplasm of the hepatocytes (H) and Kupffer cells (S). 5300×. (Spycher).

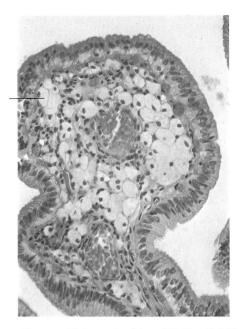

Fig. 5.50. Cholesterosis of the gallbladder; H & E, 350×.

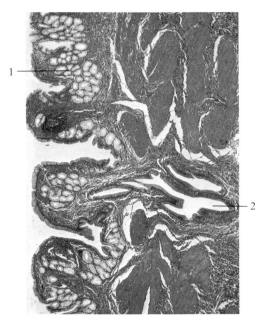

Fig. 5.51. Chronic hypertrophic cholecystitis; H & E, 80×.

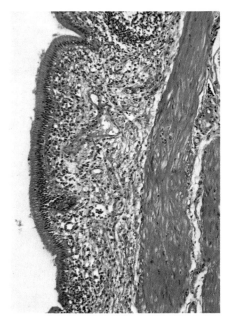

Fig. 5.52. Chronic atrophic cholecystitis; H & E, 100×.

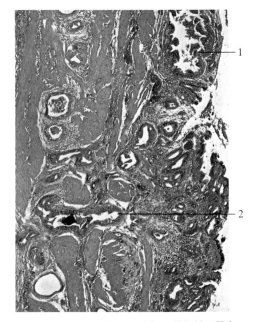

Fig. 5.53. Adenocarcinoma of the gallbladder; H & E, 60×.

Gallbladder Disease

Introduction: The gallbladder is a hollow, thin walled organ lined with mucous membrane and a net-like layer of smooth muscle. The mucosa consists of delicate stromal folds covered on the surface with a single layer of cylindrical epithelium. Occasional aberrant bile ducts *(Luschke's crypts)* occur in the outer portions of the gallbladder wall.

Cholesterosis of the gallbladder (Fig. 5.50). *This is a metabolic disorder belonging to the group of lipidoses and manifest histologically by the appearance of pseudoxanthoma cells in the mucosal folds.* Figure 5.50 shows the marked enlargement of the distended tips of a mucosal fold that is covered by cylindrical epithelium. The underlying subepithelial stroma is thick and contains large cells with central nuclei and finely granular or vacuolated cytoplasm. Macrophages (→) filled with cholesterin and cholesterin esters (dissolved during the preparatory process of parafin embedding).

Cholesterosis ("strawberry" gallbladder) is found in 5–40% of resected gall bladders. It is particularly common in women 40–70 years old. Cholesterosis has few if any clinical manifestations.

Cholecystitis (Figs. 5.51, 5.52) *in most cases is a chronic, recurrent and nonspecific inflammation of the gallbladder.* Acute inflammations characteristically show mural necrosis, hemorrhage, diffuse inflammation of the gallbladder wall (severe inflammations may be phlegmonous or gangrenous) and empyema. In chronic inflammation the mucosa may become thick (**chronic hypertrophic cholecystitis**, Fig. 5.51) and the mucosal folds broad because of lymphocytic infiltration, fibrosis and scar tissue. The surface epithelium shows transformation to mucous glands reminiscent of *Brunner's glands (intestinal metaplasia → 1)*. Increased luminal pressure in the gallbladder causes diverticulum-like mucosal outpouchings *(Rokitansky-Aschoff sinuses → 2)*. They appear as empty spaces lined with cylindrical epithelium and extend through the muscularis. In long-standing chronic cholecystitis scarring and flattening of the mucosal folds are prominent (**chronic atrophic cholecystitis**, Fig. 5.52). Finally the gallbladder wall may become completely fibrotic and rigid *(porcelain gallbladder)*.

Chronic cholecystitis occurs frequently in elderly women and in 90% of cases is accompanied by cholelithiasis. In the early stages, chronic cholecystitis is usually abacterial and results from interference with the blood supply (e.g. an impacted cystic stone). Bacterial infection develops later by way of the bile ducts, bloodstream or lymphatics.

Carcinoma of the gallbladder (Fig. 5.53) *is a malignant epithelial tumor arising from the mucosa, and occurs almost exclusively in a scarred gallbladder. Histologically it may be an undifferentiated carcinoma, a well-differentiated adenocarcinoma or an adenoacanthoma (carcinoma with a mixture of squamous and glandular epithelium).* Fig. 5.53 shows the darker staining strands of carcinoma cells replacing mucosa (→1) and infiltrating deeply into the wall (→2).

Gallbladder carcinomas form about 15% of all malignant tumors. They are diagnosed in nearly 4% of resected gallbladders. Macroscopically they are either diffusely infiltrating or nodulo-papillary.

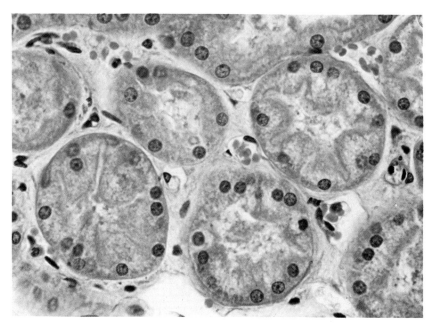

Fig. 6.1. Cloudy swelling of proximal tubules of the kidney; H & E, 600×.

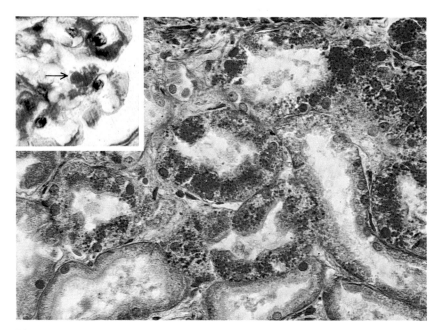

Fig. 6.2. Hyaline droplet degeneration; Azan stain, 456×. Inset: Hyaline degeneration in the investing epithelium of a glomerulus (rat); experimental glomerulonephritis; PAS, ca. 500×.

6. Kidney

Histologic examination of kidney sections should proceed according to the following guide lines. Evaluation of the *thickness of cortex and medulla* in the specimen. *Alterations of vessels:* especially at the corticomedullary junction and in the afferent arterioles. *Glomeruli:* cellularity, the condition of the basement membrane, capsular lining epithelium, focal or diffuse necrosis of the glomerulus. *Tubules:* size of lumen, size of cells, cytoplasmic deposits, segments affected. *Interstitium:* cellular and fibrous content.

Cloudy swelling (Fig. 6.1). *This is a disturbance of the ionic milieu of the cell that entails retention of water and sodium with concomitant loss of potassium from the cells, which then begin to swell.* The swelling affects mitochondria particularly. The resulting increase in the size of particulate matter leads to increased dispersion of light and, thereby, to a Tyndall effect, i.e., to cloudiness. Figure 6.1 shows proximal tubular epithelium, the cytoplasm of which is filled with fine, pale droplets (swollen mitochondria), giving rise to a finely granular appearance. Fine, granular, coagulated protein material is also seen in the narrowed lumens of the tubules. The same changes occur also in postmortem specimens and are differentiated only with difficulty from antemortem cloudy swelling. If the tissue sections are treated with dilute acetic acid, the contents of the mitochondria precipitate on the mitochondrial membrane, and the cytoplasm again becomes clear.

Macroscopic: Enlarged, soft organ with dull cut surfaces. The parenchyma bulges above the cut surface. Cloudy swelling occurs, especially with toxic injury (e.g., diphtheria).

In *hydropic degeneration,* the process is identical—free water accumulates in the cell and forms vacuoles (mitochondria, endoplasmic reticulum and ground substance). Microscopically, the cytoplasm is filled with large and small optically empty vacuoles. In some instances, perinuclear halos also appear (see p. 163). Hydropic degeneration is seen particularly in cases of acute anoxia, toxic inhibition of glycolysis (eg., cyanide poisoning), substrate depletion or inhibition of oxidative phosphorylation (e.g., barbiturate poisoning). All these conditions cause deficiency of ATP with resulting failure of the sodium pump to work.

Hyaline droplet degeneration (Fig. 6.2 and p. 168). *Proteinaceous droplets appear in the cytoplasm of the proximal tubular epithelium due to tubular reabsorption, e.g., in glomerulonephritis.* Histologically, medium magnification reveals swelling of the proximal tubular cells due to infiltration of deep red-staining and somewhat refractile protein droplets. The lumen contains hyaline casts or granular precipitates of protein. At this stage, single epithelial cells, filled with proteinaceous droplets, are also found in the lumen.

In rare cases, hyaline droplet degeneration also involves the epithelial cells of glomerular loops, which are, of course, related morphologically to the tubular epithelium. The inset in Figure 6.2 shows experimental glomerulonephritis in a rat in which there is marked thickening of the basement membrane and proliferation of epithelial and endothelial cells. The arrow points to an epithelial cell with round, hyaline droplets in the cytoplasm (see p. 186).

Macroscopic: Enlarged, pale grayish white kidneys (large, white kidney), e.g., in amyloidosis or myeloma (myeloma nephrosis).

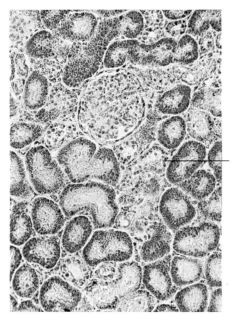

Fig. 6.3. Fatty degeneration of the proximal tubules of the cortex. Sudan-hematoxylin stain; 160×.

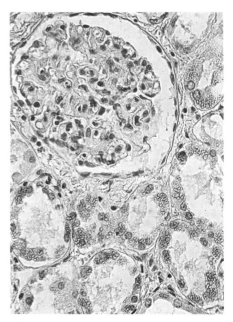

Fig. 6.4. Cholemic (bile) nephrosis. Hematoxylin; 459×.

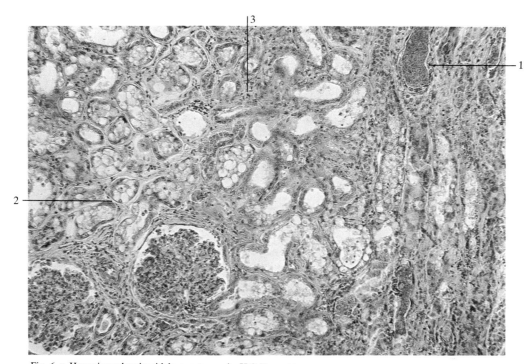

Fig. 6.5. Hypoxic nephrosis with hypopotassemia; H & E, 111×.

Noninflammatory Kidney Disease (Nephrosis)

Heretofore the term "nephrosis" has been used to describe degenerative changes in the renal tubules in inflammatory kidney disease. This limited definition is no longer tenable. At the present time the following are recognized. (a) clinically: nephrotic syndrome: kidney disease with proteinuria, hypoalbuminomia, hyperlipemia and generalized edema. Cause: chiefly glomerulonephritis, amyloidosis, diabetic glomerulosclerosis, mercury or other poisons. (b) pathologically: non-inflammatory kidney disease which may or may not be accompanied by the nephrotic syndrome, and in which there are lesions in either the glomeruli (glomerulonephrosis, e.g., Kimmelstiel-Wilson disease, amyloid disease) or the tubules (tubular nephrosis, e.g. cholemic nephrosis).

Fatty degeneration of proximal tubules of the cortex (Fig. 6.3). *Deposition of neutral fats and lipids in the tubular epithelial cells can result either from reabsorption by the tubular cells* (e.g., *lipoid nephrosis associated with diabetes*), *from hypoxia or from toxic injury.* The figure shows fatty changes resulting from the hypoxia of anemia. Scanning the section at low magnification reveals accumulation of the Sudan stain in the cortex. The medullary border is sharply delineated, and with medium high magnification (Fig. 6.3) the loops of Henle are seen to be mostly spared. Fine lipid droplets are deposited in the epithelial cells of the proximal convoluted tubules of the cortex. The lipid droplets either lie in the basal portion of the cell or completely fill it. The cells are swollen. The tubular lumen is narrowed. The portions of the distal tubules next to the glomeruli ($\rightarrow$) are not involved.

Lipoid nephrosis (see p. 181), when it occurs as an independent disease, is also characterized by marked fatty changes of the tubular system with deposition of neutral fats and lipids (doubly refractile). In addition, fatty deposits are found in the interstitium.

Macroscopic: The kidney is slightly enlarged and the cortex is yellow.

Bile, or cholemic, nephrosis (Fig. 6.4) *signifies degenerative changes and deposition of bile pigments in the proximal tubular epithelial cells during the course of jaundice (reabsorption, see p. 168).* Hematoxylin stain brings out very well the yellow-to-green color of the bile pigment. Medium magnification reveals granular deposits of bile pigment in the cytoplasm of the proximal tubular epithelium. In addition, there are degenerative changes such as cloudy swelling and slight fatty changes. Occasional shed cells can also be found in the lumens of the tubules. Bile-stained hyaline casts are present in the collecting ducts. The glomeruli are not affected.

Macroscopic: Slightly enlarged kidney, green-to-yellowish brown cortex and medulla.

Hypoxic nephrosis with hypokalemia (Fig. 6.5). *(Synonyms: hemoglobinuric nephrosis, myoglobinuric nephrosis, crush kidney, shock kidney in trauma, lower nephron nephrosis.)*

This is an acute process that may be caused by various injurious agents (trauma, poisons) and is characterized by the onset of severe shock, hemolysis or myolysis and degeneration and necrosis of renal tubules. The term vascular-tubular syndrome describes the two essential components: vascular collapse (disturbance of perfusion) and toxic tubular degeneration. Microscopically, the most striking finding is the presence of proteinaceous casts containing hemoglobin or myoglobin (brown casts in the collecting ducts, $\rightarrow$ 1) in the distal tubules, Henle's loops and collecting ducts. Proximal convoluted tubules may show focal necrosis. In addition, degenerative changes of the tubular epithelium may be seen (cloudy swelling, fatty degeneration). There is an accompanying hypokalemia (polyuric phase of the shock kidney) causing cystic dilatation of the base of the tubular epithelial cells (proximal), which microscopically gives the impression of vacuolar degeneration ($\rightarrow$ 2). Later, tubular rhexis develops (rupture of kidney tubules). The epithelium of the proximal tubules in Figure 6.5 is for the most part, flattened (a sign of insufficiency). The interstitial tissues are swollen by edema ($\rightarrow$ 3). The glomeruli are hyperemic and have wide basement membranes.

Macroscopic: Enlarged kidneys; dirty grayish brown color.

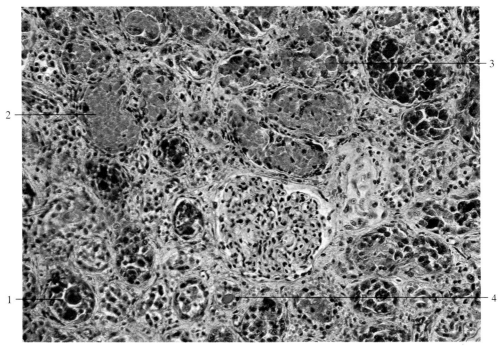

Fig. 6.6. Mercuric bichloride nephrosis; H & E, 200×.

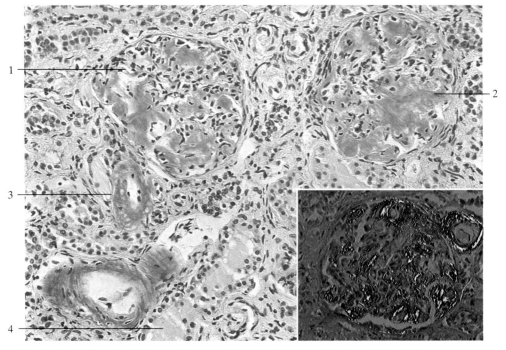

Fig. 6.7. Amyloid nephrosis; Congo red-hematoxylin, 200×. Inset, amyloid under polarized light.

Mercuric bichloride nephrosis (Fig. 6.6). *Corrosive mercuric bichloride produces a marked, necrotizing nephrosis, with secondary calcification of necrotic tubular cells.* It involves particularly the proximal convoluted tubules. There is considerable controversy concerning the pathogenesis and site of action of the mercury, but, if death occurs during the acute phase, necrosis of the proximal convoluted tubules is seen. Within a few days, deposits of calcium can be found in the necrotic areas (matrix aggregates). Regeneration of tubules follows survival of the acute phase, as evidenced by the marked proliferation of flat epithelial cells which may be the predominant feature of the microscopic picture.

Microscopic examination of the cortex in the acute and subacute stages reveals necrotic red-staining tubules and dark blue-staining deposits of calcium. Medium magnification (Fig. 6.6) shows irregular blue calcium deposits of varying size as well as calcified epithelial cells that have been partly shed into the lumen ($\rightarrow$ 1), with the result that cross sections of the tubule may appear completely filled. In other areas, tubules are filled with granular, eosinophilic masses ($\rightarrow$ 2). Here, the epithelium is necrotic and, together with the shed epithelial cells ($\rightarrow$ 3) and protein casts, forms a homogeneous concrement. Other segments of the tubules also contain casts (distal tubule, $\rightarrow$ 4). The interstitium is edematous. The glomeruli are avascular, normally cellular and have delicate basement membranes.

Macroscopic: Enlarged, soft kidney with dull red or grayish white external and cut surfaces.

Amyloid nephrosis (Fig. 6.7). *This is a glomerulonephrosis due to amyloidosis (spleen, liver, adrenal and intestine, etc., are also involved) and is manifested by deposition of abnormal protein, amyloid, in the glomeruli and afferent arterioles.*

Examination of an H & E section with a scanning lens reveals large, homogeneous, eosinophilic, hyalinized cortical glomeruli. Medium magnification shows arterioles with homogeneous, hyalinized walls. The hyalinized protein material stains readily with Congo red or methyl violet (amyloid stains red, surrounding tissue pale blue): the red stain is specific for amyloid. The amyloid accumulation appears first as a fine red streak lying between the basement membrane and the endothelium of the glomeruli ($\rightarrow$ 1, see also p. 187). With increasing deposition, the glomerular loop thickens and the lumen is narrowed. As a result, the loops take on a homogeneous, anuclear appearance. Adjacent affected glomeruli may merge to produce a uniformly red area ($\rightarrow$ 2). The end stage is an obliterated glomerulus. The same process occurs in the media of the arcuate arteries and afferent arterioles ($\rightarrow$ 3). The muscle cells deteriorate, and the media appears as a smooth red ring. Secondarily, amyloid is deposited in the pericapillary interstitial tissues and the tubular basement membranes. Many of the proximal convoluted tubules are dilated and contain casts which are Congo red negative ($\rightarrow$ 4). Amyloid stained with Congo red is doubly refractive in polarized light (Fig. 6.7, inset). Hyaline droplet degeneration occurs frequently (compare p. 160). The amyloid kidney often becomes contracted due to the glomerular involvement and the subsequent atrophy of the tubular system and the proliferation of interstitial connective tissue.

Macroscopic: The kidney is large, firm, white and waxy. The cut surface is dry and translucent; the medulla is usually reddish and the line of demarcation from the swollen cortex is preserved. The contracted amyloid kidney is small and gnarled.

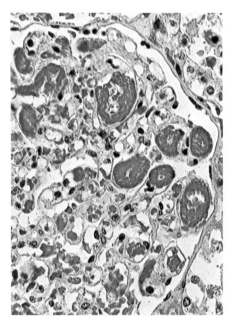

Fig. 6.8. Hyalinized fibrin thrombi in a glomerulus in shock; Goldner stain, 600×.

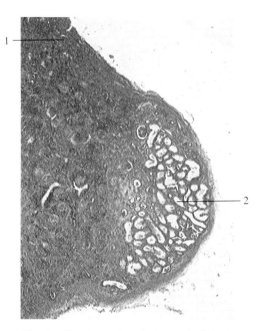

Fig. 6.9. Scar in renal cortical necrosis following shock with compensatory hypertrophy of remaining parenchyma; H & E, 20×.

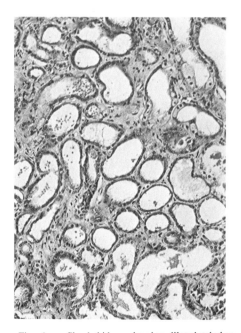

Fig. 6.10. Shock kidney showing dilated tubules; H & E, 40×.

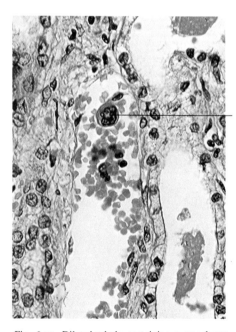

Fig. 6.11. Dilated tubule containing a megakaryocyte in shock; H & E, 280×.

Shock Kidney (See also Shock Lung, p. 84)

In all forms of shock *(endotoxic, hemorrhagic, postoperative, burn, traumatic, anaphylactic, myocardial infarction or eclampsia etc.)* renal perfusion is more or less reduced and anuria develops. Experimentally one sort of shock kidney (Type I) is easily produced in rabbits. An injection of endotoxin repeated twice within 24 hours results in bilateral necrosis of the renal cortex and formation of fibrin thrombi in the arterioles and glomeruli. This form of shock is also seen in humans. Figure 6.8 shows glomerular loops filled with fibrin thrombi which stain red with the Goldner stain. Survival is unusual in this form of shock kidney. Figure 6.9 shows the kidney of such a patient who survived unusually long—6 months (septic abortion treated with fibrinolysin and artificial kidney). The cortical tissue is completely scarred (→) except for a small area that shows compensatory hypertrophy (→ 2). The second sort of shock kidney (Type II) is by far the more common. Macroscopically the kidneys are large, soft and grayish red. Histologically (Fig. 6.10) the tubules are markedly dilated and lined with flat epithelium and the interstitium shows marked edema. Glomeruli are uninvolved and fibrin thrombi can not be seen (see also p. 163, hypoxic nephrosis-traumatic shock). A further morphological indication of shock is the finding of bone marrow cells—in this case a megakaryocyte (Fig. 6.11 →)—in the medullary venules, especially those near the corticomedullary junction.

The morphological sign of shock is almost always the presence of hyalin thrombi (fibrin, platelets). **Spherical hyalin masses** also appear commonly in shock (atypical polymerized fibrin, so-called "shock bodies", Fig. 6.12). These changes in the blood stream, as well as the development of the thrombi, can easily be observed experimentally in blood vessels by intravital microscopy, for example in the mesentery of a rabbit. Figure 6.13 shows a **finely granular platelet thrombus** in a venule (→ 1). The stasis and homogenization of the blood column is clearly visible (→2).

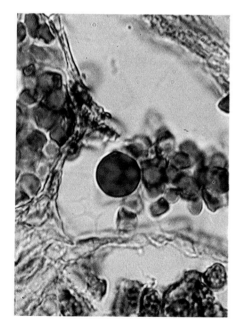

Fig. 6.12. Spherical hyaline masses in a venule in shock; Goldner stain, 500×.

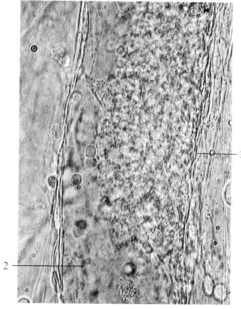

Fig. 6.13. Platelet thrombus in a mesenteric venule of a rabbit; intravital microscopy, 400×.

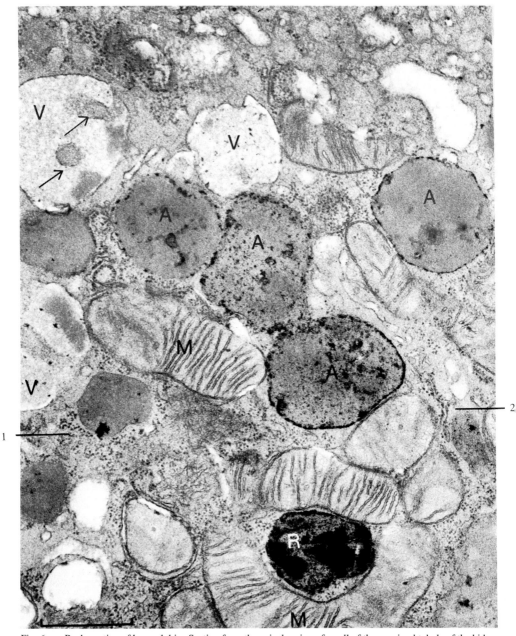

Fig. 6.14. Reabsorption of hemoglobin. Section from the apical region of a cell of the proximal tubule of the kidney (mouse, 1 hour after intraperitoneal injection of ox hemoglobin). All stages of the uptake and concentration of the hemoglobin can be followed in this picture from the top to the bottom. The vacuoles (V) contain, in addition to granular protein, hemoglobin droplets (→). In the absorption droplets (A) the hemoglobin is concentrated into bodies limited by a single membrane. The black particles are precipitates of lead phosphate (= histochemical evidence of acid phosphatase. These organelles can be thus identified as lysosomes. R = resting body with strong acid phosphatase activity and marked concentration of hemoglobin, M = mitochondria, → 1 = ribosomes and polysomes, → 2 = rough endoplasmic reticulum, 24,000 × Miller *et al.*, 1964).

Fine Structure of Tubular Reabsorption

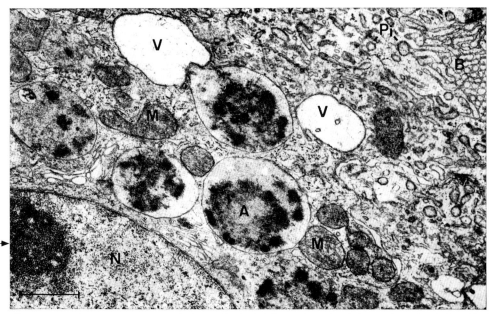

Fig. 6.15. Protein reabsorption droplets in the proximal tubule in protein nephrosis in man. Part of a tubular epithelial cell with a section of the brush border (B). There are pinocytotic vesicles (Pi) in the ground substance. These represent reabsorption vacuoles (V) of the protein. The protein reabsorption droplets (A) develop from these. M = mitochondria, N = nucleus, → nucleolus. 16,000× (Thoenes, 1965).

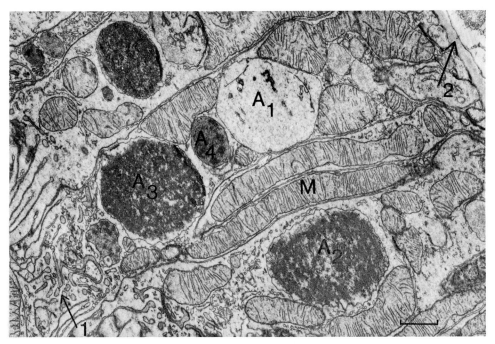

Fig. 6.16. Protein reabsorption droplets (protein storage phagoosomes) in the proximal renal tubular epithelium in lead poisoning of the rat (5 weeks after intraperitoneal administration of a single dose of 50 mg. lead acetate). Large bodies bounded by a single membrane and with a fine granularity (A 1) as well as contents of increased electron density (A 2–A 4), M = mitochondria. Numerous pinocytotic vacuoles at the base of the brush border (→1), → 2 = peritubular basement membrane. 10,500 × (Dr. Totovic).

Vascular Disorders of the Kidney

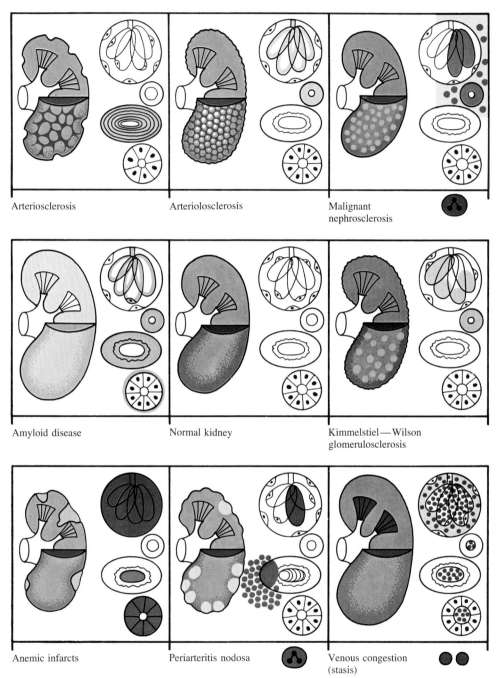

Arteriosclerosis

Arteriolosclerosis

Malignant
nephrosclerosis

Amyloid disease

Normal kidney

Kimmelstiel—Wilson
glomerulosclerosis

Anemic infarcts

Periarteritis nodosa

Venous congestion
(stasis)

Fig. 6.17. Schematic representation of the gross and microscopic changes encountered in vascular disorders of the kidney.

Vascular Renal Disorders

Vascular diseases in the kidney (Fig. 6.17) involve either large arteries or the arterioles. The glomeruli almost always become involved secondarily, and ultimately the tubules.

Arteriosclerosis (see Fig. 6.18) may uncommonly involve the main *renal arteries* at the junction with the aorta (fibromuscular dysplasia, see p. 64), and the resulting obstruction lead to ischemia of the kidney and renal hypertension *(Goldblatt mechanism)*. Involvement of arteries of the interlobular and arcuate type is manifested by concentric fibrosis and elastosis which narrows the lumen. The severity of the glomerular lesion (hyaline degeneration) depends upon the extent of the arterial sclerosis.

Macroscopic: The surface is red and shows isolated small scars.

Arteriolosclerosis or arteriolar nephrosclerosis (see p. 173) usually shows hyalinization of *afferent arterioles* with narrowing of the lumens. Decreased vascular perfusion leads to hyalinized thickening of the capillary loops, terminating in complete obliteration of the glomerulus. The hyalin is probably formed by cells of the mesangium (mesangial matrix, see glomerulonephritis). Marked involvement leads to contraction of the kidney: *red granular atrophy (primary contracted kidney)*. Arteriosclerosis and arteriolosclerosis frequently occur together (arterio-arteriolonephrosclerosis).

Macroscopic: Fine granularity of the surface with small reddish scars, resulting eventually in marked shrinkage of the entire organ, notably the cortex (primary contracted kidney, red granular atrophy). When combined with arteriosclerosis, the scars are large and red.

Malignant nephrosclerosis (see p. 175) is interpreted as an unusually intense variant of arteriolar nephrosclerosis, which has either been superimposed on pre-existing arteriolar nephrosclerosis or has arisen de novo in unaffected vessels. Characteristically, the *afferent arterioles and glomerular capillary loops show fibrinoid necrosis*.

Macroscopic: The kidney is slightly enlarged, with a variegated, spotted surface; in many cases, it is combined with an arteriolar nephrosclerosis.

Amyloidosis (see p. 165) cannot rightly be considered a vascular renal disorder, but it is considered here so as to allow comparison with the gross and histologic pictures of other renal disorders.

Kimmelstiel-Wilson glomerulosclerosis (p. 175) represents a special sort of arteriolar nephrosclerosis. It goes hand in hand with hyalinization of the afferent and efferent arterioles, as well as with diffuse hyaline thickening of the capillary loops, thereby giving rise to characteristic hyaline nodules in the glomerular loops. The gross appearance usually resembles arteriolar nephrosclerosis. Often there is also fatty degeneration of tubules giving a varigated appearance (red and yellow spots).

An **anemia infarct** (p. 175) most commonly results from embolic or thrombotic occlusion of an artery. There is a wedge-shaped, sharply demarcated, pale yellow area of necrosis that becomes depressed, contracted and white with increasing scar formation.

The acute stage of **periarteritis nodosa** (p. 69) in the kidney shows a yellowish gray mottled pattern. Eventually, fine, speckled, contracted scars develop (older areas of necrosis). There is fibrinoid necrosis of the arteries, with granulomatous inflammation and scarring.

The **congested kidney** is enlarged, dusty red, particularly in the medula, and the surface veins are spider-like. The glomeruli are congested and there are protein deposits in Bowman's space. In addition, there is interstitial edema.

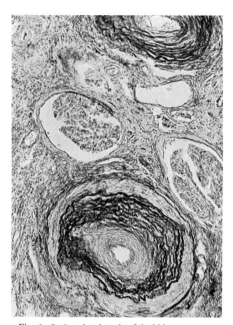

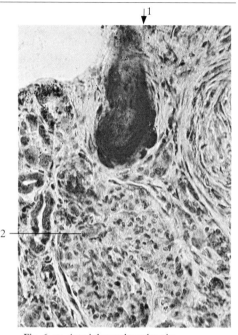

Fig. 6.18. Arteriosclerosis of the kidney; elastica-van Gieson stains, 70×.

Fig. 6.19. Arteriolar nephrosclerosis; Sudan-hematoxylin, 380×.

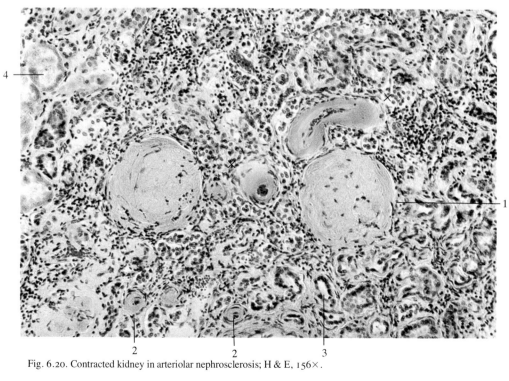

Fig. 6.20. Contracted kidney in arteriolar nephrosclerosis; H & E, 156×.

Arteriosclerosis of the kidney (Fig. 6.18). Histologically, this is actually the same process that we observed in arteriosclerosis in the heart vessels (compare with p. 62), although the lesion is not crescent-shaped, but rather has a concentric configuration. At first glance, one notices the very thick walls of the larger arteries, especially in the medulla. Medium magnification reveals hyperplastic proliferation of the elastica in the intima. This is due not only to multiplication and splitting of elastic fibers (black in the section) but also to an increase of acellular fibrous tissue (sclerosis), all of which lead to marked narrowing of the lumen. Glomeruli are partially hyalinized and the corresponding tubules have atrophied, with resulting fibrosis and lymphocytic infiltration. Local hyalinization of several glomeruli with concomitant atrophy of tubules leads to interstitial fibrosis and formation of contracted surface scars (arteriosclerotic scar). It is difficult for the beginner to differentiate arteriosclerotic scars and the associated lymphocytic infiltration from chronic pyelonephritis — but the striking arterial changes and comparatively scant lymphocytic infiltration should lead to a correct interpretation.

Arteriolosclerosis (Fig. 6.19, see also pp. 59, 171). In arteriolosclerosis (arteriolarsclerosis) hyalin appears between the intima and media with lumenal narrowing and medial atrophy. The changes are the same in the kidney as in the brain, cardiac muscle or spleen. Hematoxylin and eosin stains reveal red, homogeneous and anuclear arteriolar walls (see Fig. 6.20). The hyalinized vessels become very conspicuous when stained for fat. Inspection of the section with the scanning lens reveals several reddish dots in the cortex that can be identified, with higher magnification, as afferent arterioles ($\rightarrow$1), the wall of which is infiltrated by neutral fats. The media is markedly atrophic — isolated nuclei are still visible in the outermost parts of the media (see also Fig. 6.20, $\rightarrow$ 2). The lumen of the arteriole, barely discernible by means of a few preserved endothelial cell nuclei, is markedly narrowed. Note the deposits of fat in the glomerular connective tissue ($\rightarrow$2: mesangium). Tubules in the proximity of affected glomeruli have atrophied.

Contracted kidney in arteriolar nephrosclerosis (Fig. 6.20). If hyalinization of the afferent arterioles progresses so that a majority of the vessels are affected and if, in addition, there is concomitant sclerosis of medium-sized arteries, obliteration of large numbers of glomeruli and tubules will follow. Examination with a scanning lens discloses thinning of the cortex as well as numerous reddish discoid lesions that higher magnification shows to be glomeruli with eosinophilic concentric laminations containing a few isolated nuclei ($\rightarrow$1). The afferent arterioles surrounding these glomeruli have characteristic lesions in the wall ($\times$) — the intima is greatly thickened, the lining endothelial cells are barely discernible and the lumen is narrowed. The muscle fibers of the media are markedly atrophic or have disappeared. With hematoxylin and eosin stains, the appearance of the tissue resembles that found in amyloidosis. The Congo red stain, however, is negative, and van Gieson's stain brings out the red hyalinized glomeruli and arterioles (fresh hyalin is yellow, see page 11). Figure 6.20 shows a longitudinally sectioned lesion in an afferent arteriole ($\times$ upper right); $\rightarrow$2 and $\times$ in the center point to arteriolar lesions cut in cross section. As a result of hyalinization of the glomeruli, there is atrophy of the dependent tubular system ($\rightarrow$3), shown by shrunken tubules with narrow lumens and atrophy of lining epithelium. Several tubules have been obliterated. There is compensatory proliferation of interstitial fibrous tissue and lymphocytic infiltration (scars). Areas of the cortex that contain intact glomeruli have undergone compensatory hypertrophy ($\rightarrow$4). Grossly, such areas can be seen as projecting nodules.

Clinical: Benign hypertension (essential hypertension), in which the arteriolosclerosis is considered by some authors, but not by others, to be the result rather than the cause of raised blood pressure.

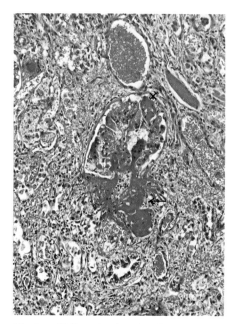

Fig. 6.21. Malignant nephrosclerosis; H & E, 120×.

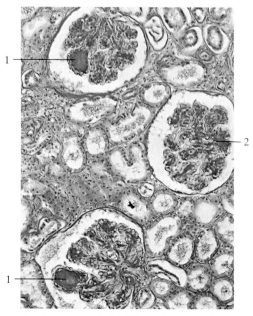

Fig. 6.22. Kimmelstiel-Wilson glomerulosclerosis; van Gieson, 120×.

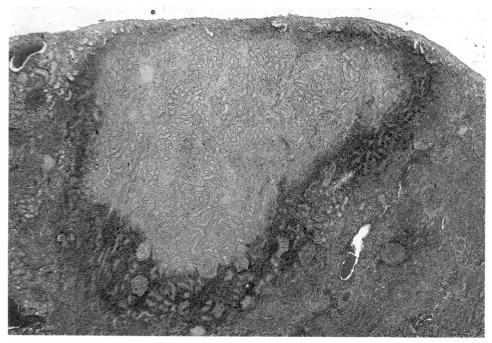

Fig. 6.23. Anemic infarct; H & E, 30×.

Malignant nephrosclerosis (Fig. 6.21) *consists of a rapidly progressive arteriosclerosis with fibrinoid necrosis of the walls of afferent arterioles and glomerular loops.*

Histologically, the arterioles seem to undergo diffuse hyalinization, so that the walls appear homogeneous and the lumens are narrowed (→). The hyaline material stains very bright red with H & E. With van Gieson's stain, it is yellow (see pages 11, 23, 29). There is nearly always an accompanying polymorphonuclear infiltration although it may be very slight. Frequently there are erythrocytes in the fibrinoid material indicative of rapid intrusion of blood into the vessel wall. The fibrinoid necrosis almost always involves adjacent glomerular loops (→), so that either single loops of the glomerulus or groups of them are affected. Should malignant nephrosclerosis be superimposed upon arterio- or arteriolonephrosclerosis, there will be a combination of sclerosis of medium-sized vessels and hyalinization of arterioles in addition to the foci of fibrinoid necrosis.

Macroscopic: Variegated, speckled kidney with indistinct gray-white foci on a reddish background. *Clinically, when malignant hypertension develops in young people it follows a rapidly fatal course, leading to uremic or apoplectic death. Older patients (50–60) may manifest malignant hypertension as a sequel to a previously benign course, in which case the histology shows a combination of arteriosclerosis and malignant nephrosclerosis.*

Kimmelstiel-Wilson glomerulosclerosis (Fig. 6.22) *occurs as a complication in approximately 20% of cases of diabetes mellitus. Typically, there is hyalinization of the glomerular loops. Clinically, the patients have proteinuria, hypertension and sometimes slight renal failure.*

Histologically, there is a very characteristic lesion. Numerous glomeruli show hyalinization of single or several capillary loops, resulting in the formation of rounded ball-like structures (van Gieson red or yellowish red, →1). The remaining glomerular loops are either free of any changes or else show the early stages of hyalinization. Some glomeruli also exhibit a diffuse thickening of the capillary wall (→2). The basement membranes are often frayed. In addition, the hyalinization frequently involves the afferent and *efferent arterioles.* Electronmicroscopically there is thickening of basement membranes, especially in the mesangium.

Macroscopic: Finely granular, slightly contracted kidney.

Anemic infarct (Fig. 6.23). *This is caused by embolic obstruction of a branch of the renal artery, resulting in a wedge-shaped area of coagulation necrosis.*

Examination of the section with a scanning lens reveals a pale red, wedge-shaped area, surrounded by a bluish, highly cellular zone outside of which there is a thin red rim. Observation of the central portion of the wedge-shaped area reveals the typical signs of *necrosis:* the nuclei are achromatic and the cytoplasm is homogeneous or finely granular. The nuclei in the interstitium and the glomeruli appear as shadows of their former selves. On the whole, early infarcts will still show the faint outlines of tubules and glomeruli. Higher magnification reveals *polymorphonuclear leukocytes* in the *peripheral cellular zone* as well as all the phases of nuclear disruption: pyknosis, rhexis, lysis and finely scattered nuclear debris. Surrounding the cellular zone there is usually a *zone of reactive hyperemia:* however, this is not conspicuous in our section. Note the thin, subcapsular strip of preserved parenchyma which receives its blood supply from the capsular vessels.

Macroscopic: Yellow, dry firm area. Older foci are contracted (reabsorption by granulation tissue), the final result being a deeply contracted, white scar. The emboli most frequently come either from a verrucous endocarditis, a mural thrombus in the heart (e.g., myocardial infarct) or from the aorta. Other causes: thrombotic arteriosclerosis, periarteritis nodosa.

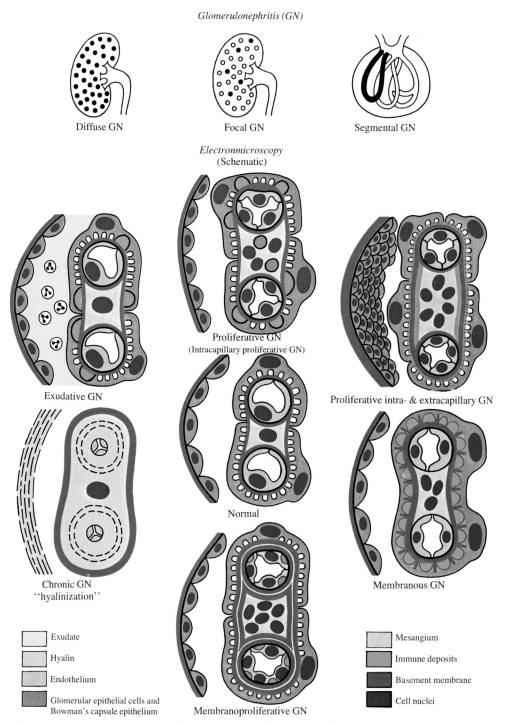

Glomerulonephritis (GN)

Diffuse GN   Focal GN   Segmental GN

Electronmicroscopy
(Schematic)

Proliferative GN
(Intracapillary proliferative GN)

Exudative GN   Proliferative intra- & extracapillary GN

Normal

Chronic GN
"hyalinization"   Membranous GN

Exudate
Hyalin
Endothelium
Glomerular epithelial cells and
Bowman's capsule epithelium

Mesangium
Immune deposits
Basement membrane
Cell nuclei

Membranoproliferative GN

Fig. 6.24. Electronmicroscopy of the different types of GN, shown diagramatically.

Table 6.1. **Classification of Glomerulonephritis (GN)**[1]

Type	Morphology	Pathogenesis Immunology	Clinical Features
Exudative GN (acute exudative & proliferative GN)	Granulocytes Exudation and slight mesangial & endothelial proliferation.	**Postinfectious** (streptococcal infection, scarlet fever, sore throat) Also serum sickness. **Immunecomplex nephritis** Subepithelial immune body deposits ("humps")	Raised antistreptolysin O titer, BP + Albuminuria. Prognosis usually good, but may progress to proliferative GN.
Proliferative GN (intracapillary GN) acute → chronic	Proliferation of mesangium & endothelium.	**Postinfectious** (streptococcus) IgA-, IgG-nephritis, Immunecomplex nephritis. Subepithelial immune deposits on glomerular loops ("humps") and/or mesangium.	Hematuria, Proteinuria. Most common type of GN. Steroid therapy + Good prognosis, Frequently a nephrotic course.
Proliferative intra-extracapillary GN (extracapillary GN) rapid progression	Proliferation of parietal capsular epithelial cells, semilunar crescents. Often proliferation of both endothelium & mesangium. Variant: necrotic type.	**Antibasement membrane nephritis,** e.g., in Goodpasture's syndrome. Immunoglobulins line basemembrane diffusely.	**Poor prognosis** Rapid progression, subacute, BP++
Membranous GN	Basement membrane much thickened, so-called spikes. No cellular proliferation	**Immune complex nephritis** (autoantibodies?), subepithelial immune deposits, spikes. Virus? (Aleutian mink).	**Nephrotic syndrome.** Steroid therapy (+). 30% heal, 50–70% persist.
Membranoproliferative GN	Basement membrane thick (double contour), proliferation of mesangium.	**Hypocomplementemia,** conspicuous subendothelial immune deposits.	60% have nephrotic syndrome, steroid therapy +. Prone to heal.
Lipoid nephrosis ("minimal changes")	Glomeruli not remarkable with light microscopy or only minimal mesangial proliferation.		True lipoid nephrosis Steroid therapy (+), 60% heal.
Focal and/or segmental GN	Single glomeruli affected and/or single groups of loops. Proliferative or sclerotic[2]	Includes connective tissue diseases: Schönlein-Henoch purpura, lupus erythematosus. Goodpasture syndrome, Idiopathic cases.	Proliferative form: chiefly favorable prognosis. Sclerotic form: chiefly lipoid nephrosis.

[1]Modified from W. Thoenes: Nieren- und Hochdruckkrankenheiten 5, 199, 1973; H. U. Zollinger: Beitr. Path. 143: 395, 1975; P. Royer, R. Harib, H. Mathieu: Nephrologie im Kindesalter, C. Thieme, Stuttgart, 1967.
[2]Sclerotic = thickening of mesangial matrix.

Inflammations of the Kidney (other than GN)

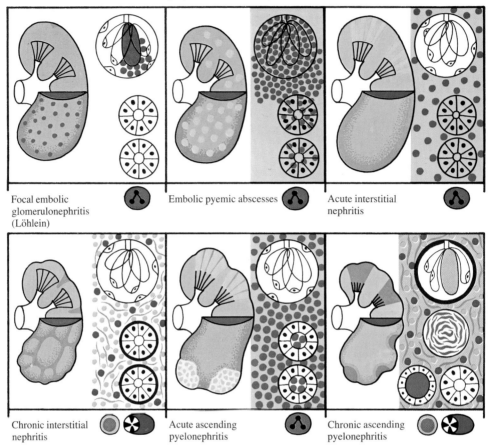

Focal embolic glomerulonephritis (Löhlein)

Embolic pyemic abscesses

Acute interstitial nephritis

Chronic interstitial nephritis

Acute ascending pyelonephritis

Chronic ascending pyelonephritis

Fig. 6.25. Diagrammatic survey of the gross and histological characteristics of inflammatory renal diseases.

Focal embolic glomerulonephritis (see p. 182) shows patchy fibrinoid necrosis of single or groups of glomerular loops.

Macroscopic: Slightly enlarged kidney with discrete petechiae.

Embolic pyemic kidney abscesses (see p. 182) appear as small abscesses in the region of a single glomeruli.

Macroscopic: Diffusely scattered yellow foci surrounded by a zone of hyperemia.

If the bacteria have gained access to the medullary parenchyma, there are numerous yellow, linear streaks which microscopically resemble elongated abscesses with bacterial colonies.

Acute interstitial nephritis may be either *suppurative or nonsuppurative* (see p. 185). The interstitial tissues are distended by exudate (e.g., in burns, see shock kidney) or show streak-like infiltration of lymphocytes and histiocytes.

Macroscopic. Enlarged, yellowish gray kidney.

Chronic interstitial nephritis (see p. 185) is characterized by the infiltration of lymphocytes and histiocytes. There is accompanying proliferation of connective tissue.

Macroscopic: Grayish red, gnarled, contracted kidneys.

Ascending pyelonephritis, acute or chronic (p. 185), results in damage to one or more kidney segments. The inflammation spreads upward from the tips of the pyramids. In the acute stage, there are widely scattered focal abscess formation and yellow streaks of exudate in the parenchyma. The necrotic areas are replaced by contracted grayish white scars in the chronic stage.

Glomerulonephritis (GN)

Glomerulonephritis is an inflammation of glomeruli that affects either all the glomeruli of both kidneys uniformly (diffuse GN) or single glomeruli (focal GN, see p. 176). Most frequently all the glomerular loops are involved and less frequently only a part of the loop (segmental involvement), as for example in focal embolic glomerulonephritis.

The inflamed glomeruli show the usual signs of inflammation: exudation due to leakage of blood plasma and migration of granulocytes (exudative GN). Cells of the mesangium and endothelium proliferate either alone (mesangial or intracapillary proliferative GN) or in association with proliferation of the glomerular and capsular epithelial cells (intra/extra capillary proliferative GN). In so-called membranous GN the basement membrane is conspicuously thickened. Cellular proliferation is very limited. The basement membrane is abnormally permeable. In membranoproliferative GN there is both thickening of the basement membrane and cellular proliferation.

Because immune complexes can be detected either in or on the basement membrane, at some stage in nearly all forms of GN, it is thought that an antigen-antibody reaction is the chief underlying cause of the injury. Activation of complement (c_1-c_9) takes place at the same time. These facts seem to explain many of the morphological features, such as exudation, accumulation of granulocytes and even necrosis.

In chronic glomerulonephritis, regardless of the form of GN from which it develops, there is thickening of the mesangial matrix which advances beneath the endothelium until the lumina of the capillary loops are completely obstructed (damaged glomeruli become hyalinized) resulting in diminution and finally loss of glomerular filtration.

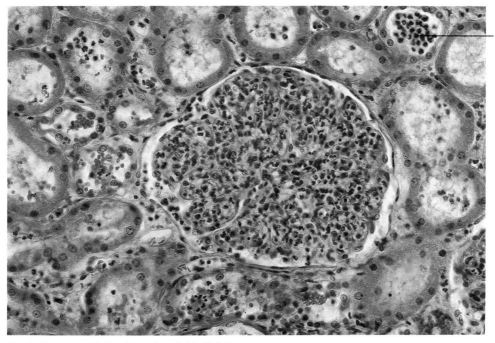

Fig. 6.26. Acute exudative glomerulonephritis; H & E, 300×.

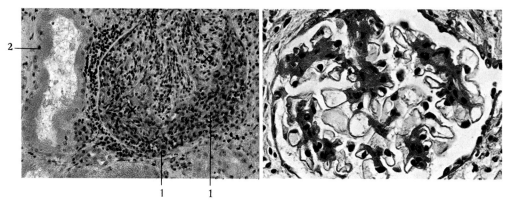

Fig. 6.27. Proliferative intra- and extracapillary glomerulonephritis; H & E, 160×.

Fig. 6.28. Proliferative glomerulonephritis; PAS & H, 160×.[1]

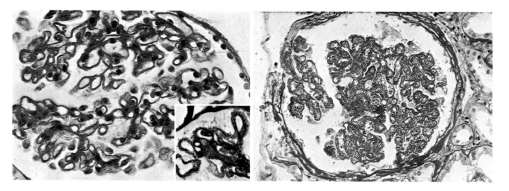

Fig. 6.29. Membranous glomerulonephritis; PAS & H, 160×.
Inset: Jones-chromotrope R, 400×.[1]

Fig. 6.30. Membranoproliferative glomerulonephritis; PAS & H, 100×.[1]

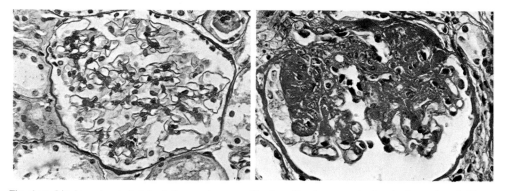

Fig. 6.31. Lipoid nephrosis (minimal change glomerulonephritis); PAS & H, 150×.

Fig. 6.32. Focal segmental sclerotic glomerulonephritis; PAS & H, 150×.[1]

---

[1] Professor Thoenes of Mainz has kindly lent Figures 6.28 thru 6.32.

Acute exudative glomerulonephritis. Figure 6.26 shows the **acute stage of exudative glomerulonephritis.** Only the magnification provided by a scanning lens is needed to see the enlarged, highly cellular glomeruli. The glomerular tuft fills Bowman's space completely; capillary loops are dilated and filled with neutrophils. The glomerular basement membrane is swollen. Erythrocytes, protein and polymorphonuclear leukocytes are present both in the capsular space and the tubules ($\rightarrow$). Interstitial tissues are edematous and swollen and contain a few neutrophils (slight periglomerulitis). Tubular epithelial cells are enlarged and often show cloudy swelling.

Macroscopic: The kidneys are swollen and the cut surfaces bulge beyond the edges of the tense capsule. Fleabite hemorrhages on the surface.

Proliferative intra- and extracapillary glomerulonephritis (Fig. 6.27). This form of GN was formerly called extracapillary GN. The glomeruli appear richly cellular because of great increase in size and number of the epithelial cells on the parietal capsular membrane with semilunar crescent-like proliferation of greatly elongated cells with oval nuclei ($\rightarrow$ 1 and X-X show the extent of the crescent). The capillary loops are compressed by the cellular overgrowth. The loops themselves are cellular and show proliferation of the endothelial cells and mesangium. As the disease progresses the crescents become hyalinized and eventually the glomeruli become partially or completely hyalinized. Serous exudate and slight infiltration of lymphocytes have caused the interstitium to swell. The proximal tubules show hyaline degeneration ($\rightarrow$2) and often fatty degeneration. This type of glomerulonephritis can be reproduced experimentally in rabbits (Masugi-nephritis. Antibasement membrane nephritis, Goodpasture syndrome in man).

Macroscopic: Large, variegated kidneys, flecked red and yellow.

Proliferative glomerulonephritis (formerly: intracapillary GN). Figure 6.28, which is stained with PAS to show mucopolysaccharides, clearly shows the important points of the disease: prominent, thick mesangium with thin, delicate basement membranes in the capillary loops. The nuclei of the mesangial cells are increased in number and the endothelial cells appear slightly enlarged and more numerous. The parietal capsular membrane is unchanged. As is indicated in Table 6.1 this type of GN may be either acute in which case the patients have hematuria and proteinuria, or the disease either with or without renal failure may have a chronic course (nephrotic stage). The prognosis with steroid treatment is good.

Membranous GN. Inspection of Figure 6.29 may make one wonder where the evidence of inflammation is, because a cellular response is completely lacking. In its place there is marked widening of the basement membrane of all the glomerular loops without cellular proliferation. In addition, spiny projections may be soon on the basement membrane (so-called "spikes") that are most easily seen with special stains (inset in Fig. 6.29). Immune complexes can be detected between the spikes. The basis both for morphological and clinical features is membrane damage with resulting nephrotic syndrome.

Membranoproliferative glomerulonephritis (Fig. 6.30). As the name suggests this form of the disease is marked by thickening of the basement membrane and simultaneous proliferation of intracapillary cells in the mesangium. When sections of tissue are stained with silver the basement membrane appears to have a double contour (splitting.) Clinically the patients have a nephrotic syndrome, frequently with hypocomplementemia.

Lipoid nephrosis (minimal change GN, Fig. 6.31). The glomerular changes are so slight that differences from the normal glomerulus are scarcely detected by the uninitiated. At the very most there is thickening of the mesangium. Despite such minimal histological changes, clinically there is marked proteinuria with a high content of lipid.

181

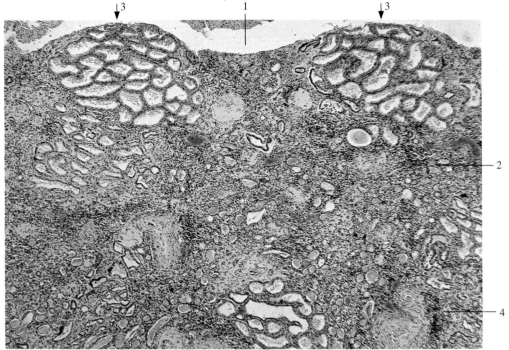

Fig. 6.33. Chronic glomerulonephritis; H & E, 40×.

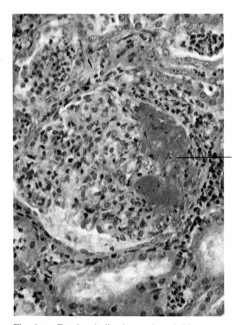

Fig. 6.34. Focal embolic glomerulonephritis; H & E, 280×.

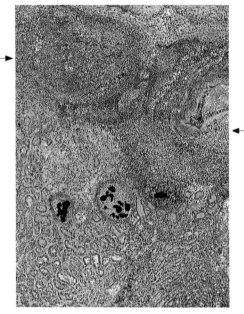

Fig. 6.35. Embolic renal abscess; H & E, 72×.

Focal segmental glomerulonephritis (Fig. 6.32). In this type of GN only parts of some glomeruli or groups of capillary loops are damaged. The figure shows distortion (sclerosis and hyalinization) of many but not all of the glomerular loops. Their cellularity is only slightly increased. The hyalinization and resulting distortion of the glomerular loops is caused by thickening of the mesangial matrix (so-called sclerotic form). Clinically the patients frequently have the nephrotic syndrome.

Chronic glomerulonephritis (Fig. 6.33). Survey of the preparation with a scanning lens reveals noticeable thinning of the cortex. Some areas show scarring of the surface accumulations of inflammatory cells, while other areas show small cystic spaces and cellular paucity. Under medium magnification, most of the glomeruli are seen to have been replaced by hyalinized nodules. Frequently, the crescent-shaped lesions of *extracapillary* glomerulonephritis are still preserved. The attached tubules are markedly atrophic ($\rightarrow$ 1), lined with flattened epithelium and filled with hyaline casts ($\rightarrow$ 2). The interstitial tissue is correspondingly increased in amount and infiltrated by lymphocytes. In addition to areas of scarring (resulting in irregularity of the surface, $\rightarrow$ 1), there are also areas of compensatory hypertrophy ($\rightarrow$ 3), with fully preserved glomeruli and dilated tubules lined with cuboidal epithelium. Aside from the completely hyalinized glomeruli, there are also some in which the inflammatory changes are recent. The vessels often show arterio- and arteriolosclerosis ($\rightarrow$ 4). In the end stages, the various types of glomerulonephritis cannot be differentiated. Kidneys contracted by arterio- or arteriolonephrosclerosis may also be difficult to differentiate.

Macroscopic: Small, firm kidneys with yellow or gray granular surfaces. Sometimes, the surface may be smooth, especially in cases of chronic intracapillary glomerulonephritis.

In **focal embolic glomerulonephritis** (Fig. 6.34), *there is inflammation of isolated loops of single glomeruli. It is seen particularly in cases of subacute bacterial endocarditis.* In the acute stages, there is fibrinoid necrosis of isolated capillary loops. They appear as homogeneous, anuclear, eosinophilic masses ($\rightarrow$). Erythrocytes can often be seen in the fibrinoid material. This material involves the wall of the glomerular loops and also actually lies in the loops (fibrin thrombi). The unaffected loops are intact, showing, at most, slightly increased cellularity and thickening of the basement membrane. Bowman's space and the tubules contain granular casts, possibly containing erythrocytes and polymorphs. Healing of the lesions leads to focal scar formation and fusion of the loops with the parietal epithelium.

Macroscopic: The kidneys are slightly enlarged and present a flea-bitten appearance.

Embolic renal abscesses (Fig. 6.35). *Hematogenous spread in septicemia or pyemia leads to the formation of abscesses in the cortex and focal, streak-like suppuration in the medulla.* The scanning lens reveals scattered, highly cellular lesions in the cortex. Medium high power reveals near individual glomeruli, focal agglomerations of polymorphs invaded by wisps of connective tissue ($\rightarrow$: abscesses). In other parts, there are clusters of bacteria in the capillary loops, and the surrounding parenchyma is infiltrated by leukocytes and invaded by connective tissue. The interstitial connective tissue also contains leukocytes. The proximal tubules contain granular casts.

The *foci of suppuration in the medulla* result from passage of bacteria through the glomeruli and their accumulation in the medulla, where they form streak-like abscesses containing central bacterial colonies (blue), frequently surrounded by an area of necrosis and a peripheral zone of leukocytes.

Macroscopic: Yellow or gray abscesses (1—2 mm) are scattered throughout the cortex, on the surface of the kidney and as streaks along the medullary rays.

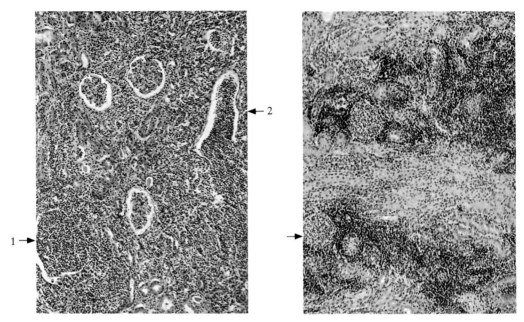

Fig. 6.36. Ascending pyelonephritis;
H & E, 9×.

Fig. 6.37. Interstitial nephritis in scarlet fever;
H & E, 66×.

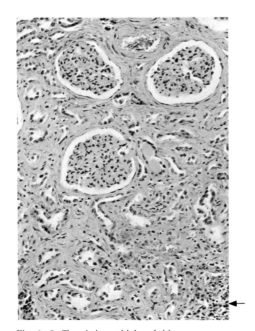

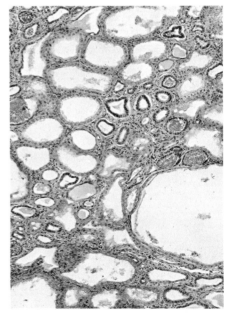

Fig. 6.38. Chronic interstitial nephritis;
H & E, 144×.

Fig. 6.39. Cystic kidney;
H & E, 72×.

Ascending pyelonephritis (acute interstitial nephritis (Fig. 6.36). *Lower urinary tract infection (e.g., E. coli) may ascend to the kidney via the tubules or lymphatics. It usually results from obstruction, e.g., in prostatic hypertrophy or ureteric constriction and leads to suppurative inflammation of the cortex and the medulla. Pyelonephritis can also follow hematogenous spread from a distant infection.* Very low magnification reveals streak-like areas in one or more of the medullary pyramids and increased cellularity of the adjacent cortical segments. Higher magnification shows numerous polymorphonuclear leukocytes in the collecting tubules (→ 2) and interstitial tissues. The exudate is distributed in a streaked pattern. The tubular epithelium is largely flattened and the lumen contains protein. As the disease progresses, abscesses develop in the cortex (→ 1). Healing of the acute stage may result in the complete deterioration of both glomeruli and tubules, accompanied by proliferation of interstitial connective tissue and lymphocytic infiltration. The process is always limited to a pyramid and its corresponding cortical segment, so that, in contrast to hematogenous renal abscesses, the lesions are focal.

Macroscopic: Clusters of abscesses or flat, depressed, gray scars, depending upon the age.

The disease proceeds at a lingering pace for years, with secondary renal insufficiency and hypertension developing in 40% of cases. Uremia appears in 30% of cases. Peri- and paranephric abscess can occur as complications.

Interstitial nephritis in scarlet fever (Fig. 6.37). Nonsuppurative inflammation with serous exudation and emigration of lymphocytes in the interstitial tissues occurs mainly *during* infectious diseases, e.g., in about 7 days after onset of scarlet fever; in contrast to glomerulonephritis which occurs 3 weeks after onset. Microscopically, the interstitial tissues are focally or diffusely infiltrated with lymphocytes and later with histiocytes and plasma cells which displace the renal tubules. The glomeruli are not affected (→). For the most part, it is a serous interstitial inflammation.

Macroscopic: Enlarged, dull, grayish white kidney.

Chronic interstitial nephritis (Fig. 6.38). The connective tissue surrounding the tubules is infiltrated by a chronic inflammatory exudate. There is interstitial fibrosis. The tubules are pushed apart and their lumens, which are compressed, are lined with flattened epithelium. The basement membrane of the tubules is frequently thickened. Localized collections of lymphocytes and histiocytes are seen, especially at the corticomedullary junction (→). This type of nephritis can also be observed in cases of phenacetin poisoning. The pathogenesis of these cases is usually accounted for on the basis of toxic renal damage concomitant with ascending or descending inflammation. The chronic sclerosing form is thought to have a hematogenous origin.

Macroscopic: Gnarled kidney surface.

Cystic kidney (Fig. 6.39). *This is most commonly a bilateral, congenital disorder, with formation of multiple cysts. Cases with small cysts have been observed in neonates.* Microscopically, the prominent feature is the presence of numerous cysts in the medulla or cortex which may be either empty or filled with homogenous, eosinophilic material. The larger cysts have a flat, endothelium-like lining and the smaller cysts a lining of cuboidal tubular epithelium. In some cysts, glomeruli can still be made out although disrupted by pressure atrophy. A few strips of intact, but atrophic, parenchyma are still evident between the cysts.

Macroscopic: In juveniles and adults, the cysts are large and closely clustered. The parenchyma shows varying degrees of atrophy. Recent research (Potter and coworkers, 1964) has disclosed that either isolated tubular segments may undergo cystic dilatation (small cystic kidney of the neonate, uremic death) or the ureteric buds may undergo partial obstruction at an early stage, leading to cyst formation in every part of the nephron (cystic kidney of the adult).

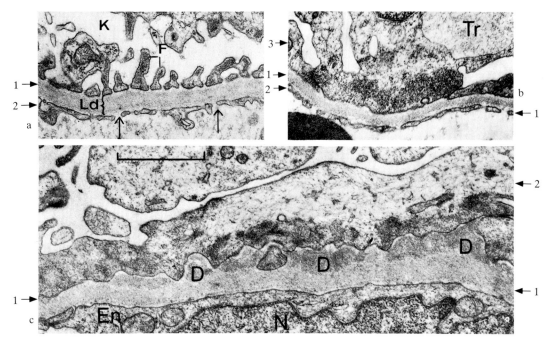

Fig. 6.40. a) *Normal rat glomerulus.* → basement membrane with lamina densa (Ld), endothelial cell (→ 2) with pores (→), foot processes (F) of the epithelial cells (podocytes) and capsular space (K). 22,000× (Dr. Thoenes). b) *Aminonucleoside nephrosis* in the rat illustrates the glomerular changes in glomerulonephrosis. Unaltered basement membrane (→1) and endothelial cell projection (→2, swollen epithelium (→3) with marked thickening of the foot processes, Tr. = droplets of absorbed protein in the epithelium (see also the inset in Fig. 6.2). 22,000× (Dr. Thoenes). c) Human *membranous glomerulonephritis* (clinically a case of pure nephrosis) with marked dense deposits (D) (see Fig. 6.29) on the epithelial side (→2 epithelial cell) of the thickened basement membrane (→1). Below is a section of an endothelial cell (En) with nucleus (N). The endothelial cells in this particular specimen have remained unchanged for a long time, while the epithelial cells (→2), because of the transformation of the foot processes, have formed broad obstructing plaques. 22,000× (Dr. Thoenes).

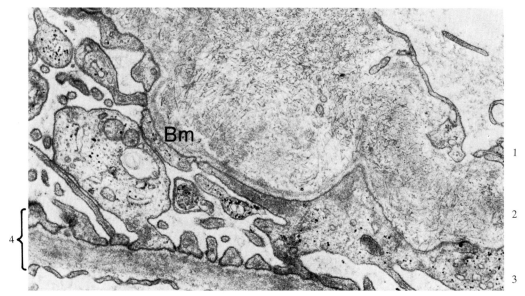

Fig. 6.41. *Amyloidosis of a human glomerular loop* (renal biopsy). Finely fibrillar amyloid (2) lies between the endothelium (1) and the basement membrane (middle of figure). Epithelium with wide lamina comparable to a normal capillary loop (4). 25,000×.

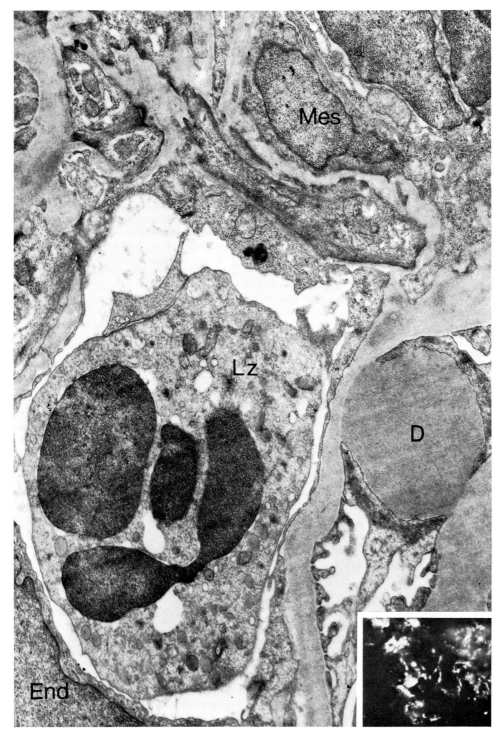

Fig. 6.42. *Acute proliferative mesangial postinfectious glomerulonephritis* (needle biopsy). The conspicuous histological features are swelling of endothelial (End) and an increase in mesangial cells (Mes). Numbers of neutrophilic granulocytes fill the capillary lumen (Lz). To the right there is a large immune deposit (D, ''hump'') on the outer side of the delicate basement membrane. 163,000×. Human gamma globulin (white areas) can be demonstrated by fluorescence microscopy (inset at lower right of the figure), which with the simultaneous demonstration of complement is further evidence of the presence of an immune complex disorder. (Thoenes).

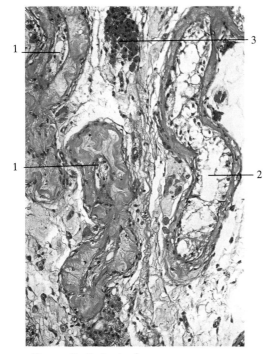

Fig. 7.1. Testicular atrophy;
H & E, 100×.

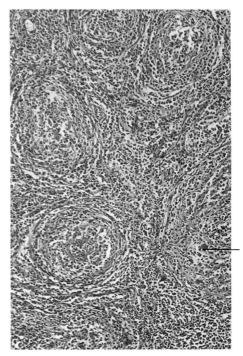

Fig. 7.2. Granulomatous orchitis;
H & E, 80×.

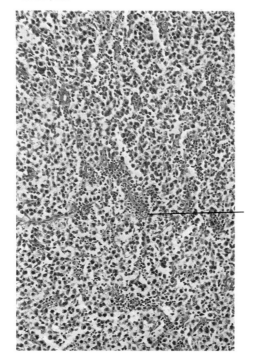

Fig. 7.3. Seminoma;
H & E, 100×.

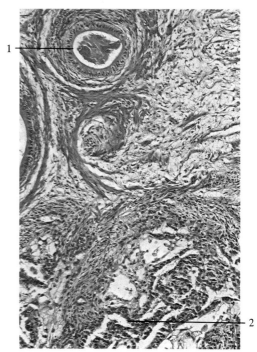

Fig. 7.4. Malignant teratoma of testes, intermediate
type (M.T.I.); H & E, 90×.

7. Genitalia—Pregnancy

Male Genitalia: Testis

Testicular atrophy (Fig. 7.1) *results from either local or generalized injury which causes wasting of testicular tubules and either partial or complete arrest of spermatogenesis.* Figure 7.1 shows two completely hyalinized and wasted tubules (→ 1). A third testicular tubule (→ 2) has a thick basement membrane that is only partially lined by *Sertoli interstitial cells* and no longer contains spermatozoa. The loose and relatively increased connective tissue resulting from the testicular atrophy contains islands of hyperplastic, eosinophilic *Leydig cells* (→ 3).

The testis is one of the most sensitive of organs. It reacts with marked, irreversible atrophy to mechanical (trauma), chemical (chemotherapy), and thermal (heat-intra-abdominal or inguinal testes) stimuli; inflammations (gonorrhea), hormones (e.g., hyperestrogenism of liver cirrhosis or hormone therapy for prostatic carcinoma) and irradiation. In the aged testicular involution develops *(involution—physiological process, atrophy—pathological process!).* Testicular atrophy may also be genetically conditioned, as for example in Klinefelter syndrome (men with a eunuchoid stature, gynecomastia, sterility, XXY chromosomes).

Granulomatous orchitis (Fig. 7.2) *is a chronic inflammation of the testis, presumably of multiple causes, that is manifest pathologically by granulomatous inflammation with giant cells and clinically simulates a tumor.* Histologically the normal structure of the testis is completely destroyed and replaced by granulomatous inflammation with lymphocytes, plasma cells, histocytes and solitary, multinucleated giant cells (→) that occasionally resemble *Langhans giant cells*.

Granulomatous orchitis occurs preferentially in the 50–60 age group. Causes include escape of spermatozoa from the tubules (sperm granuloma make up 40% of cases), specific and nonspecific bacterial and mycotic inflammations, trauma and autoimmune disorders as well as primary vascular lesions.

Preliminary remarks about testicular tumors: the most frequent tumors arise from germinal epithelium among which are seminomas and teratomas. Among the nongerminal tumors are androgen-producing *Leydig cell tumors* (sexual precocity when they arise in children), *Sertoli cell tumors,* tubular adenomas (adenoma tubulare testis, corresponding to *Sertoli cell hyperplasia* in cryptorchism) as well as lymphomas and mesenchymal tumors. Tumors of the testis may appear at all ages. About 6% of tumors arise in an undescended testis.

Seminoma (Fig. 7.3) *typically consists of clear cells arranged in islands or cords surrounding collections of lymphocytes* (→).

Testicular tumors showing only a seminomatous component (cut serial sections to exclude a teratocarcinoma) have a relatively good prognosis. They mestastasize preferentially by way of the lymph stream.

Teratoma of the testis (Fig. 7.4) *is composed of tissue of various degrees of maturity and organoid structure derived from the 3 germ layers.* Teratoma, differentiated (T.D.) containing adult type tissues such as differentiated glands, respiratory epithelium, smooth and stripped muscle fibers, cartilage and bone. Malignant teratoma, anaplastic (**MTU** - embryonic or undifferentiated carcinoma) shows no evidence of differentiation. An in-between form, malignant teratoma, intermediate type (**MTI**) is shown in Figure 7.4 in which there are differentiated glands (→ 1) and cords of solid, anaplastic tumor (→ 2).

Malignant trophoblastic teratoma (**MTT**) has a different clinical and prognostic significance. It consists of multinucleated giant cells and macroscopically is hemorrhagic. Clinically it is characterized by gonadotropin production and a high grade of malignancy (early hematogenous metastasis). Seminoma, teratoma and chorionepithelioma may present in combination (see p. 199).

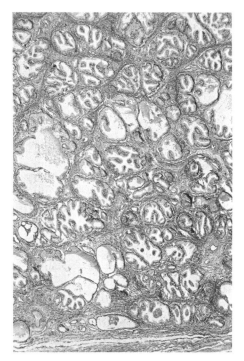

Fig. 7.5. Adenomyosis of prostate (so-called prostatic hypertrophy); H & E, 20×.

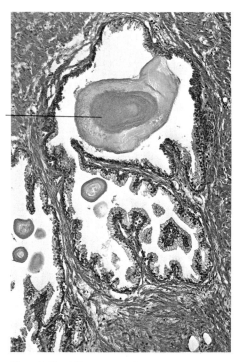

Fig. 7.6. Prostatic concrement; H & E, 120×.

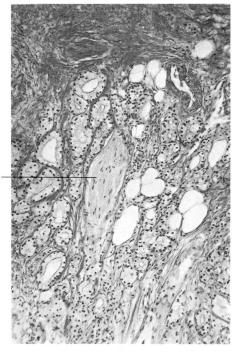

Fig. 7.7. Well-differentiated carcinoma of prostate; H & E, 100×.

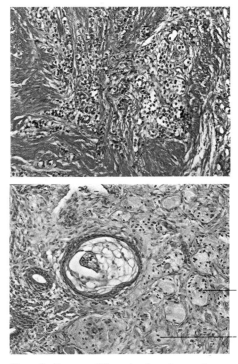

Fig. 7.8. Above: undifferentiated carcinoma of prostate. Below: involution of a prostatic carcinoma with squamous metaplasia after estrogen therapy; H & E, 100×.

Adenomyosis of the prostate (so-called prostatic hypertrophy, Figs. 7.5, 7.6) *is a hormone conditioned[1] hyperplasia and hypertrophy of the periurethral glands of the prostate (so-called internal prostatic glands) accompanied by either diffuse or nodular increase in the smooth muscle fibers.* The external prostatic glands (site of origin of prostatic carcinoma!) are pushed to the periphery and form the so-called "surgical capsule." Histologically under **low magnification** (Fig. 7.5) the apparently hyperplastic and dilated glands are easily seen. **High magnification** (Fig. 7.6) show irregularly shaped lumens resulting from pseudopapillary infolding of the lining epithelium, which is composed of cylindrical cells with clear cytoplasm and basally situated nuclei. The single cell layer is preserved. The stroma contains elongated eosinophilic muscle fibers. Often a prostatic nodule will show a purely leiomyomatous pattern (stony hard consistency clinically is highly suggestive of carcinoma). The lumens of the glands contain amorphous, eosinophilic secretory masses, inflammatory cells and occasional concentrically layered, calcified protein bodies *(corpora amylacea or prostatic concrements →)*.

Adenomyomatosis is a disease of elderly men. Macroscopically both lateral lobes are enlarged and commonly a pseudo-middle lobe develops. Not infrequently adenomyomatosis is accompanied by *sclerosis of the sphincter.* *Histologically* this shows band-like hypertrophy of the musculature of the sphincter by connective tissue rich in collagen fibers. Only rarely does malignancy develop in adenomyosis.

Introductory remarks about carcinoma of the prostate. Carcinoma of the prostate likewise is a disease of older men. For all practical purposes it appears at about 50 years of age and thereafter increases progressively with age. *Histologically,* for prognostic and therapeutic purposes, the following kinds are distinguished: *well-differentiated carcinomas* (clear or occasionally eosinophilic cell adenocarcinoma), *moderately well-differentiated* and *undifferentiated carcinomas* (see p. 337).
Less usual types are cribriform carcinoma (Fig. 9.31), squamous cell carcinoma (very rare), transitional cell carcinoma (corresponding to carcinoma of the urinary bladder) and mucinous carcinoma (suspect a rectal carcinoma!). Mesenchymal and metastatic tumors of the prostate are rare.

Well-differentiated carcinoma of the prostate (Fig. 7.7) shows a diffuse spreading and infiltrating growth pattern with cords of closely packed glands with narrow lumens and composed of clear cells. Perineural invasion by the tumor is typical but not pathognomonic (the arrow points to a nerve). Well-differentiated adenocarcinoma has the best prognosis. Frequently it is discovered accidentally in older men (after 70 years of age) during prostatectomy for adenomyomatosis. If they are silent clinically they are described as *latent carcinoma* (in *occult carcinoma* the site of a primary tumor which has produced metastases is now known. Examples: carcinomas of stomach, breast, prostate and lung).

Undifferentiated carcinoma of the prostate (Fig. 7.8, above) *consists of solid masses or cords of tumor cells with cytological signs of wild growth (pleomorphic cells and nuclei, hyperchromatic nuclei, mitoses).*

Undifferentiated prostatic carcinoma appears frequently before the 60th year and runs a progressive and malignant course. It infiltrates the prostatic capsule (stage T_2), invades neighboring organs (T_3 invasion of the urinary bladder and T_4 invasion of periprostatic organs). Later there is lymphatic (N_1) and hematogenous (M_1) spread with distant metastasis (especially osteoplastic metastases to bones).

Squamous metaplasia (Fig. 7.8, below) *develops in the prostate particularly in the region of an infarct or after estrogen therapy for carcinoma.* In the middle of Figure 7.8 there is an island of epithelium showing squamous epithelial differentiation. Surrounding it there are groups of degenerating carcinoma cells resulting from hormone therapy (shrivelled glands with pyknotic nuclei). Originally this was a well-differentiated clear cell prostatic carcinoma (→).

---

[1]Probably not (or not only) estrogens, but androgens (5α-dihydroxytestosterone).

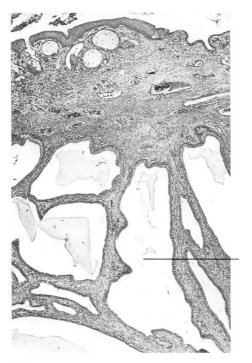

Fig. 7.9. Ectropion;
H & E, 20×.

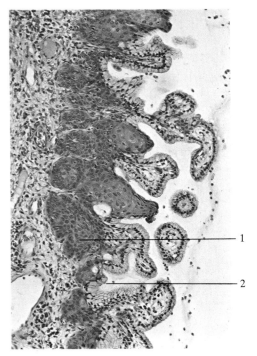

Fig. 7.10. Squamous metaplasia of the cervical mucosa; H & E, 110×.

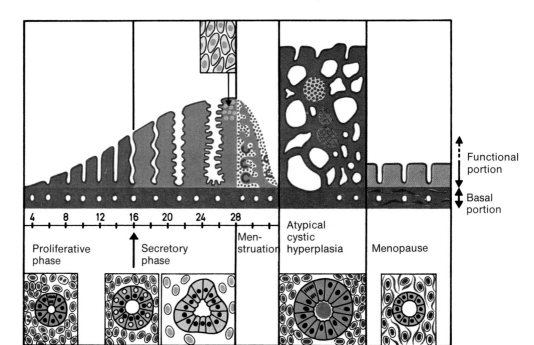

Fig. 7.11. Diagram of cyclical endometrial changes.

Female Genitalia: Ectropion—Squamous Metaplasia—Menstrual Cycle

Ectropion of the external os (Fig. 7.9). *This is eversion of the cervical mucosa in the direction of the surface of the cervical os.* The cylindrical epithelium of the endocervical mucosa, which is very sensitive to mechanical and chemical stimuli, is gradually replaced by squamous epithelium. Such transformation may take place by extension from the periphery *(ascending overgrowth)* as well as developing locally. A fully developed **squamous covering of a pseudoerosion** *(ectropion with contiguous overgrowth* Fig. 7.10) shows multilayered noncornified squamous epithelium on the surface with extension into the cervical glands (→). As a result secretion of mucous by the cervical glands is obstructed and retention cysts develop *(Nabothian follicles)*.

In an **erosion** there is a true defect of the mucosa which, however, seldom causes reddening of the surface of the os. More commonly the mucosal defect is only incidental. The hyperemic blood vessels and cervical glands are clearly visible through the thin everted cervical mucosa. This is called a *glandular pseudoerosion* and is the consequence of papillary transformation caused by chronic irritation *(glandulo-papillary pseudoerosion)*.

As a result of chronic local irritation (e.g., chronic inflammation) the normal cylindrical epithelium of the cervical mucosa may change to **metaplastic squamous epithelium** (Fig. 7.10). This metaplasia results from an increase of the basal reserve cells that normally are present in the mucosa and progressively lift up and finally push off the cylindrical epithelium. Figure 7.10 shows the bulky, villous structure of the cervical mucosa and the inflamed stroma which in the deeper parts is replaced (→ 1) or invaded by (→ 2) metaplastic squamous epithelium.

Normal cyclical changes in the endometrium (Fig. 7.11). The endometrium is made up of a *functional portion* (with a superficial compact layer and an underlying spongiosa), both the structure and function of which are under the control of the ovarian hormone, and a narrow basal layer lying on the myometrium which remains after menstruation and so acts as a base for regeneration. In the **normal menstrual cycle** between the 4th and 15th day following activation of the follicular hormone *(estradiol)* the **proliferative phase** appears. The endometrial glands increase and thicken and cytogenic stroma becomes prominent. At 15 days rupture of the follicle occurs. Between the 15th and 28th day of the cycle the influence of the corpus luteum (progesterone) is established—the **secretory phase.** On the 28th day the period of **menstruation** takes place, generally lasting for 3 days. During a normal cycle the tissue and cellular changes in the different phases are quite characteristic.

Proliferative phase (4–14 day): the tubular glands elongate and the stromal cells are compact. In cross sections the glands are seen to have small rounded, optically empty lumens lined by dark, cubical to cylindrical cells. Mitoses are common in both glands and stromal cells.

Secretory phase (15–18 day). Small vacuoles containing glycogen situated basally or retronuclearly in glandular epithelium are the first sign of secretion. During the secretory phase, the endometrial glands become tortuous, thin and irregular. The cytoplasm of the epithelium is clear and the nuclei migrate to the bases of the cells. The stromal cells are loosened and large (pale stroma). At the end of the secretory phase the compact layer (under the mucosa) shows large pseudodecidual cells (pseudodecidual transformation, see Fig. 7.22).

Menstruation (1–3 day): after the secretory phase, bleeding occurs and all but the basal layers of the endometrium are shed. The glandular epithelium and stromal fragments can be easily identified in the blood. There are no evidences of coagulation (fibrin thrombi).

Senile involution: a physiological process (not to be confused with atrophy) which sets in with the menopause. The entire uterine mucosa becomes thin. The stromal cells and fibers are compactly arranged and the glands small, round and numerically increased. Frequently the lumens of the glands are dilated, filled with eosinophilic material and lined with bevelled cuboidal epithelium.

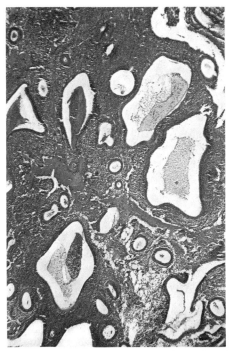

Fig. 7.12. Cystic hyperplasia (glandular-cystic) of the endometrium; H & E, 32×.

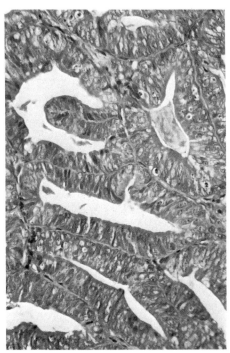

Fig. 7.13. Adenomatous hyperplasia of the endometrium; H & E, 200×.

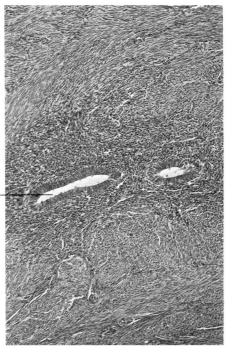

Fig. 7.14. Endometriosis of the myometrium; H & E, 80×.

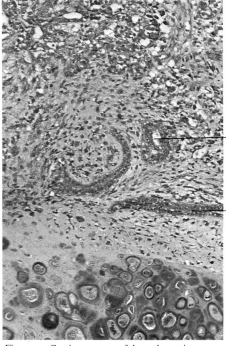

Fig. 7.15. Carcinosarcoma of the endometrium; H & E, 90×.

Diseases of the Endometrium

Cystic hyperplasia of the endometrium (Fig. 7.12) *is a stromal and glandular hyperplasia induced by hyperestrogenism*. The diagnosis is usually made by curretage which yields large pieces of tissue embedded in blood. Naked eye inspection of the microscopic section is remarkable for the abundance of the material and the large size of the individual fragments. Higher magnification shows endometrium in the proliferative stage and a compact stroma. Cystic dilatation of the endometrial glands that are lined by a single layer of cylindrical epithelial cells is a prominent feature. Intermingled with the intact endometrium are small fragments of aglandular stroma as well as loosened and detached glands and epithelium which may have resulted from the surgical scraping. Of diagnostic significance, if present, are small, eosinophilic, homogeneous or finely granular fibrin thrombi which are the substrate of a hemorrhagic disorder.

Cystic hyperplasia is caused by hormonal imbalance as a result of which estrogen secretion is both increased and prolonged. The commonest cause of this estrogen excess is *persistence of the follicle* which is especially prominent in the premenopausal period (after 40 years of age). In young women changes similar to cystic hyperplasia may be seen in the first period after a preceding pregnancy (so-called *adjustment hyperplasia*). In older women in the menopause a hormone producing ovarian tumor (granulosa cell tumor or thecoma) may be present.

Following prolonged estrogen stimulation cystic hyperplasia can change to **adenomatous** or **atypical hyperplasia** (Fig. 7.13). Histologically the endometrial glands are small and not dilated, lying "back to back." Individual glands consist of a disorderly layer of tall epithelium showing many mitoses. Adenomatous hyperplasia is a "precancerous" condition and—especially in very marked cases—cannot be distinguished from a well-differentiated adenocarcinoma. Particularly in young women the differential diagnosis is important both for prognostic and therapeutic reasons, because in this age group adenomatous hyperplasia has the potential of recurrence. Carcinomas of the fundus of the uterus are either glandular or anaplastic carcinomas. *Adenoacanthoma* has a glandular pattern plus areas of squamous metaplasia.

Uterine endometriosis (adenomyosis uteri, Fig. 7.14) *indicates either deep endometrial penetration or ectopic endometrium in the uterine wall*. Histologically there are small collections of endometrial glands (→) in the myometrium surrounded by stroma. The quiescent appearance of the cells in the glands and surrounding stroma rule out a diagnosis of carcinoma.

Endometriosis occurs most frequently in the myometrium where it may cause focal *(adenomyosis)* or more often *diffuse muscular hyperplasia* (thickness of wall in excess of 20mm). Endometriosis, however, may occur in other organs (external endometriosis), e.g., ovary (chocolate cysts), small intestine, navel and dermal scars. It is a benign lesion which very seldom becomes malignant (adenoacanthoma in the floor of an endometrial cyst of the ovary).

Carcinosarcoma (Fig. 7.15) *is a malignant neoplasm with both carcinomatous and sarcomatous components*. Histologically there are ill-defined cords of glandular carcinomatous tissue (→) lying in a polymorphocellular stroma. In the lower third of the figure the stroma shows cartilaginous differentiation.

Carcinosarcomas are very rare tumors. Adenomyosarcoma or Wilms' tumor of the kidney is one of the best-known malignant mixed tumors and carcinosarcomas also are known to occur in the endometrium, lung, esophagus, breast and thyroid. These carcinomas are all age and sex conditioned. Distant metastases—of frequent occurrence—can be purely sarcomatous or a mixture. Pathogenetically one should differentiate among *collision tumors* (accidental collision of a sarcoma and a carcinoma), *compositional tumors* (simultaneous origin from the stroma and the parenchyma of an organ) and *combination tumors* (origin from the same neoplastic parent tissue but with different differentiation, e.g., Wilms' tumor).

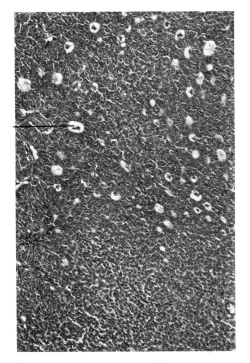

Fig. 7.17. Granulosa cell tumor of the ovary;
H & E, 30×.

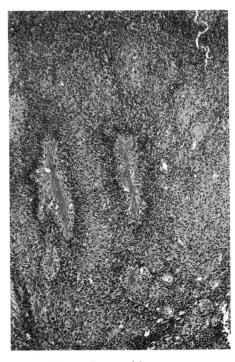

Fig. 7.18. Theca cell tumor of the ovary;
H & E, 80×.

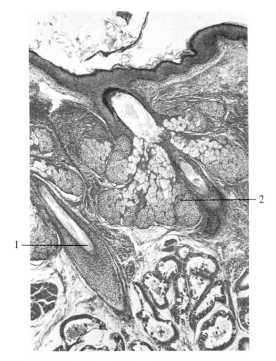

Fig. 7.19. Dermoid cyst of the ovary;
H & E, 45×.

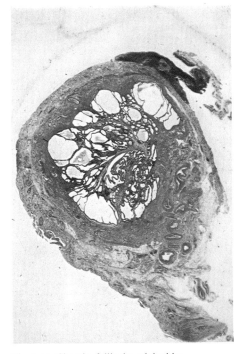

Fig. 7.20. Chronic, follicular salpingitis;
H & E, 15×.

Ovarian Cysts—Tumors—Salpingitis

Ovarian cysts (Fig. 7.16) are of very common occurrence but are uncommonly a cause of clinical illness. The cysts can be derived from follicles, corpora lutea, embryonal rests (epoophoron) or the peritoneum (serous cysts). Usually, however, the origin of an ovarian cyst can not be determined at the time of its discovery and so it is called a *simple ovarian cyst*. Figure 7.16 shows three cysts of the ovary: both of the upper ones are **follicular cysts,** the lower one is a **corpus luteum cyst** (the distinction between a cystic corpus luteum and a corpus luteum cyst is arbitrary). As a rule ovarian cysts are a chance finding. Complications are unusual, e.g., rupture, hemorrhage or torsion with infarction of the cyst. If the organ is studded with cysts it is called a polycystic ovary. *Stein-Leventhal syndrome:* large, white polycystic ovaries with a thickened capsule, absence of a corpus luteum, sterility and hirsutism.

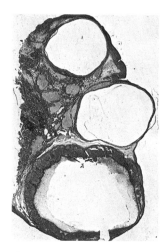

Fig. 7.16. Follicle and corpus luteum cysts in an ovary; H & E, 15 ×.

Introductory remarks on ovarian tumors: systematic consideration of ovarian tumors takes into account the numerous variants in their pathological and clinical aspects. There are tumors that arise from *paramesonephric coelomic epithelium* (e.g., cystoma, *Brenner tumor*), tumors that arise from *undifferentiated gonadal mesenchyme* (benign and malignant mesenchymal tumors), tumors that arise from *sexually differentiated gonadal mesenchyme* (granulosa and theca cell tumors, androblastoma, hilus cell tumor, gynandroblastoma); tumors that arise from *embryonic cells* (dermoid cyst, teratoma) and from the *mesonephric system* (mesonephroma). In addition metastatic tumors may occur in the ovary, especially from stomach *(Krukenberg tumor)* and breast carcinomas.

Granulosa cell tumor of the ovary (Fig. 7.17) *belongs to a group of facultative malignant tumors that are derived from differentiated ovarian mesenchyme and usually manifest endocrine activity (estrogen secretion).* Histologically the tumors are richly cellular and have solid trabeculi, microfollicles or a sarcoma-like structure. Characteristically the tumor cells form rosettes surrounding hollow spaces, *(Call-Exner bodies, →).*

Granulosa cell tumors occur at any age. About 30% of them show evidences of malignancy (metastases are uncommon), in the remaining 70% recurrence may occur. Histologically a diagnosis of granulosa cell tumor cannot always be made with certainty (p. 287).

Theca cell tumors (Fig. 7.18) are also germinal tumors (differentiated ovarian mesenchyme) showing endocrine activity. Histologically elongated cells are arranged in whirls surrounded by abundant collagen fibers. Marked fatty change is typical and gives these fibroma-like tumors a yellow color. About 3% become malignant.

Dermoid cyst of the ovary (Fig. 7.19) *is a dysontogenetic neoplasm arising from embryonic cells and containing epidermis, skin appendages and not infrequently bone and teeth.* Histologically there is a large empty cystic space lined with a layer of epidermal-like squamous epithelium beneath which there are hair follicles (→ 1) and sebaceous glands (→ 2). In the lower third of the figure there are dilated sweat glands.

Salpingitis isthmica nodosa (Fig. 7.20): *the end product of previous chronic interstitial salpingitis and is the result of growth of remnants of the mucosa into the wall with formation of a labyrinth of epithelial sinuses.* Histologically with low power the tube is made up of numerous glandular spaces of various sizes.

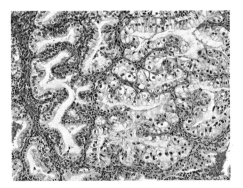

Fig. 7.21. Secretory endometrium in extrauterine pregnancy (Arias-Stella phenomenon); H & E, 80×.

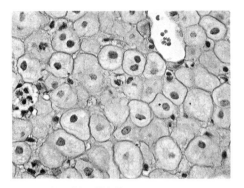

Fig. 7.22. Decidua; H & E, 250×.

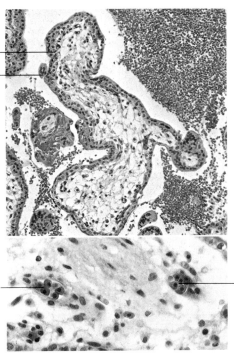

1
2

Fig. 7.23. Placental villi, H & E, 100×. Below: nucleated erythrocytes; H & E, 250×.

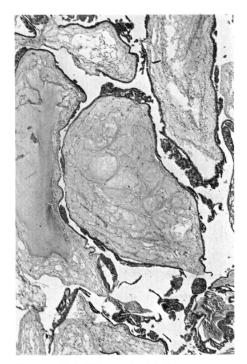

Fig. 7.24. Hydatidiform mole; H & E, 20×.

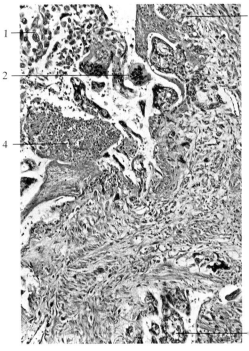

1
2
4

Fig. 7.25. Choriocarcinoma; H & E, 100×.

Pregnancy: Abortion–Hydatidiform Mole–Choriocarcinoma

Abortion or miscarriage (Figs. 7.21–7.23): intrauterine death and expulsion of an embryo before the 28th week of pregnancy. Histologically the aborted material shows secretory or postsecretory endometrium returning to the resting phase (Fig. 7.21), decidual reaction of the stroma (Fig. 7.22) and placental villi (Fig. 7.23). Frequently there is also marked infiltration of polymorphonuclear leukocytes, which as a rule are not a response to bacteria but rather to disintegration and separation of the endometrium.

In pregnancy the endometrium is in the secretory phase—due to the presence of a gravid corpus luteum—and returns to normal after death of the embryo. At this time star-shaped glands are seen having projecting cells with clear cytoplasm and dark, pyknotic nuclei. Such changes, particularly when marked are referred to as the **Arias-Stella phenomenon** (Fig. 7.21) and are solely the result of delayed expulsion of an embryo which has been the cause of the pregnancy. When the curettage shows evidence of incomplete expulsion but no placental villi, then the possibility of an extrauterine pregnancy must be considered. NOTE: extrauterine pregnancy can neither be excluded or established safely by histological examination of endometrium.

Decidual cells (Fig. 7.22) are large stromal cells having distinct borders, abundant cytoplasm and a round, centrally placed nucleus. They make up the maternal portion of the placenta. Since placental cells are influenced also by exogenous hormones, they are not pathognomonic evidence of pregnancy.

Placental villi (Fig. 7.23) are histological evidences of abortion which can be lacking in extrauterine pregnancy and delayed miscarriages. The villi are composed of a delicate, cell poor stroma that contains capillaries. In the mature placenta these capillaries contain nucleated erythrocytes (Fig. 7.23, lower arrows). The surface of the placental villi consists of an inner layer of cuboidal cells (cytotrophoblasts-Langhans cells → 1) and an outer layer of large, multinucleated giant cells without definable borders (syncytial trophoblasts → 2).

Hydatidiform mole (Fig. 7.24): it is presumed that this results from absent or defective formation of fetal vessels leading to ballooning of the stroma of the villi and marked proliferation of trophoblasts. Histologically there are markedly enlarged villi showing lake-like transformation of the stroma which is poor in cells and fibers and shows nodules of proliferated chorion epithelium on the surface (Figs. 7.24, 7.26).

Choriocarcinoma (Fig. 7.25) is a malignant tumor of placental chorionic villi. The tumor has cytohistolytic trophoblastic activity giving rise to destructive growth and early metastases. In Figure 7.25 the myometrium is invaded by large masses of cells (→ 1). Polymorphous, multinucleated giant cells (→ 2) as well as small clusters of cuboidal cells (→ 3: derived from the Langhans cells) are also seen. Finally there are areas of necrosis and fibrin deposition (→ 4). Of diagnostic significance is invasion of veins (→ 5: tumor in a vein).

Most choriocarcinomas arise from the base of a hydatidiform mole (about 60% of cases). Both the primary tumor and its metastases are unusually hemorrhagic. The tumor produces gonadotropin (its detection is important for both diagnosis and prognosis). Choriocarcinomas also occur in the testis in men.

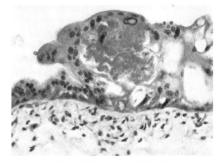

Fig. 7.26. Hydatidiform mole; H & E, 200×.

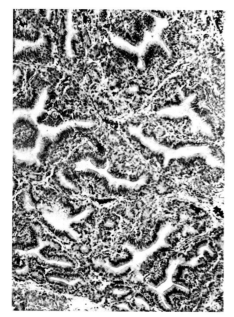

Fig. 8.1. Simple goiter; H & E, 99×.

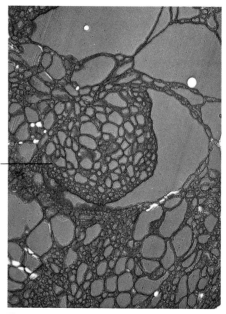

Fig. 8.2. Nodular colloid goiter; H & E, 38×.

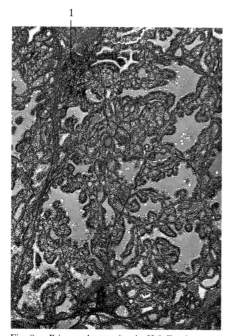

Fig. 8.3. Primary thyrotoxicosis; H & E, 38×.

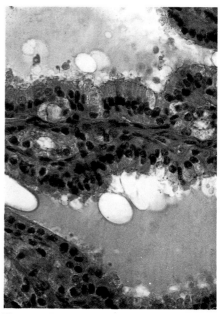

Fig. 8.4. Primary thyrotoxicosis; H & E, 396×.

8. Endocrine Glands

Consideration of disturbances of the endocrine glands will be limited to illustrations of a few typical cases, since a thorough description would exceed the scope of this book. Hyperfunction is ordinarily associated with hyperplasia, the proliferation and enlargement of the cells and nuclei ultimately bringing about an adenomatous appearance. Hypofunction, on the other hand, is associated with atrophy of the organ, hypoplasia of cellular elements and interstitial fibrosis.

Goiter: *Any enlargement of the thyroid in excess of the normal weight for adults of* 20–25 g. *The enlargement may result from disturbances of thyroid function (decrease or increase), inflammations or tumors.*

Diffuse colloid goiter in the adult (euthyroid nodular goiter) develops from simple goiter, i.e., simple diffuse hyperplasia of the thyroid (Fig. 8.1) which is common during childhood to puberty (especially in females). Microscopically the thyroid lobules are enlarged and consist of either colloid-free follicles and branching glands lined by tall cylindrical epithelium or of solid cell masses.

Nodular colloid goiter (Fig. 8.2). *Nodular thyroid hyperplasia and thyroid adenomas appear to be endemic in certain regions (e.g., the Great Lakes region, Switzerland) but may also be sporadic and are usually regarded as compensatory hyperplasia due to iodine insufficiency* (amino acid deficiency?, inhibition of thyroxin synthesis?). Colloid goiter shows a variety of morphological features. The illustration (Fig. 8.2) shows a section of a macrofollicular nodular colloid goiter. A survey of the microscopic section with the scanning lens shows that the nodules are composed of many different-sized follicles and are surrounded by a dense fibrous capsule. The follicles are filled with colloid and lined with flat cuboidal epithelium. Higher magnification reveals cushionlike excrescences of epithelium, which may be so pronounced that new follicles arise within the excrescence (→). Degenerative changes (e.g., central necrosis, cysts, hemorrhages, scars, calcifications) arise as a result of vascular insufficiency and compression of the proliferating colloid nodules against the connective tissue capsule in which lies the nutrient vasculature (oxygen deficiency).

Macroscopic: Enlarged, nodular thyroid. The cut surface shows glistening nodules and focal yellow lesions (degenerative changes). Chiefly occurs in men. *Pathogenesis:* iodine deficiency leads to diffuse hyperplasia (excess TSH)–with increase in iodine certain areas develop enriched colloid → colloid nodules. The reason for focal distribution is not clear. *Toxic adenomatous goiter* is a hormone-producing adenoma. Histologically there is no correlation between I^{131} activity and the morphological signs of activity (tall, clear epithelium and decreased colloid).

Primary thyrotoxicosis or exophthalmic goiter (Figs. 8.3, 8.4). *In this condition, hyperfunction of the gland produces increased amounts of thyroid hormones* (thyrotoxicosis). With the scanning lens, the histological section (Fig. 8.3) reveals large and small, highly branched follicles of various shapes with little or no colloid. The irregular configuration of the follicles is due to the cushion-like overgrowth of the epithelium (pseudopapillary proliferation) which, in places, shows fibrous stalks (papillary proliferation). The colloid, particularly near the surface of the epithelial cells, contains numerous vacuoles. Isolated foci of lymphocytes, in which there are some plasma cells, are quite characteristic (→ in Fig. 8.3). **High magnification** (Fig. 8.4) shows tall columnar epithelium with pale cytoplasm and basally placed nuclei. In some places, the epithelium is stratified (→ in the picture). The so-called resorption vacuoles stand out clearly in this picture. These are artifacts of fixation, indicating that the colloid has a thin consistency.

The cause of hyperthyroidism is not known. An increase in production of thyrotropin releasing factor (TRF) in the midbrain inhibits thyroid stimulating hormone (TSH). Meanwhile a long acting thyroid stimulator, an IgG (immunoglobulin), is produced which becomes bound to cell membranes of the thyroid glands and, like TSH, increases activity. Circulating antibodies against thyroglobulin and the presence of lymphocytes and plasma cells in thyrotoxicosis (Graves' disease, Basedow's disease) suggest an autoimmune disorder.

Macroscopic: The thyroid is enlarged, and the cut surfaces resemble pancreas.

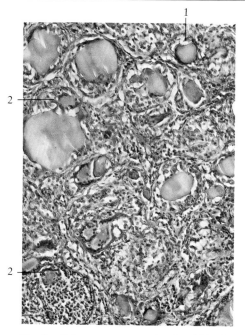

Fig. 8.5. Subacute, nonsuppurative thyroiditis (de Quervain); H & E, 160×.

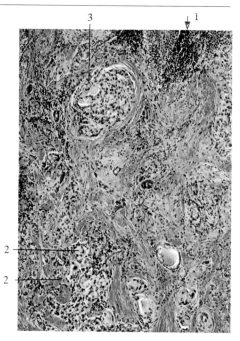

Fig. 8.6. Riedel's struma; van Gieson, 102×.

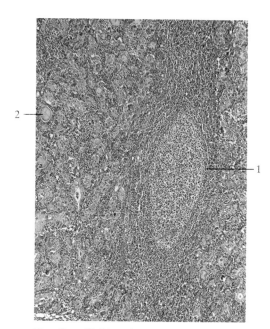

Fig. 8.7. Hashimoto's struma (struma lymphomatosa); H & E, 60×.

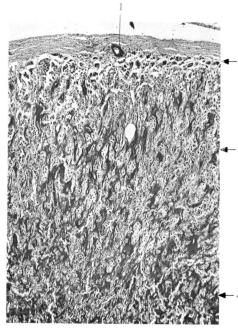

Fig. 8.8. Amyloidosis of the adrenal gland; Congo red, 120×.

Thyroiditis

The nonspecific inflammations of the thyroid, although rare, do present an impressive and characteristic histological picture. In addition to *acute or subacute suppurative and nonsuppurative inflammations* (*thyroiditis* of de Quervain, 1936), there are two types of *chronic thyroiditis* — chronic hypertrophic thyroiditis or *Riedel's struma* (Riedel, 1896) and *struma lymphomatosa* (Hashimoto's disease or lymphadenoid goiter, 1912).

Subacute nonsuppurative thyroiditis (de Quervain) (Fig. 8.5). Histologically, there are follicles of different sizes lined by cuboidal to columnar epithelium, which, in part, has a cushion-like appearance. Scattered about are smaller follicles without colloid. The relatively viscous colloid and colloid masses (→1) have been resorbed by giant cells partly derived from epithelium and partly from mesenchyma (→2, a foreign body reaction). Small numbers of lymphocytes, plasma cells and occasional polymorphonuclear leukocytes can be seen between the follicles.No hypothyroidism. Often a past history of viral infection (mumps).

Chronic hypertrophic thyroiditis or Riedel's struma (Fig. 8.6). This form of chronic thyroiditis is accompanied by thyroid enlargement. The organ is firm and the cut surface reveals dense, white sclerotic scar tissue. The predominant features, microscopically, are hyalinized streaks of scar tissue and focal lymphocytic infiltration (→ 1). The follicles, except for some small remnants, are destroyed. A few isolated groups of intact follicles (→ 2) may undergo regenerative proliferation, thus giving rise to small adenomata (→ 3). An important diagnostic feature is the extension of the chronic sclerosing inflammation into the soft tissues of the neck, in particular, the muscles. Sometimes only a single thyroid lobule is affected.

Struma lymphomatosa (Hashimoto) (Fig. 8.7). This is a chronic, progressive inflammation characterized by lymphocytic infiltration and atrophy of thyroid follicles and destruction of follicular epithelium. Figure 8.7 shows diffuse interstitial lymphocytic infiltration (often there are plasma cells), with formation of a typical lymphoid follicle having a reaction center (→ 1). The thyroid follicles are small and some contain inspissated colloid (→ 2) and others are empty.

Clinical: Hypothyroidism, sometimes myxedema.

Macroscopic: Slightly swollen, firm, brownish cut surface flecked with white.

Pathogenesis: 65% of the cases of chronic thyroiditis show autoantibodies against thyroid tissue when tested immunologically (autoimmunity). It can be shown in animal experiments that injection of thyroid extract causes a thyroiditis that histologically resembles very closely struma lymphomatosa (Witebsky, 1962). Also antibodies against gastric parietal cells and intrinsic factor (40% of all patients have pernicious anemia). Thyroid carcinoma occurs in 3% of the cases. A similar mechanism (autoaggression) has been suggested for many other diseases: allergic encephalitis, lupus erythematosus, immune hemolytic anemia, agranulocytosis, thrombocytopenia, chronic glomerulonephritis, cirrhosis of the liver, myasthenia gravis, ulcerative colitis.

Amyloidosis of the adrenal gland (Fig. 8.8). *Amyloid deposition in the adrenal cortex occurs regularly in cases of general amyloidosis (kidney, spleen, liver). Clinical adrenal cortical insufficiency can develop in severe cases.* The section shows a small artery (→ 1) in the capsule, in the wall of which a homogeneous, red-stained deposit can be seen. In the cortex, the amyloid is deposited around capillaries. The zona glomerulosa is unaffected (→ 2). Broad bands of amyloid in the zona fasciculata (→ 3) and reticularis (→ 4) have caused pressure atrophy of the cortical cells.

Macroscopic: The adrenals are enlarged and appear glassy.

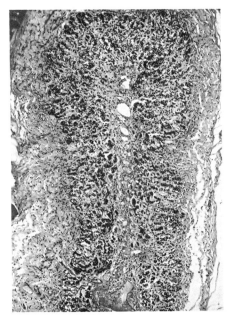

Fig. 8.9. Atrophy of the adrenal cortex; H & E, 66×.

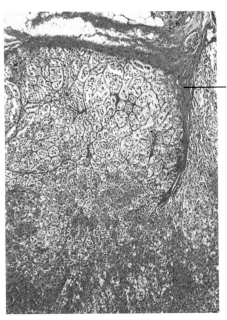

Fig. 8.10. Hyperplasia of the adrenal cortex in Cushing's disease; H & E, 64×.

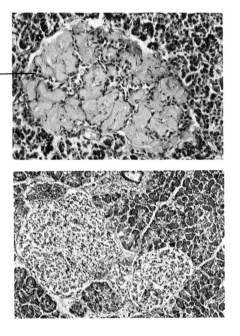

Fig. 8.11a. Hyalinization of an islet of Langerhans (diabetes mellitus); H & E, 170×.
Fig. 8.11b. Islet hyperplasia (newborn of a diabetic mother); H & E, 127×.

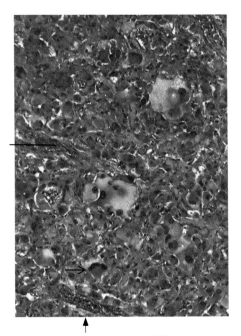

Fig. 8.12. Pheochromocytoma; H & E, 130×.

Atrophy of adrenal cortex (Fig. 8.9). Adrenal insufficiency may result from primary disease of the adrenal cortex (tuberculosis, cytotoxic contraction, hemorrhage, etc.), so-called *primary adrenal insufficiency.* Clinically, the picture is that of *Addison's disease.* On the other hand, adrenal insufficiency may be *secondary to insufficient hypophyseal stimulation* (ACTH deficiency) as in postpartum pituitary necrosis or scarring (Sheehan, 1955), or after infections or trauma.

Figure 8.9 is from a patient with *Sheehan's syndrome and secondary cortical atrophy.* The cortex is much reduced and the various zones are completely disorganized. The cortex consists solely of clumps and groups of cells, the arrangement of which is faintly reminiscent of the zona glomerulosa. There is also proliferation of interstitial fibrous tissue.

Macroscopically, the adrenal gland is paper-thin. *Clinically,* there is panhypopituitarism, so-called Simmond's disease.

Adrenal cortical hyperplasia in Cushing's disease (Fig. 8.10): In Cushing's syndrome, there is overproduction of adrenocortical hormone (glucocorticoid), with metabolic transformation from protein manufacture to production of glucose and fat. In 30% of cases, the adrenal cortex shows hyperplasia which is dependent upon increased ACTH production by a basophilic or chromophobic pituitary adenoma. Usually, however, no pituitary tumor can be found, (primary hyperplasia of unknown cause). True adrenal cortical adenomas (or carcinoma in children) may also cause the syndrome.

Figure 8.10 shows great widening of the adrenal cortex (compare this with Fig. 8.9, which is at the same magnification), which is so great that only a portion of the cortex can be shown. The zona fasciculata extends to the connective tissue capsule →, in the upper part of which there are fat-laden cells (the fat has been dissolved in preparation of the section), arranged in ball fashion, →: radiating septum of connective tissue (beginning adenoma formation, nodular hyperplasia).

Macroscopic: Enlarged adrenals, showing a wide, yellow cortex and nodular hyperplasia or adenomas. *Clinical:* Obesity of the trunk, full-moon visage, thick neck, striae, hypertonus, osteoporosis, diabetes.

Islet hyalinization in diabetes mellitus (Fig. 8.11a). Hyalinization of the capillaries of the islets of Langerhans may be found, particularly in diabetes in elderly persons (not in young persons!). Whether this is the cause or the consequence of the diabetes is disputed. The hyaline material (amyloid?) is deposited in the wall of the capillaries, obstructs the lumen and secondarily causes atrophy of the islet cells (→).

Islet hyperplasia (newborn of a diabetic mother) (Fig. 8.11b). This is considered an adaptation hyperplasia of the islets of Langerhans of the fetus to the hyperglycemia of the diabetic mother. The richly cellular giant islets can be easily seen under low magnification. Higher magnification shows, in addition, greatly enlarged nuclei and often multinucleated giant cells (β-cell hyperplasia).

Pheochromocytoma (Fig. 8.12, 8.13). This is usually a benign tumor (malignant examples are rare) of the adrenal medulla (most unilateral, 40–50 years). Most have endocrine activity (periodic outpouring of adrenalin and noradrenalin. *Clinical:* Increase in blood pressure, hyperglycemia).

The histological picture shows epithelial tumor tissue arranged in strands or cellular balls, often situated perivascularly (→: vessel). The cells are large, round or polygonal and pleomorphic and frequently have eccentrically situated nuclei. Giant cells are seen frequently. Expanding hemorrhage is common. The brown color produced by the chromate reaction (dichromate salts) demonstrates adrenalin (fine granules) and noradrenalin-producing cells (large granules) (Fig. 8.13). Noradrenalin can be identified with potassium iodide (Kracht *et al.*, 1958; Weber, 1949; Sherwin *et al.*, 1965). Commonly there is hemorrhage and resulting deposition of hemosiderin (Fig. 8.13).

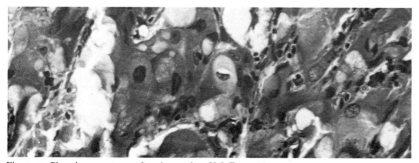

Fig. 9.13. Pheochromocytoma after chromation; H & E, 375×.

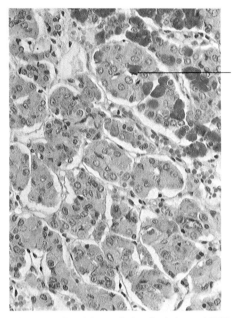

Fig. 8.14. Focal hyperplasia of pituitary ACTH cells; H & E, 400×.

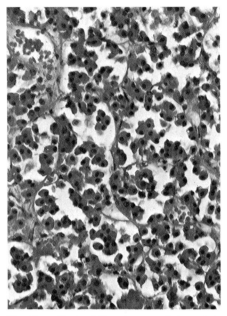

Fig. 8.15. Eosinophilic adenoma of the anterior lobe of the pituitary; H & E, 130×.

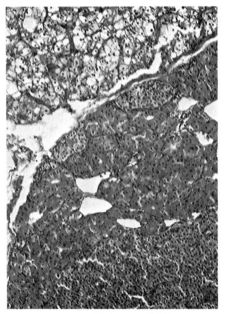

Fig. 8.16. Parathyroid adenoma; H & E, 130×.

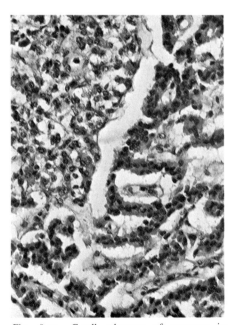

Fig. 8.17. G-cell adenoma of pancreas in Zollinger-Ellison syndrome; H & E, 400×.

Focal hyperplasia of pituitary ACTH cells in primary adrenal cortical insufficiency (Fig. 8.14). The illustration is of the margin of a hyperplastic focus of ACTH stimulating cells. Stained by H & E the cells appear large and polygonal and have granular gray appearing cytoplasm. Since the ACTH granules do not stain clearly they have been called chromophobe cells, amphophiles or neutrophiles. The ACTH cells for the most part show a follicular arrangement (→) and enclose a drop of colloid. In the upper right hand corner of the figure there are some bright red acidophilic STH cells (growth hormone).

The classical division of cells of the anterior lobe of the hypophysis (adenohypophysis) into acidophiles, basophiles and chromophiles, which was based on H & E stains (Schönemann, 1892), no longer is appropriate for our modern functional and morphological ideas. With the help of fluorescence antibody techniques and new histological staining methods (Pearse, 1950, Adams and Sweetenham, 1958; Herlani, 1960) it is possible to make a truly functional classification of the different types of cells of the anterior lobe of the hypophysis. Thus the classical "basophiles," which are identical to the periodic acid positive mucoid cells, can be subdivided into TSH-cells (thyroid stimulating hormone, alizarinian blue positive "S-cells"), FSH (follicle stimulating) and LH cells (luteinizing hormone alizarinian blue negative, purple staining cells), ACTH cells (alizarinian blue negative, faintly purple staining "R" cells) and MSH cells (melanocyte stimulating hormone, Willkowski, 1971).

Eosinophilic adenoma of the anterior lobe of the pituitary (Fig. 8.15). About 30% of anterior pituitary adenomas are composed either entirely or predominantly of eosinophilic (acidophilic) cells. Histologically, in sections stained with H & E, they are compactly arranged, medium sized, uniform, polygonal cells with bright red cytoplasm (Fig. 8.15). The spaces between the cell groups are artifacts due to shrinkage during preparation.

Eosinophilic adenomas may show increased hormone activity and thus cause *acromegaly* or *gigantism*.

Parathyroid adenoma (Fig. 8.16). Histologically adenomas of the parathyroid glands, in contrast to hyperplasia, are nodules consisting of the three cell types that compose the glands: 1. small chief cells (bottom of picture), 2. oxyphil cells with abundant eosinophilic cytoplasm (middle of picture), 3. water clear chief cells (top of picture). The chief cells contain glycogen which has been washed out by the aqueous fixatives and stains. Water clear chief cells constitute the functionally active parathormone producing cells, while oxyphil cells are thought to be involutional forms of chief cells. (Castleman, 1952).

Autonomous, benign parathyroid adenomas are the cause of 90% of all cases of *primary hyperparathyroidism*. The remaining 10% are due to primary hyperplasia and hypertrophy of the parathyroids or to a functionally active parathyroid carcinoma.

G-cell tumors of pancreatic islets in the Zollinger-Ellison syndrome (Fig. 1.17). Histologically they are solid tumor nodules composed of nests and cords of uniform epithelium with eosinophilic cytoplasm. Usually pseudoacini are prominent, in contrast to true glands, and contain scanty, shrunken stroma (→). In the top left hand part of the picture there is exocrine pancreas.

G-cell tumors are tumors of gastrin secreting cells which occur chiefly in the pancreatic islets. *Gastrin* is a polypeptide hormone with the cytochemical properties of polypeptide secreting endocrine cells (APUD-series[1]) to which, among others, belong ACTH cells, MSH cells, α cells (glucagon), β cells (insulin) of the islets of Langerhans, C cells of the thyroid (calcitonin) as well as argyrophiles (cholecystokinin, pancreozymin) and the enterochromaffin cells of the small intestine (Pearse, 1969). G-cell tumors with *Zollinger-Ellison syndrome* (clinical triad: pancreatic tumor, hypersecretion and hyperacidity of gastric juice, therapeutically intractable, and commonly recurrent ulcers typically located in stomach or duodenum or atypically in jejunum).

---

[1] APUD = amine precursor uptake decarboxylation.

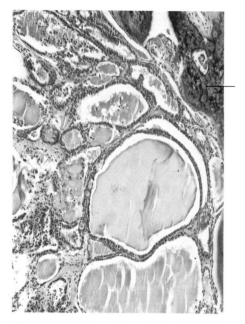

Fig. 8.18. Follicular carcinoma of thyroid; H & E, 80×.

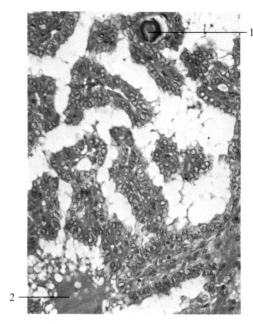

Fig. 8.19. Papillary carcinoma of thyroid; H & E, 200×.

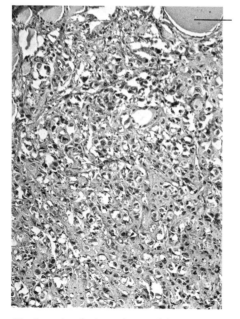

Fig. 8.20. Anaplastic carcinoma of thyroid; H & E, 100×.

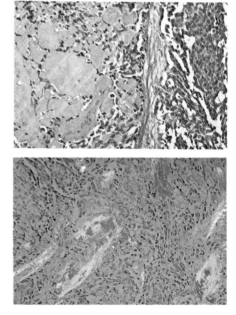

Fig. 8.21 a) Medullary carcinoma of thyroid with amyloid stroma; H & E, 100×. b) Doubly refractive amyloid in polarized light; Congo red stain, 80×.

Malignant Thyroid Tumors

Malignant tumors of the thyroid may arise either from follicular or parafollicular epithelium or calcitonin-producing C-cells. Tumors derived from follicular epithelium include well differentiated, organoid carcinomas as well as undifferentiated or anaplastic carcinomas. Oncocytoma is a cytological variant of these. Malignant thyroid tumors make up 0.5% of deaths from all malignant tumors and are about eleventh in the tumor fatality list. They appear mostly between 40 and 60 years of age: organoid neoplasms earlier, undifferentiated carcinomas later. Women are affected 2–3 times more frequently than men.

Follicular carcinoma (Fig. 8.18) *belongs to the organoid malignant neoplasms of the thyroid and frequently is first detected by the presence of a metastasis from a seemingly normal thyroid gland or encapsulated thyroid nodule or adenoma.* (For this reason it was formerly called "metastasizing adenoma"). Figure 8.18 shows a vertebral metastasis of a follicular carcinoma of the thyroid having follicles of different sizes which are filled with homogeneous eosinophilic colloid (the metastases may store I^{131}). The arrow points to the bluish staining bony trabeculae of the vertebra (decalcified).

Papillary thyroid carcinoma (Fig. 8.19) consists of ramifying, broad, branch-like, stromal septa covered by a single layer of epithelium. The nuclei of these cells are poor in chromatin and occasionally enclose a large, round, faintly acidophilic vacuole (invagination of cytoplasm). The stroma (Fig. 8.19) contains bluish, concentrically layered calcium deposits (psammoma bodies 1→). Small colloid masses lie between the strands of tumor (2→).

Papillary carcinoma of the thyroid chiefly occurs in children and young persons. At first it grows very slowly and metastasizes to cervical lymph nodes, not uncommonly only after a long time (months), which may be the first and only clinical sign of the tumor. *Note:* solitary thyroid nodules are more frequently malignant in the young than in adults. For prognostic and therapeutic purposes papillary tumors should always be diagnosed as malignant tumors.

Anaplastic thyroid carcinoma (Fig. 8.20) *is an undifferentiated tumor showing no organoid structure.* Histologically the tumor shows all the signs of malignancy: cellular and nuclear pleomorphism and many mitoses, some of which are atypical. Occasionally anaplastic thyroid carcinoma can not be differentiated from a spindle cell carcinoma (sarcoma-like growth of a carcinoma). Figure 8.20 shows a very pleomorphic carcinoma which has invaded and destroyed the thyroid follicles (→).

Anaplastic thyroid carcinomas are particularly malignant. They occur preferentially in older men (after 60), invade the capsule, blood vessels (→ hematogenous metastases → lung) and trachea very early. Histologically the following types are recognized: spindle cell, round cell, pleomorphic (polymorphous) and clear cell (corresponding to hypernephroid renal carcinoma).

Oncocytomas are composed of large cells with finely granular eosinophilic cytoplasm (rich in mitochondria) and round chromatic nuclei. Oncocytomas develop from an adenoma or carcinoma and show no clinical manifestations different from follicular or anaplastic carcinomas. Oncocytes (= swollen cells) appear also in other organs (e.g., in parathyroid and salivary glands, trachea, liver, etc.) Thyroid oncocytomas formerly were called *Hürthle cell tumors*.

Medullary thyroid carcinoma with amyloid stroma (Fig. 8.21) *is a slow-growing, late-metastasizing carcinoma which arises from C-cells.* The tumor forms large medullary islands surrounded by homogeneous, eosinophilic stroma (Fig. 8.21a). Preparations stained with Congo red and examined with polarized light show the greenish-yellow double refraction characteristic of amyloid.

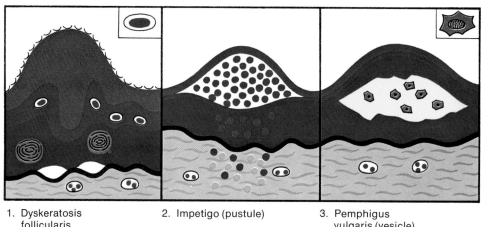

1. Dyskeratosis
   follicularis

2. Impetigo (pustule)

3. Pemphigus
   vulgaris (vesicle)

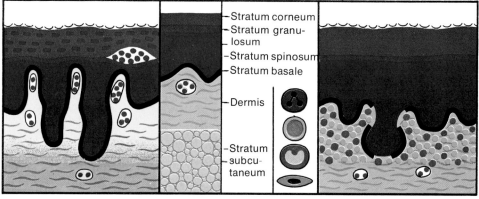

4. Psoriasis vulgaris   Normal skin   5. Lichen ruber

—Stratum corneum
—Stratum granu-
 losum
—Stratum spinosum
—Stratum basale

—Dermis

—Stratum
 subcu-
 taneum

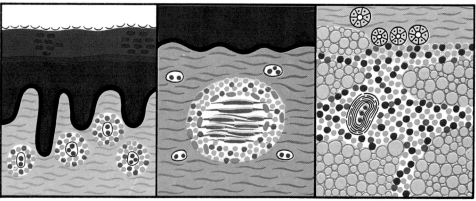

6. Chronic eczema
   (neurodermatitis)

7. Granuloma annulare

8. Erythema nodosum

Fig. 10.1. Diagram of examples of different sorts of skin lesions.

9. Skin–Breast

The histopathology of the skin constitutes a difficult and complicated area of knowledge. As a rule the tissue changes can only be interpreted correctly with knowledge of the clinical (age, sex, duration) and gross findings (localization, onset, appearance, color, etc.). Only a few skin diseases, chosen for their clinical or theoretical significance, can be discussed in this chapter because of limitations of space.

1. Disturbances of cornification. There are numerous congenital and acquired skin and allergic lesions. In *ichthyosis congenita,* which differs from ichthyosis vulgaris only in the severity of the changes, hyperkeratosis and atrophy of the prickle cell layer are conspicuous. Hyperkeratosis also occurs in local chronic irritation *(callouses)* or in viral warts, cutaneous horns, in chronic arsenic poisoning (palmar and plantar hyperkeratosis) and from other causes.

In **dyskeratosis follicularis of Darier** (Fig. 9.1/1) there is both hyperkeratosis and dyskeratosis leading to subbasal splitting (acantholysis) with formation of vesicles and lacunae. Typically there are "corps ronds" (large eosinophilic cells with distinct borders and basophilic nuclei in the stratum granulosum and stratum spinosum) as well as "grains" (small cells with elongated nuclei) localized in the horny layer.

2. Epidermal lesions. Impetigo (Fig. 9.1/2) is a bacterial skin infection (staphylococci and streptococci) manifested by vesicle formation in the horny layer. The vesicles contain polymorphonuclear leukocytes. Vesicle formation (bullous eruption) is also a prominent feature of **pemphigus vulgaris** (Fig. 9.1/3). There are intraepidermal acantholytic cells with degenerate prickle cells (so-called Tsanck cells). The dermal papillae in the floor of the vesicles are hyperplastic and covered with a layer of persistent basal cells.

3. Disturbances of epidermis and corium: psoriasis vulgaris (Fig. 9.1/4). A familial, progressive disease which presents as sharply delimited erythematous, maculopapillary eruptions overlaid with pale silver scales. The microscopic picture shows parakeratosis (nucleated scales), acanthosis (prolongation of the epidermal columns) and papillomatosis (extension of dermal papillae nearly to the horny layer). Dilated vessels, perivascular edema and infiltration of lymphocytes, histiocytes and leukocytes are seen in the stratum papillare and stratum reticulare. Microabscesses, which are not always found, contain compacted neutrophilic leukocytes in the epidermis.

Lichen ruber planus (Fig. 9.1/5). This is a dermatitis accompanied by marked itching, irregularly marginated, livid red papules. The principal histological features are thickened, hyperkeratotic epidermis (→ 1) and a band-like infiltrate composed predominantly of lymphocytes. It occurs in the basal cell layer, which shows vacuolar degeneration and has a moth-eaten appearance.

Chronic eczema (Fig. 9.1/6) is a common form of dermatitis and is classified according to either etiology, course or morphology. Histologically there are chiefly hyperkeratosis, lichenification and occasional islands of parakeratosis. Rete pegs are elongated, the corium showing a prominent perivascular infiltrate.

4. Disturbance of corium and subcutis. In this category are inflammatory, degenerative diseases as well as infiltrations (e.g., amyloidosis of skin). **Granuloma annulare** (Fig. 9.1/7) shows nodular degeneration of collagen in the corium together with inflammation and fibrosis. The nodules result from coagulation necrosis, homogenization and fragmentation of collagen fibers and are infiltrated with lymphocytes, histiocytes and fibroblasts. The lesion must be differentiated from lipoid necrobiosis and rheumatic nodules. **Subcutis: erythema nodosum** (Fig. 9.1/8). The lesions appear on the extensor surfaces of the lower legs. They are raised, discoid, reddish, infiltrated lesions covered with smooth skin and sensitive to pressure. The essential histological findings are localized in the subcutaneous fat tissue. In the early stages there are only small collections of neutrophiles and lymphocytes. Small blood vessels, particularly veins, are chiefly affected showing inflammatory infiltration of the wall and proliferation of the endothelium. In a later stage small nodular collections of histiocytes and multinucleated foreign body giant cells are present. Small, radially arranged collections of regimented histiocytes and fibroblasts may also be seen. Here and there, blood vessels are involved in the inflammatory process.

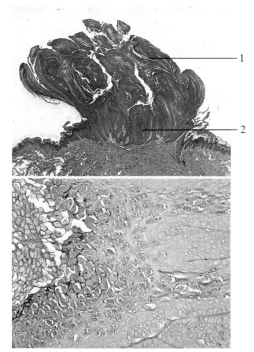

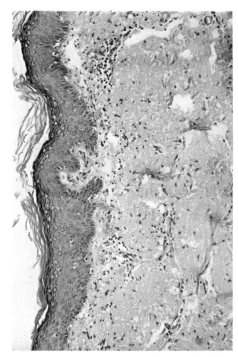

Fig. 9.2. Above: common wart; H & E, 8×. Below: molluscum contagiosum; H & E, 80×.

Fig. 9.3. Senile elastosis; H & E, 100×.

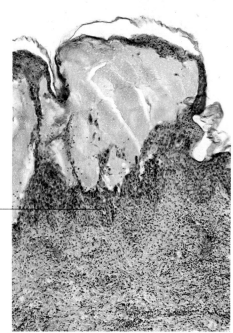

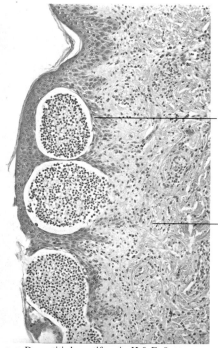

Fig. 9.4. Vesicular eruption in chickenpox (varicella); H & E, 60×.

Fig. 9.5. Dermatitis herpetiformis; H & E, 80×.

Verruca vulgaris (common wart, Fig. 9.2) *occurs chiefly in children and young persons. It is a benign, virus-caused neoplasm of the skin, manifested by hyperkeratosis, acanthosis, papillomatosis and cellular inclusions.* Histologically there is a mixture of hyperkeratotic and parakeratotic (persistence of nuclei in the horny layer) cornification (→ 1). The underlying epidermis shows acanthosis and papillomatosis (→ 2), and prominent kerato-hyaline granules. In the upper layers of the stratum spinosum and corneum many cells are ballooned by edema. Verruca vulgaris shows two types of inclusions: basophilic, intranuclear, DNA-containing (positive Feulgen reaction) inclusions and eosinophilic, Feulgen negative, cytoplasmic inclusions that derive from kerato-hyaline granules.

There are several types of viral warts which differ in their localization and morphology. *Verruca plantaris,* the plantar wart, develops beneath the surface of the skin. *Horny mucous warts* (e.g., on the lip) show only slight cornification. *Verruca plana juvenilis* shows prominent acanthosis and hyperkeratosis, lacks papillomatosis and may convert to verruca vulgaris. **Molluscum contagiosum** or venereal wart (Fig. 9.2, below) may be described as an infectious acanthoma lying beneath the skin surface. Typically there are molluscum bodies (corps ronds): cornified epithelial cells containing nuclear remains and viral elementary bodies. They are eosinophilic and at first show septa but later are homogeneous.

Senile elastosis (Fig. 9.3) *consists of homogeneous degeneration of collagen fibers in the upper corium.* The tissue has a uniform appearance and stains intensely with elastica stains. The overlying epidermis is distinctly widened with slight hyperkeratosis.

Senile elastosis is a degenerative lesion and should be distinguished from **senile keratoma** (senile keratosis) in which there are marked epidermal changes: parts are atrophic and other parts hypertrophic. There is pronounced superficial hyperkeratosis and the underlying epidermis shows cellular atypia and mitoses (so-called dysplasia). These changes occurring particularly in the elderly and in persons exposed excessively to the sun or weather (farmers, seamen, etc.) may be precancerous lesions.

Vesicular eruption in chickenpox (Fig. 9.4). *This is a virus disease characterized by a generalized vesicular and pustular exanthem.* Histologically, there is intraepidermal vesicle formation just as in variola, smallpox, herpes zoster and herpes simplex. Figure 10.2 shows such a vesicle containing homogeneous protein material. The uppermost epidermal layer forms the outer margin, and a thin basal layer (→) delimits the vesicle from the dermis. The dermis is slightly infiltrated with lymphocytes. The intraepidermal vesicle is formed from the deterioration of epidermal cells. Intranuclear inclusion bodies are present. Similar vesicles, but without inclusion bodies, are seen in the skin in burns and freezing.

Dermatitis herpetiformis (Fig. 9.5). *This is a dermatitis of allergic origin which causes an irritating pruritus. The disease involves particularly the trunk, buttocks and scalp.* In contrast to pemphigus vulgaris (= intraepidermal vesicles), the microscopic picture of dermatitis herpetiformis consists of subepidermal vesicles or bleb formations (→ 1). In the vesiculobullous eruptions, many eosinophilic leukocytes are found. The dermal connective tissue forming the floor of the vesicles show an inflammatory reaction (→ 2). Edema, dilated blood vessels, eosinophilic leukocytes and lymphocytes are present.

Macroscopic: The clinical picture is pleomorphic. Erythema, urticaria, vesicles and bullae occur. Often, the eruption is herpetiform. A symmetrical distribution is often apparent.

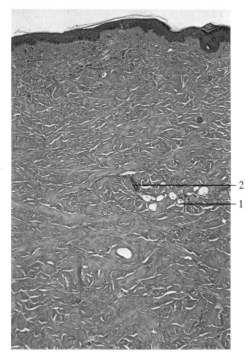

Fig. 9.6. Scleroderma; H & E, 40×.

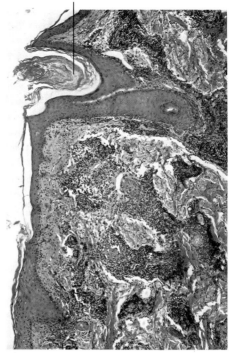

Fig. 9.7. Chronic discoid lupus erythematosus; H & E, 30×.

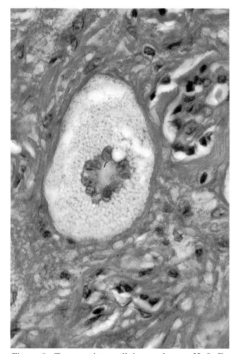

Fig. 9.8. Touton giant cell in xanthoma; H & E, 320×.

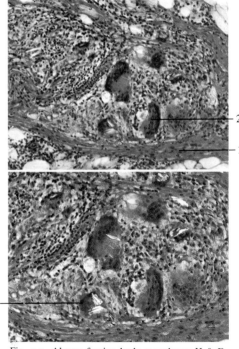

Fig. 9.9. Above: foreign body granuloma; H & E, 80×. Below: doubly refractile foreign bodies in polarized light. H & E, 100×.

Scleroderma (Fig. 9.6) *may be either isolated or generalized and belongs to the group of collagen or more properly connective tissue diseases. Clinically it is manifested by thickening of the corium due to increase in collagen fibers.* Histologically there is distinct thinning of the epidermis. The underlying corium contains bundles of numerous thick and sclerotic collagen fibers. Fibroblasts are numerically diminished and skin appendages are absent (atrophy). Trapped fat cells (→ 1) and sweat glands (→ 2) suggest that the corium is increased in thickness at the expense of the fat panniculus.

Clinically a distinction is made between *circumscribed, localized benign scleroderma* and the *progressive, diffuse, generalized form* with involvement of internal organs (heart, muscle, intestine, esophagus, nerve). Transitions between the two forms do not occur. They are indistinguishable histologically. *Macroscopically* there is an irregularly shaped nodule of thick and retracted skin. It occurs particularly on the hands and face *(acrosclerosis)*.

Disseminated **lupus erythematosus** (Fig. 9.7) also belongs to the group of connective tissue diseases. It can be manifest as an acute, generalized disorder or as a chronic ailment limited to the skin. In *chronic discoid lupus erythematosus* the following changes in the skin are seen: 1. hyperkeratosis of *epidermis,* hypergranularity (increase in keratohyaline granules), atrophy of prickle cells and focal liquefaction of basal cells. 2. Atrophy of *skin appendages* as well as follicular plugging by keratin (→). 3. Lymphocytic infiltration in the *corium* extending into the epidermis and hair follicles. Telangiectasis, edema and destruction of elastic fibers are also present.

In acute lupus erythematosus there is fibrinoid degeneration of the collagen fibers of internal organs (heart, kidney, spleen) and involvement of the skin is seldom prominent.

Touton giant cells (Fig. 9.8) are multinucleated foam cells (resulting from fine fat droplets in the cytoplasm). Characteristic of these cells are the centrally placed, cross-shaped nucleus and the surrounding eosinophilic cytoplasm. Foam cells are seen in numerous metabolic disturbances and inflammatory and neoplastic diseases, e.g., in primary hypercholesterolemic xanthomatosis, xanthoma and fibroxanthoma, histiocytoma, giant cell tumors of bone, in fatty deposits (xanthelasia of the eyelids), in cholesterosis and inflammation of the gallbladder, and in the pelvis of the kidney and other organs.

Foreign body granuloma (Fig. 9.9) *has a peripheral zone of scarring* (→) *and a central zone rich in inflammatory cells* (lymphocytes, histiocytes, blood vessels) as well as *typical foreign body giant cells.* They contain *foreign bodies* (→ 2) of various sizes. Doubly refractive foreign bodies (talc crystals) can be clearly demonstrated in polarized light (Fig. 9.9, below). Other foreign bodies include *endogenous material* (cholesterin crystals, extruded epithelial mucous, horny lamellae from a ruptured atheroma) as well as *exogenous* material (wood, talcum, metal, oily materials, paraffin). Fat-soluble foreign bodies often appear as crystal-like spaces.

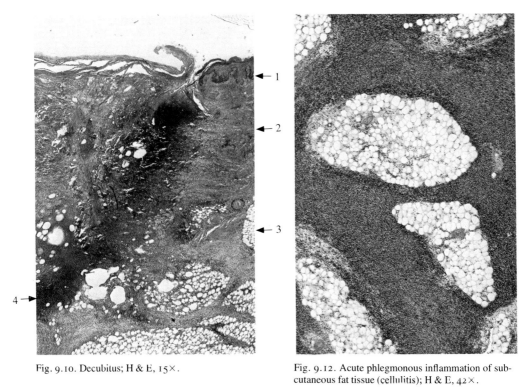

Fig. 9.10. Decubitus; H & E, 15×.

Fig. 9.12. Acute phlegmonous inflammation of subcutaneous fat tissue (cellulitis); H & E, 42×.

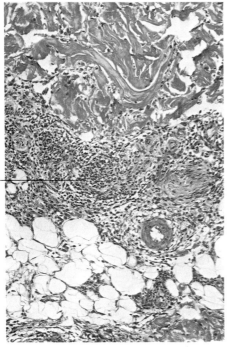

Fig. 9.12. Anaphylactoid purpura; H & E, 80×.

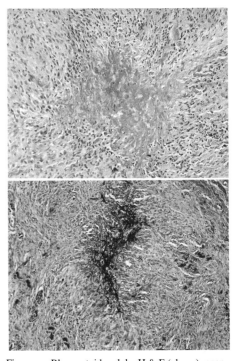

Fig. 9.13. Rheumatoid nodule; H & E (above), azan (below), 80×.

Decubitus (Fig. 9.10). *This is an example of cutaneous necrosis due to local tissue death resulting from prolonged pressure. This type of necrosis occurs most frequently over the ischium in bedridden patients or patients with spinal cord injuries and is due to compression of blood vessels and eventual ulceration.* The histological picture reveals preserved epidermis ($\rightarrow$1), corium ($\rightarrow$ 2) and subcutaneous tissues ($\rightarrow$ 3). A blue-staining zone of leukocytes and cellular debris cuts transversely through the section ($\rightarrow$ 4). This blends into another necrotic, anuclear zone. Later, granulation tissue will infiltrate and replace the necrotic tissue, producing an ulcer.

Acute phlegmonous inflammation (cellulitis) of subcutaneous fat tissue (Fig. 9.11). Diffuse leukocytic inflammation of the skin has developed mainly in the loose subcutaneous fat tissue, in which it can easily spread. Histologically, there is a diffuse, dense, streak-like infiltration of polymorphonuclear leukocytes that surrounds islands of remaining fat cells. Streptococci are the usual causative agent.

Anaphylactoid purpura (Henoch-Schönlein, Fig. 9.12) *is an inflammatory vasculitis of the skin of infectious, drug allergy or not uncommonly an unknown origin manifested by skin hemorrhages (petechiae and ecchymoses) and frequently also by involvement of internal organs (intestine, kidney, joints).* Histologically in a **fresh nodule** the vascular endothelial cells are swollen, the vessel walls are necrotic and there are dense collections of neutrophiles (occasionally eosinophils or lymphocytes) surrounding them ($\rightarrow$). Typically there are nuclear fragments derived from destruction of neutrophiles. Older lesions are recognized by the appearance of erythrocytes.

Purpura occurs in several infectious bacterial diseases (e.g., meningococcal meningitis, subacute bacterial endocarditis). Purpura caused by drug and therapeutic allergy shows the same histological picture as anaphylactoid purpura.

Rheumatoid nodule (Fig. 9.13). *In both acute rheumatic fever (see p. 49) and chronic rheumatoid arthritis (see p. 269) skin nodules may develop with central zones of fibrinoid necrosis and a palisade-like arrangement of histiocytes.* In an H & E stained section (Fig. 9.13, above) it is easy to see the central zone of eosinophilic, anuclear necrosis surrounded by a wall-like arrangement of histiocytes with elongated nuclei. The fibrinoid necrosis characteristically stains red with azan (Fig. 9.13, below).

Rheumatic skin nodules occur preferentially at the elbow, knee joint and ankle. They may attain a diameter of 2 cm or more. Rheumatic nodules develop usually in the deeper layers of the skin, i.e., in the panniculus adiposus. Granuloma anulare occurs in the corium or surface layers and there is extensive, diffuse tissue involvement.

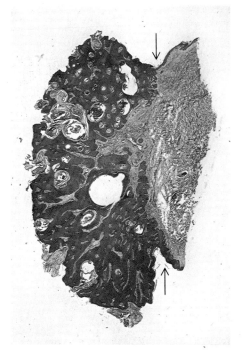

Fig. 9.14. Seborrheic wart; H & E, 5×.

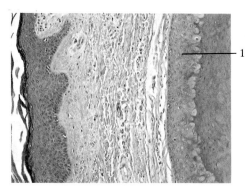

Fig. 9.15. Cyst of skin hair follicle; H & E, 80×.

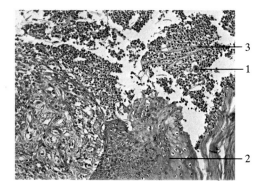

Fig. 9.16. Epidermal cyst; H & E, 80×.

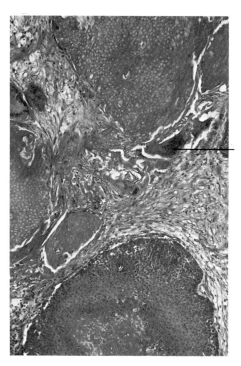

Fig. 9.17. Benign calcifying epithelioma of Malherbe (trichoepithelioma); H & E, 80×.

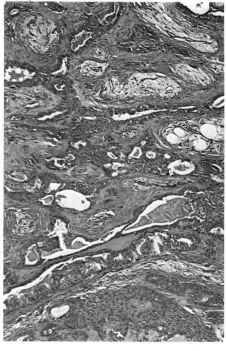

Fig. 9.18. Sweat gland adenoma; H & E, 80×.

Seborrheic wart (seborrheic keratosis, basal cell papilloma, verruca senilis, senile wart Fig. 9.14). *This is a common benign neoplasm which develops in areas of non-exposed skin in older men* and is manifest by proliferation of the cells of the basal layer and horny keratosis. Histologically there is a cap-like tumor located on the surface of the skin (← →) that is composed of proliferated basal cells (hence the marked basophilia). Superficially and between the cells there is cornification which is derived from the granular cell layer. The basal portion of the tumor shows marked melanin pigmentation. The stroma of chronically irritated lesions show inflammatory cellular infiltration.

Seborrheic warts are one of the commonest of skin neoplasms. In younger men there are often engulfed islands of prickle cells (baso-prickle cell acanthoma). Basal cell carcinoma is seldom cornified and invades more deeply than seborrheic wart from which it must be differentiated.

Dermal cysts are of two types: 1. **hair follicle cysts** (Fig. 9.15, above), derived from the epithelial sheath of hair follicle. Histologically the cyst is lined by multilayered epithelium (→ 1) and shows amorphous, acidophilic, frequently centrally calcified masses containing cholesterin crystals. 2. **Epidermal cysts** (Fig. 9.16, below), in contrast to hair follicle cysts, are lined by keratotic, cornified epithelium and contain layered horny lamellae. When a dermal cyst ruptures a *foreign body reaction* develops with accumulation of inflammatory and giant cells (→ 1) about the remaining epithelium (→ 2) and the cornified lamellae (→ 3).

Dermal cysts are among the commonest tumors of the skin. True dermoid cysts are uncommon—apart from *pilonidal sinus* or *sacral dermoid* which is a dermal foreign body reaction caused by broken and impacted hairs in the corium.

Benign calcifying epithelioma of Malherbe (Fig. 9.17) *is a benign tumor of squamous epithelium of the matrix of the hair follicle*. Histologically the tumor consists in part of bands of intact basophilic epithelium (bottom of Fig. 9.17) and in part of necrotic epithelium without nuclei (so-called shadow cells: top of Fig. 9.17). The necrotic parts may calcify or occasionally even ossify. A foreign body reaction in the stroma with multinucleated giant cells (→) is typical.

Sweat gland tumors can show a variety of architectural patterns. **Syringoma** (Fig. 9.18) will serve as an example. There is a double layer of epithelium and a fibrous stroma. In general the cells have a uniform appearance.

There are numerous variants of *benign sweat gland tumors* which can merely be mentioned here: papillary syringoma, eccrine spiradenoma (myoepithelioma), eccrine acrospiroma (clear cell myoepithelioma), chondroid syringoma with cartilaginous stroma, eccrine dermal cylindroma and hidradenoma. Mucinous adenocarcinoma of the skin is a special, malignant variant of sweat gland tumors.

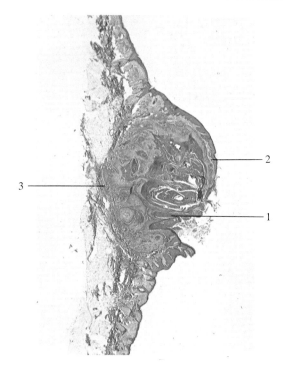

Fig. 9.19. Keratoacanthoma; H & E, 8×.

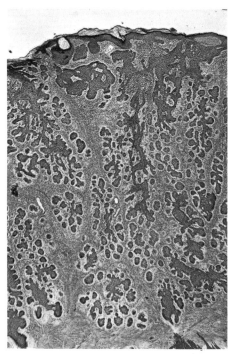

Fig. 9.20. Basal cell carcinoma; H & E, 25×.

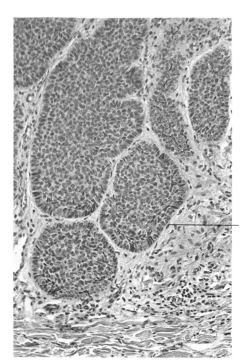

Fig. 9.21. Basal cell carcinoma; H & E, 80×.

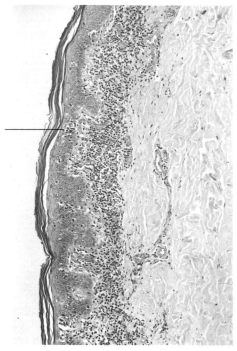

Fig. 9.22. Mycosis fungoides; H & E, 80×.

Keratoacanthoma (molluscum sebaceum, Fig. 9.19) *is a benign, rapidly growing skin tumor, probably virus produced, which develops on the face of elderly men. Most are self-healing in a few months.* The histological picture is very characteristic. The tumor is a sharply defined, superficial plaque composed of proliferating squamous epithelium. The surface is depressed, bowl shaped (→ 1) and is markedly hyperkeratotic and partially covered by overlapping contiguous epidermis (→ 2). Deeper portions of a keratoacanthoma show distinct stromal invasion (→ 3).

Keratoacanthoma is usually a solitary lesion, developing within a few months and then regressing spontaneously. If only a part of the tumor is examined histologically it may be very difficult to differentiate from a well-differentiated squamous cell carcinoma.

Basal cell carcinoma (Figs. 9.20 & 9.21, synonyms: basiloma, rodent ulcer, basal cell epithelioma) *is a locally destructive, expanding skin tumor comprised of basal cells. It very rarely metastasizes.* Histologically it is chiefly located beneath the level of the skin and shows a decidedly deep pattern of growth (Fig. 9.20). Under **high magnification** (Fig. 9.21) there are solid nests of tumor composed of dark cells (scanty cytoplasm). In the periphery of the nests the cells show a typical palisade arrangement reminiscent of the basal layer of the epidermis (→). The surrounding stroma is abundant and infiltrated by inflammatory cells.

Basal cell carcinoma occurs chiefly in elderly men in areas of the skin exposed to light and the weather. They are also seen in younger persons in chronic arsenic intoxication, xeroderma pigmentosum and the nevoid basal cell carcinoma syndrome (Gorlin-Goltz syndrome: multiple pigmented basal cell carcinomas in squamous epithelial lined maxillary cysts and other incidental anomalies or malformations). *Histological variants of basal cell carcinomas:* there are solid, cystic, fibroepithelial (Pinkus tumor) and superficial multicentric forms. Clinically it is important to differentiate the sclerosing type (morphea type) which should not be irradiated. Basal cell carcinoma showing disorderly cytology, squamous differentiation and cornification (basosquamous carcinoma) is considered to be a separate tumor since it occasionally metastasizes.

Mycosis fungoides (Fig. 9.22) *is a lymphohistiocytic disease of the skin with an intermittent course that is thought to be a non-Hodgkin type of lymphoma (lymphomas of low-grade malignancy) and thus a true neoplasm.* In the first or erythematous or premycosis stage the disease, both clinically and histologically, is not characteristic. Only the appearance of an infiltrate in the deeper layers of the corium gives a hint of the diagnosis. In the second or plaque stage (Fig. 9.22) typical tissue changes occur. The epidermis is thick, acanthotic and hyperkeratotic and contains small collections of lymphohistiocytic cells (→) or *microabscesses.* In the subepidermis (corium) pleomorphic and atypical lymphoid cells form a band-like layer. These co-called *mycosis fungoides cells* have hyperchromatic nuclei of various sizes (see also Fig. 15.2).

Mysosis fungoides occurs after the 40th year. After a long course of 5–10 years the disease progresses from the second or plaque stage to the third or tumor stage in which there is an increased number of atypical cells, mitoses, and deeper invasion of corium and subcutis. In about 60–80% of cases not only are subcutaneous lymph nodes involved but also internal organs (liver, lung, spleen, kidney).

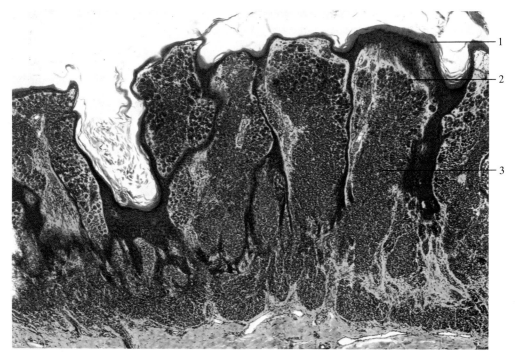

Fig. 9.23. Pigmented intradermal nevus; H & E, 50×.

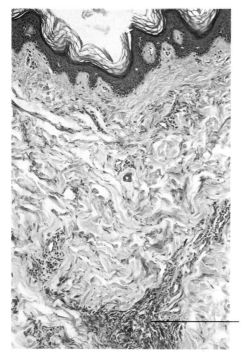

Fig. 9.24. Blue nevus; H & E, 80×.

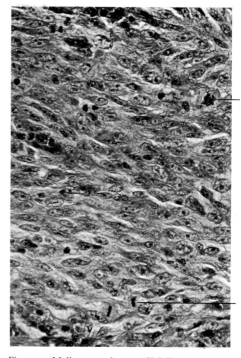

Fig. 9.25. Malignant melanoma; H & E, 350×.

Pigmented Tumors

Introductory remarks. The term nevus (mole) describes a number of tumor-like malformations (hamartomas) of the skin that may arise either from newly formed capillaries *(vascular nevus)*, hyperplastic sebaceous glands *(sebaceous nevus)*, papillomatous and hyperplastic epidermis *(verrucous nevus)* or melanin producing cells *(pigmented nevus)*. Nontumorous disorders of pigmentation that are concerned with increase in numbers of the pigment producing cells include *lentigo* (infantile and senile forms) and *mongoloid spots*. Among the benign tumors are *pigmented nevi* and *blue nevi*, while *malignant melanomas* belong to the group of malignant pigmented tumors.

Pigmented intradermal nevus (Fig. 9.23) *consists of ball-shaped collections of nevus cells localized in the dermal papillae. As they are derived from melanoblasts they are of neuroectodermal origin.* Histologically (Fig. 9.23) they have a papillary structure and show marked cornification of the superficial epidermis (→ 1). Between the elongated rete pegs can be seen the dark blue staining nevus cells (→ 3). Beneath the epidermis there is a zone of connective tissue (→ 2) containing no tumor cells. The nevus cells show distinct melanin pigmentation.

Different sorts of pigmented nevi are recognized—nevi with *proliferative activity at the junction between dermis and epidermis (junctional nevus)* occurring most commonly in children and able to convert to a compound nevus. A *combination nevus* is a pigmented intradermal nevus that simultaneously shows border activity. Pure pigmented *intradermal or corium nevi* correspond to the type described above. They can be flat, raised or verrucous.

Blue nevus (Fig. 9.24) *forms a round ill-defined skin nodule of dark blue color comprised of elongated, markedly melanin-pigmented cells* (melanocytes of mesodermal origin). Histologically, beneath a normal epidermis and in the region of the mid-corium there are elongated cells containing granular brown pigment (→). This pigment is iron negative and when stained by **Masson's silver stain** shows black, intracytoplasmic desposits (Fig. 9.24a).

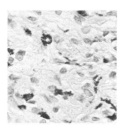

Fig. 9.24a. Blue nevus, Masson silver stain; 320×.

Malignant melanoma (Fig. 9.25) *is the malignant variant of pigmented tumors and biologically is characterized by the frequency with which it metastasizes.* Histologically it is formed of cells that resemble in part carcinoma and in part sarcoma. This part sarcoma-like and part carcinoma-like structure is absolutely typical of malignant melanoma (sarcomatous-like carcinomas also occur in thyroid and hypernephroid renal carcinomas). The cytological evidences of malignancy are present: cell atypia (cells of different sizes), mitoses (→) and invasion of epidermis. The stroma shows an inflammatory reaction as well. About 10% of malignant melanomas are not pigmented (amelanotic melanoma).

Malignant melanoma occurs most frequently in men after 40 years of age. It is especially frequent in white men in the tropics. The commonest sites are skin (face, extremities), genitalia, eye, oral cavity and colon. Among melanomas of the skin it is important to distinguish *superficial spreading melanoma* (intraepidermal metastasis), *the infiltrating, nodular type* and melanoma in the base of *malignant lentigo* (diffuse infiltration of the epidermis by pigment cells without infiltration of the *corium-melanoma in situ-melanosis praeblastomatosa circumscripta of Dubreuilh).*

For the most part malignant melanoma develops only after puberty. Occasionally in small children pigmented tumors are seen that have marked cellular polymorphism and sometimes invasive growth. These pigmented tumors are benign and are referred to as *benign juvenile melanomas* or *Spitz-Allen tumors.*

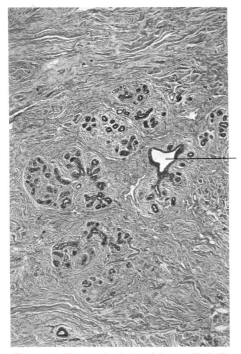

Fig. 9.26. Fibrous dysplasia of breast; H & E, 32×.

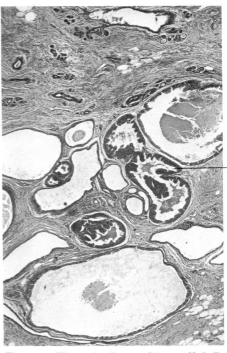

Fig. 9.27. Fibrocystic disease of breast; H & E, 32×

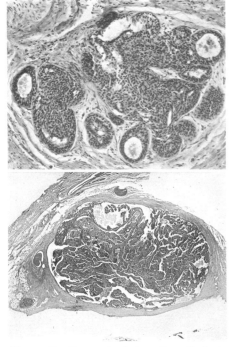

Fig. 9.28. Above: dysplasia with epitheliosis; H & E, 80×. Below: dysplasia with intraductal proliferation; H & E, 10×.

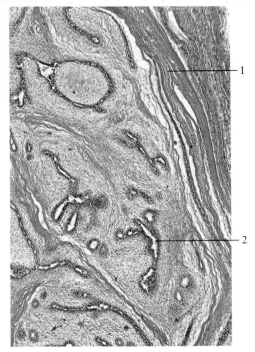

Fig. 9.29. Intracanalicular fibroadenoma; van Gieson stain, 50×.

Breast

Dysplasia is a disorder of the female breast in which there are simultaneously atrophy, hyperplasia and meta-plasia as well as various clinical signs. It is due to dysfunction of sex hormones, but the pathogenesis is still un-known. For prognostic and therapeutic reasons a distinction is made between *simple mammary dysplasia* and *proliferative dysplasia*.

In *simple mammary dysplasia* proliferation of intra- and perilobular fibrous connective tissue predomi-nates, hence the name **fibrous dysplasia** (Fig. 9.26). The mammary lobules are encased by collagenous stroma and the acini are pressed together. The arrow points to a dilated excretory duct. In **fibrocystic dysplasia** (fibrocystic disease, Fig. 9.27) cysts lined by flattened epithelium dominate the histological picture. In part they are dilated pre-existing excretory ducts and in part newly formed cysts lined with tall eosinophilic epithelium showing apocrine secretion and reminiscent of sweat glands (therefore the designation **sweat gland metaplasia** →). The fibrous component of the dysplasia is seen in the upper third of the picture.

The myoepithelial cells (basket cells) are also hypertrophied in simple dysplasia of the breast. They are large cells, seen in the region of the acinar epithelium, with distended vesicular cytoplasm and distinct dark nuclei. Frequently they form a discrete, solid nodule, the center of which may be sclerotic. Such lesions are described as *adenosis* or *sclerosing adenosis*. They are of diagnostic significance since they can be mistaken for a scirrhous carcinoma when seen under low magnification or in frozen sections.

In **proliferative dysplasia** (Fig. 9.28) *there is marked intraductal epithelial proliferation with forma-tion of solid, adenomatous or papillary structures*. In **epitheliosus** (Fig. 9.29, above) small excretory ducts are filled with proliferated epithelium, which may show a **papillary structure**, i.e., they consist of branching stroma covered by epithelium (*pseudopapillary growth,* in contrast, only consists of epithelium). Of particular prognostic significance is the presence of cell atypia (polymorphic cells with hyperchromatic nuclei, increased mitoses) which is found in *atypical proliferating breast dysplasia*.

Simple dysplasia of the breast is common and develops in practically every breast after age 25 and should not be considered precancerous. On the other hand *atypical proliferative breast dysplasia* has an increased risk of cancer. Women with this lesion have up to 30 times the chance of developing breast cancer than do "normal women." Other cancer risk factors are: early menarche, late menopause, child-lessness, still births, prolonged estrogen therapy and mammary carcinoma in sisters.

Fibroadenoma of the breast (Fig. 9.29) *is a benign, true mixed tumor with both epithelial and mesen-chymal components, that occurs preferentially in young women.* Figure 9.29 shows an **intracanalicu-lar fibroadenoma** with branching tube-like structures lined by deeply stained epithelium and having slit-like lumens (→ 2). The connective tissue in the immediate neighborhood of the epithelium is myxomatous and does not stain as intensely with van Gieson stain as normal connective tissue (→ 1). In some fibroadenomas the connective tissue surrounds in concentric fashion differentiated tubules show-ing epithelial proliferation (*pericanalicular fibroadenoma*).

Fibroadenomas are solid, greyish white, coarsely lobulated nodules of firm consistency. They are easily enucleated. Rarely there is marked atypical cellular proliferation, particularly of the mesenchy-mal component. Such tumors can reach considerable size and are then called *cystosarcoma phylloides*. They are usually only locally malignant and seldom have distant metastases.

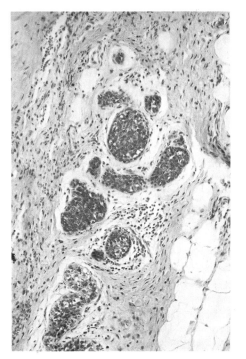

Fig. 9.30. Lobular carcinoma in situ of breast; H & E, 100×.

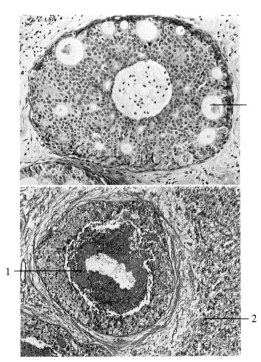

Fig. 9.31. Above: Cribriform carcinoma of breast; H & E, 50× Below: Comedocarcinoma, H & E, 50×.

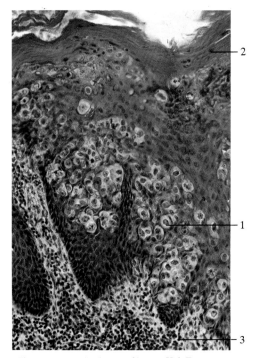

Fig. 9.32. Paget's disease of breast; H & E, 200×

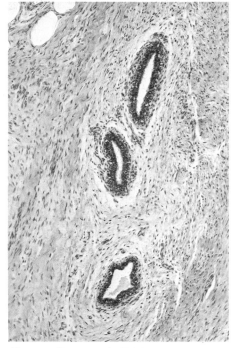

Fig. 9.33. Gynecomastia; H & E, 80×.

Mammary Carcinoma–Gynecomastia

In women, carcinoma of the breast is the chief cause of death from malignant tumors (about 20% of all malignant neoplasms). The average age of these women is 60 years. The WHO international classification of carcinoma of the breast contains the following groups. Group I: non-infiltrating intraduct and lobular carcinoma. Group II: infiltrating carcinoma (scirrhous, solid carcinoma simplex, medullary carcinoma). Group III: special types of carcinoma (papillary, cribriform, mucinous, medullary carcinoma with lymphoid infiltration of stroma, squamous carcinoma, Paget's disease, carcinoma arising in a fibroadenoma). Carcinomas of Group II make up about 92% of breast cancers and the other 2 groups 8%.

Lobular carcinoma in situ (Fig. 9.30) as a rule is discovered by chance on histological examination of the breast. The figure shows solid islands of atypical cells replacing and filling the lobule. The basement membrane is preserved which is an indication of lack of stromal invasion.

Most authors are of the opinion that *lobular carcinoma in situ* of the breast is a precancerous lesion and not a true carcinoma growing in situ (see p. 315).

Other breast tumors with an intraductal pattern of growth are: papillary, cribriform and comedocarcinomas. In **cribriform carcinoma** (Fig. 9.31) the tumor cells fill large and medium sized excretory ducts producing multiple small lumens (→ "glands within glands") thus giving the tumor a characteristic sieve-like appearance. In **comedocarcinoma,** the ducts are also distended by the solid growth of the carcinoma. Typical of this carcinoma are eosinophilic, central areas of necrosis (→ 1)—often with granular calcium deposits—and marked polymorphism of the tumor cells. Comedocarcinoma usually shows invasion of the stroma (→ 2).

Paget's disease of the breast (Fig. 9.32) *refers to intradermal spread of an intraduct carcinoma and is manifested clinically by an eczematous lesion of the nipple.* Figure 9.32 shows the large, clear carcinoma cells (→ 1), which are to be found in all layers of the epidermis. The cells are distinctly polymorphic and there are many mitoses. The overlying surface epidermis is hyperkeratotic (→ 2) and the underlying stroma contains chronic inflammatory cells (→ 3).

The non-dependence of the prognosis of mammary carcinoma on therapy: in the last years it has become clear that the prognosis of various malignant tumors (in particular mammary carcinoma) finally depends on the pathological anatomical findings rather than the therapy. The final fate of a women with mammary carcinoma is not determined by the primary tumor itself, but rather by the development of lymphogenous (axillary, supraclavicular) and hematogenous (lung, liver, bones) distant metastases. If lymph node metastasis is already present, then only a small percentage of these women will survive beyond 5 years. Lymph node metastases occur chiefly with primary tumors of infiltrative type (Group II) having a diameter greater than 2 cm. In contrast the 5- and 10-year survival rate is relatively high for mucinous carcinoma, medullary carcinoma with lymphocytic stroma and non-infiltrating carcinomas of Group I.

Gynecomastia (Fig. 9.33) *is a hormonally conditioned hyperplasia of the ducts and stroma in the male breast.* Histologically there is mild proliferation of duct epithelium. The connective tissue is increased and in the region of the excretory ducts shows a concentric and myxomatous arrangement. There is practically no formation or differentiation of acini. In *pseudogynecomastia* enlargement of the breast is attributable to overgrowth of fat.

Gynecomastia is seen regularly at the onset of puberty and regresses spontaneously. Otherwise it occurs in men with liver cirrhosis and following prolonged estrogen therapy (e.g., for prostatic carcinoma). *Carcinoma of the breast in males* is a rarity (less than 1% of all breast carcinomas). It is usually observed after estrogen therapy and in the Klinefelter syndrome.

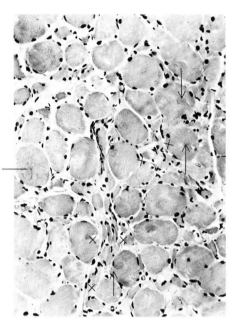

Fig. 10.1. Recent atrophy with degeneration of muscle fibers occurring in acute polyneuritis; H & E, 170×.

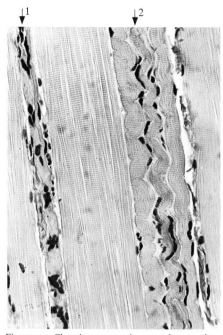

Fig. 10.2. Chronic neurogenic muscular atrophy in polyneuritis; H & E, 320×.

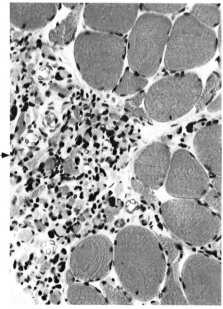

Fig. 10.3. Progressive spinal muscular atrophy (infantile form); H & E, 233×.

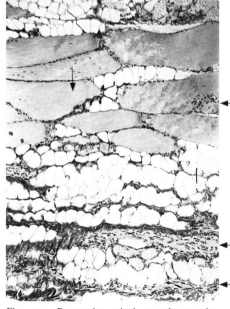

Fig. 10.4. Progressive spinal muscular atrophy (pseudomyogenic form); van Gieson, 60×.

10. Muscles

Skeletal muscles can be affected in *generalized disease states* or they can be *affected independently*. In both cases, the result is either *degeneration of the muscle fibers* themselves or secondary involvement of the muscle from extension of primary disease of the *interstitial tissues*. In primary degenerative muscle disease, acute degenerative changes occur and lead to necrosis. They must, of course, be differentiated from chronic atrophies of muscle fibers.

Muscular atrophies are the result of neurogenic or of myogenic disease. The basis of *neurogenic atrophies* is peripheral denervation, due either to a primary lesion in the anterior horn cells *(spinal muscular atrophy)* or to a lesion along the course of the *peripheral motor nerves*.

The early stages of **neurogenic muscular atrophy** are well seen in cases of polyneuritis. Figure 10.1 **(recent muscular atrophy in acute polyneuritis)** illustrates the atrophy of individual muscle fibers in cross-section (between the crosses). The fibers are smaller and the nuclei lie closer together. Although the other muscle fibers seem unchanged in size, they already show early degeneration, as evidenced by the loss of their regular fibrillary cytoplasmic structure (compare this with Fig. 10.3) and the very characteristic localized clumps of contractile material, the so-called target fibers (→).

If neurogenic atrophy develops slowly, the histological picture will consist of groups of markedly atrophic muscle fibers intermixed with essentially intact fibers. The former represent areas innervated by affected motor axons or their branches **(chronic neurogenic muscular atrophy in polyneuritis).** Figure 10.2 is a longitudinal section showing typical groups of atrophic muscle fibers. It can be seen that the fibers about → 1 are more severely atrophied than those about → 2. The atrophy in this case affects only small groups, corresponding to the so-called subunits of a motor unit.

Motor unit = anterior horn cell with its corresponding peripheral motor axon, its collaterals, the motor end plates and the muscle fibers. Depending upon the type of muscle involved, a motor unit is composed of 800–1,700 or more muscle fibers.

Spinal muscular atrophy, as a result of destruction of anterior horn cells of the spinal cord, always involves entire motor units and not just subunits, leading to atrophy of all the muscle fibers supplied by a particular unit. Figure 10.3 **(the infantile form of progressive spinal muscular atrophy)** shows more widespread involvement of larger groups of muscle fibers (→). The cross-sectional view reveals the very thin fibers and closely placed nuclei so that they seem to have multiplied (frustrated regeneration). The other muscle fibers are unaffected and have retained the integrity of their intracytoplasmic structure.

Spinal progressive muscular atrophy of adults (pseudomyogenic type) (Fig. 10.4). This lesion progresses very slowly so that adaptation and regeneration are prominent. The figure shows a longitudinal section of a muscle bundle (→ 1) surrounded by tongues of connective tissue and proliferated lipomatous tissue. The groups of intact muscle fibers undergo compensatory hypertrophy as a result of increased demand. There are increased numbers of nuclei, as well as centrally located multinuclear muscle cells (→ 2). This fibroadipose transformation and replacement of muscle is a nonspecific manifestation of chronic, progressive wasting of muscles. Similar changes to these are also seen in chronic muscular atrophy having an inflammatory or degenerative basis (Fig. 10.5).

I am indebted to the late Prof. Erbslöh (Director of the Neurology Clinic, University of Giessen) for Figures 10.1–10.7 and for his suggestions.

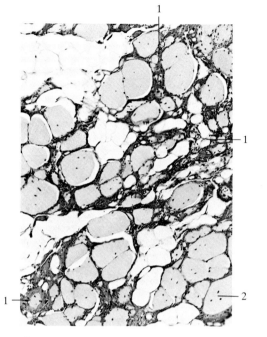

Fig. 10.5. Progressive muscular dystrophy (Erb); van Gieson, 80×.

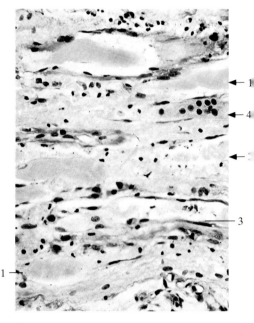

Fig. 10.6. Early muscular necrosis in acute polymyositis; H & E, 200×.

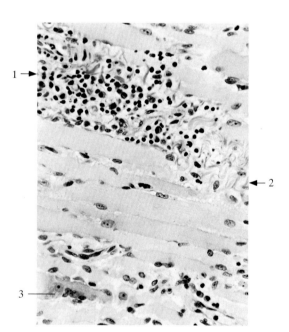

Fig. 10.7. Dermatomyositis; H & E, 250×.

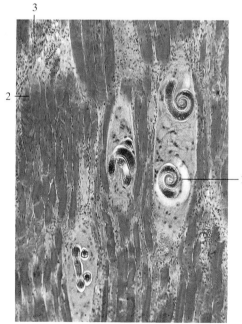

Fig. 10.8. Trichinosis; H & E, 78×.

Progressive muscular dystrophy (Erb) (Fig. 10.5). In contrast to spinal progressive muscular atrophy, *the primary disturbance in progressive muscular dystrophy (myogenic atrophy) resides in the muscle cells themselves* (hereditary metabolic disorder of unknown origin). Thus, the atrophic manifestations do not correspond to a motor unit distribution. Instead, they represent disseminated atrophy of individual fibers without regular distribution.

The section shows atrophic fibers ($\rightarrow$ 1) adjoining numerous normal as well as hypertrophic fibers. Many have central nuclei ($\rightarrow$ 2). In addition, the muscle fibers are surrounded by connective tissue and the degenerated and atrophic fibers have been replaced by fat tissue *(fibro-adipose replacement)*. The scar ring can produce secondarily a lobular arrangement of muscle bundles, giving a cirrhosis-like appearance.

Dystrophic muscles frequently show early stages of muscle fiber degeneration, such as occur in systemic diseases, e.g., the progressive degeneration of the abdominal musculature in typhoid. Figure 10.6 **(early muscular necrosis in acute polymyositis)** shows several types of degeneration that may lead to necrosis. The first change is often progressive waxy degeneration ($\rightarrow$ 1) leading to dissolution of the fibrous proteins and cross-striations. Gradually, as the nuclei degenerate, lumpy aggregates ($\rightarrow$ 2) become evident and as the sarcoplasm comes apart and vanishes, only empty sarcolemmal sheaths are left behind ($\rightarrow$ 3) (compare p. 40). Focal groups of muscle nuclei can be seen indicating a regenerative activity ($\rightarrow$ 4).

Acute muscular degeneration of such severity often results in development of the so-called *crush-syndrome* in the kidney (p. 163). Not only does it occur with necrotizing myositis but also with *intoxications* (e.g., CO poisoning) or in severe muscle trauma.

Dermatomyositis (Fig. 10.7) is a *necrotizing panmyositis with dermatitis* which in the acute stages prominently displays the degenerative and necrotizing changes described above. In addition, the tissues are densely infiltrated with lymphocytes and plasma cells. In the subacute and chronic stages of this intermittently progressive disease, there is mainly interstitial infiltration ($\rightarrow$ 1), scarring ($\rightarrow$ 2) and tissue replacement. Additionally, there may be marked regeneration of the muscle fibers themselves ($\rightarrow$ 3).

The clinical course of *necrotizing polymyositis* consists of extensive paralysis of the peripheral muscles, which, because of its resemblance to the muscular paralysis of trichinosis, is at times referred to as pseudotrichinosis.

Trichinosis of muscle (Fig. 10.8). *The embryos of* Trichinella spiralis *pass through the lacteals of the intestine into the blood stream, and so reach striated muscle, where they develop into spiral-shaped larvae.* Sexually immature thread worms live in the small intestine (man, swine, dogs, etc.). When the trichina reach the stomach they develop into sexually mature worms. In massive trichinal infestation intestinal manifestations are prominant (diarrhea) followed by muscle pains (myolysis). Later, prolonged complaints of muscular rheumatism may develop. Histologically, the cross-cut or tangentially cut, spiral-shaped trichinellae are surrounded by a hyaline capsule ($\rightarrow$ 1) and can be easily seen even at low power. Adjoining muscle fibers show considerable alteration, e.g., granular and waxy degeneration ($\rightarrow$ 2). The interstitial tissue contains aggregations of eosinophils and chronic inflammatory cells.

Macroscopic: Small white nodules.

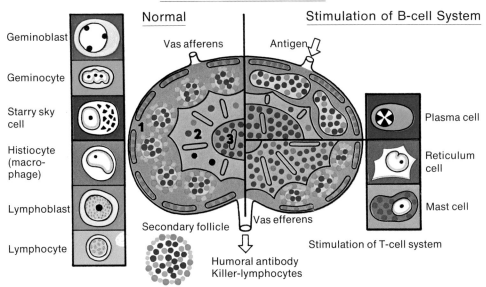

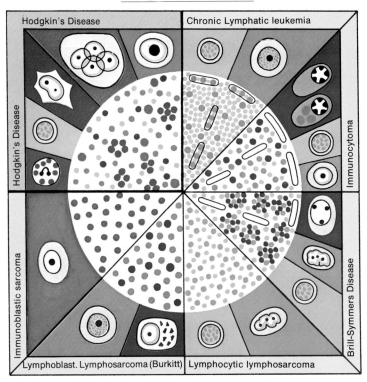

Fig. 11.1. Schematic illustration of normal lymph nodes, nonspecific lymphadenitis and malignant lymphomas.

11. Lymph Nodes – Spleen

Lymph nodes: Recent advances in immunology have made clear that the immunological aspects of the various lymphomas must be coordinated with their morphology (Fig. 11.1 above). When an antigen reaches lymph nodes by way of the vas afferens, it may stimulate either *humoral antibody production* (**B-cell system** = bone marrow dependent system) or the *cell-bound immune system* (**T-cells** = thymus dependent system). The B-cell system is represented by the secondary follicles with germinal centers in the cortex (1 in Fig. 11.1, above) and medulla (3 in Fig. 11.1, above) of lymph nodes. The T-cell system is represented by the paracortical zone (lying between medulla and cortex: 2 in Fig. 11.1, above). Experimentally after thymectomy in newborn animals there is no paracortical zone.

On **stimulation of the B-cell system** (Fig. 11.1, above, right) the addition of antigen causes an intensified reaction, especially of the germinal centers of the secondary follicles which may become enormously enlarged and contain increased numbers of germinoblasts and germinocytes as well as phagocytes containing nuclear fragments (so-called starry sky cells). It is assumed that the antigen is taken up and manufactured by cells of the germinal center. Production of humoral antibody takes place in the plasma cells of the medulla of lymph nodes. The medulla then increases in width because of the numerous masses of plasma cells. In this way the immunological message of the cortex is transmitted to the medulla (cellular, lymphogenous?). If the **T-cell system** (Fig. 11.1, above, right) is stimulated by antigen then the paracortical zone increases as do the T-lymphocytes, reticulum cells and mast cells. In the spleen the follicles correspond to the B-cell system and the pulp to the T-cell system. In the past these different sorts of reaction in lymph nodes have been shown to have practical significance: in the area of drainage of a carcinoma (breast, uterine cervix) if stimulation of T-cells (paracortical zone) was observed the patient's prognosis was better than in patients showing activity in the B-cell region or no lymph node reaction at all.

In **nonspecific lymphadenitis** there is an increase in sinus histiocytes which are the probably first site of uptake of antigen. The lymphatic tissue may respond by follicular hyperplasia (enlarged reaction centers) and an increase in the medulla (B-cell stimulation) or by lymphoid hyperplasia (increase of the paracortical zone). Both of these reactions may occur simultaneously.

Special sorts of lymph node reactions. Focal epithelioid cell reaction (Piringer): small nodules of clustered epithelioid cells in the cortex with sinus histiocytosis accompanying nonspecific lymphadenitis occurs in toxoplasmosis and also is seen with carcinomas and in the very early stages of lymphogranulomatosis. *Sarcoid:* an epithelioid cell granuloma (larger than in Piringer). *Caseous tuberculosis:* caseation (necrosis surrounded by epithelioid cells and Langhans' giant cells). *Pseudotuberculosis:* 1. *Pasteurella pseudotuberculosis* (pseudotuberculosis of Masshoff) chiefly in mesenteric lymph nodes. 2. *Tularemia (Pasteurella tularensis)* contracted from wild game (pelt and game handlers). 3. *Cat scratch fever* (viruses of the Miyaga group). All these forms have a similar appearance. At first there is focal overgrowth and fusion of reticulum cells and then demarkation by epithelioid cells, especially reticulum cells.

Tumors of lymph nodes (Fig. 11.1, lower): primary tumors of lymph nodes as a rule are malignant (exception: *benign lymphocytoma of Castleman,* arising preferentially in the mediastinum and showing germinal centers with onion layer-like arrangement of lymphocytes) and are classified under the general heading of **malignant lymphomas.** Among such tumors **Hodgkin's disease** has been separated as an independent disease process and the remaining tumors have been classified as **non-Hodgkin lymphomas** (see p. 241).

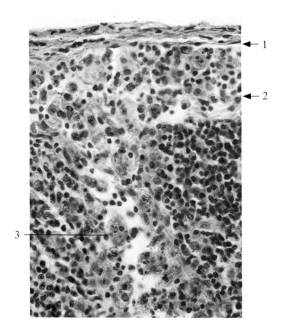

Fig. 11.2. Acute nonspecific lymphadenitis (sinus catarrh); H & E, 360×.

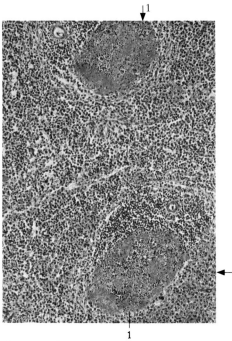

Fig. 11.3. Follicular necrosis in diphtheria; H & E, 108×.

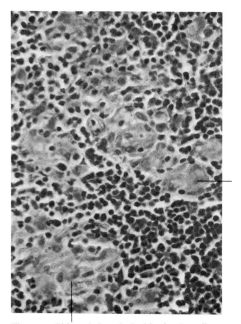

Fig. 11.4. Piringer's lymphadenitis (focal small epithelioid cell reaction); H & E, 420×.

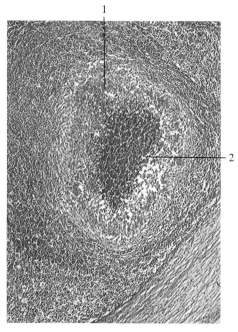

Fig. 11.5. Suppurative reticulocytic lymph-adenitis; H & E, 80×.

Forms of Lymph Node Reactions

Acute nonspecific lymphadenitis (sinus catarrh) (Fig. 11.2) is one histological form of lymphadenitis (see p. 233). The histological feature of sinus catarrh is proliferation of the reticulum cells (histiocytes) of the sinus due to their exposure to increasing amounts of resorbable substances (protein breakdown products, as from nearby cancers, bacteria, toxins, etc.). The proliferating reticuloendothelial cells become detached in large numbers and lie in the lumen of the sinus as isolated, round or oval histiocytes with a pale eccentric nucleus: *sinus histiocytosis*. Figure 11.2 shows the cortical sinus of a lymph node with nonspecific lymphadenitis. The sinuses are wide (→ 1 and → 2: border of the sinus) and filled with large cells with abundant cytoplasm which are detached reticulum cells containing cytoplasmic nuclear fragments (→ 3). Single lymphocytes and leukocytes are also present.

Follicular necrosis is diphtheria (Fig. 11.3). A particularly pronounced lymphadenitis with necrosis of the germinal centers of the secondary follicles occurs in diphtheria (direct toxic effect). Histologically, the reactive centers of the follicles are changed into necrotic eosinophilic masses (→ 1) in which nuclear debris can still be seen. A narrow margin of lymphocytes is preserved at the periphery of the follicles. The remainder of the lymph node is acutely inflamed and frequently hemorrhagic (→ 2). Also seen in the mesenteric lymph nodes of small children with acute enteritis (nondiphtheritic).

Piringer's lymphadenitis (Fig. 11.4). In most cases, Piringer's lymphadenitis (Piringer-Kuchinka, 1953) is due to toxoplasmosis (see p. 279), and occurs preferentially in the lymph nodes of the neck (75%). The characteristic histological changes are small focal collections of epithelioid cells, proliferation of immature histiocytes in the sinuses, hyperplasia of lymphoid follicles having large germinal centers, and perilymphadenitis. Figure 11.4 shows several groups of 4–8 large epithelioid cells with abundant pale eosinophilic cytoplasm (→). The nuclei of these cells are oval or shaped like a cat's tongue and possess a loose chromatin structure.

Similar foci of small epithelioid cells may be found in lymph nodes in the early stages of Hodgkin's disease, in infectious mononucleosis, and in lymph nodes draining degenerating tumors.

Suppurative reticulocytic lymphadenitis (Masshoff, Fig. 11.5). This type of lymphadenitis occurs in various infections: Yersinia or Pasteurella pseudotuberculosis infection of mesenteric and ileocecal lymph nodes which, in children, mimics the clinical picture of appendicitis (Masshoff, 1953): infections with Pasteurella tularensis and the agent of cat scratch fever (virus) which attack the lymph nodes regional to the infection (primary complex), especially in juveniles.

All these infections of lymph nodes show a similar histological picture. In the fully developed stages, there is extensive focal reticulum cell proliferation (→ 1) with areas of destruction of tissue (abscess → 2) surrounded by polymorphonuclear granulocytes. Next to the abscess and the cuff of reticulocytes there is a secondary follicle with a distinct reaction center (→ 3) and several so-called stellate cells (→ 4), phagocytes containing nuclear fragments). Other changes seen in this disease—not represented in the illustration—are considerable perilymphadenitis, endophlebitis and endarteritis of neighboring blood vessels.

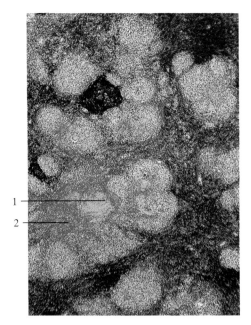

Fig. 11.6. Hyperplastic (epithelioid cell) tuberculous lymphadenitis; van Gieson stain, 44×.

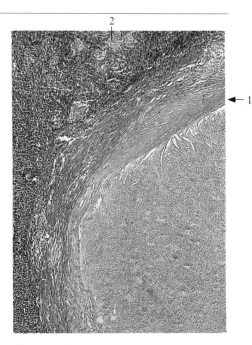

Fig. 11.7. Caseous tuberculous lymphadenitis; H & E, 20×.

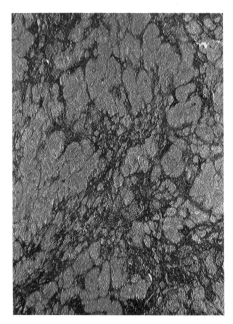

Fig. 11.8. Sarcoidosis of hilar pulmonary lymph nodes; H & E, 40×.

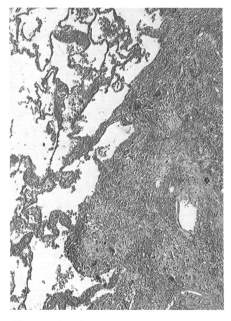

Fig. 11.9. Sarcoid scar in the lung; H & E, 100×.

Specific Inflammation of Lymph Nodes

In hyperplastic tuberculous lymphadenitis (Fig. 11.6), the microscopic section shows numerous, closely packed tubercles containing chiefly epithelioid cells. The rounded, frequently confluent lesions are conspicuous under low-power magnification. Slightly higher magnification reveals typical epithelioid cells (see p. 30) and solitary Langhans type giant cells. There can be secondary central necrosis (→ 1). In older lesions, a good deal of hyaline connective tissue may appear (→ 2) and finally lead to scar formation.

In **caseating tuberculosis of lymph nodes** (Fig. 11.7), necrosis completely dominates the histological picture, and the specific granulation tissue is visible only as a narrow border or, as in this illustration, is for the most part replaced by a fibrous capsule (→ 1). With the unaided eye, large homogeneous eosinophilic masses (caseation) are seen to have replaced the lymphoid tissue. Higher magnification shows extensive finely granular areas of necrosis without remnants of the original tissues. Peripheral to the focus of caseation there are noncaseating granulomas of epithelioid cells (→ 2).

Macroscopic: Compartmented cut surface with focal or map-like, dry, yellow areas.

Sarcoidosis (Boeck's sarcoid, Besnier-Boeck-Schaumann disease, Figs. 11.8, 11.9 and 11.10) is a disease entity that arises sui generis. The morphological substrate is an epithelioid cell tubercle without caseation. Practically any organ can be affected; lymph nodes in the pulmonary hilus are involved at the beginning of the disease (clinical stage I, 40% heal).

Figure 11.8 shows a pulmonary hilar lymph node under a scanning lens. There are numerous epithelioid cell granulomas which in part are confluent. Higher magnification shows the same histological picture as Figure 3.43 on p. 106: a thick layer, chiefly of plump epithelioid cells with oval or cat's tongue shaped nuclei as well as Langhans' giant cells. In contrast to tuberculosis there is no caseation and the granulomas tend to fibrose from the periphery toward the center. Frequently the epithelioid cells contain small conchoid-shaped calcified bodies, (Fig. 11.10), so-called *conchoid* bodies or Schaumann bodies (cell inclusions: calcified lysosomes? are detected in 80% of sarcoidosis cases and in only 6% of tuberculosis). Figure 11.10 shows these small bodies with doubly refractive centers in polarized light.

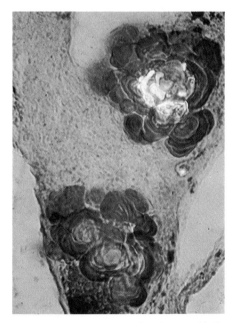

From the lymph nodes in the pulmonary hilus the granulomas spread by lymphatics to the lungs (inter- and intra-alveolar, perivascular and in the bronchial wall). Stage II, 40% heal. Figure 11.9 shows the beginning of Stage III (fibrosis of lung, death from dyspnea) with scarring of the granuloma and solitary giant cells of Langhans type. The surrounding tissue shows emphysema (scar emphysema). Distant organs may be seeded hematogenously (see p. 138).

Note: epithelioid cell granulomas occur in tuberculosis, sarcoidosis, after beryllium exposure, accumulation of dye stuffs, in lymph nodes draining malignant tumors, in terminal ileitis, toxoplasmosis etc. The granulomas are thus a relatively nonspecific tissue reaction to the most varied agents. The diagnosis of sarcoidosis must be clinically confirmed.

Young women are chiefly affected. Frequency 1:1000

Fig.11.10. Schaumann bodies in sarcoidosis (polarized light); H & E, 700×.

237

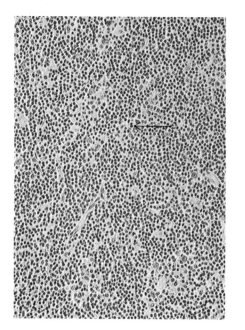

Fig. 11.11. Hodgkin's disease, lymphocytic predominance; H & E, 250×.

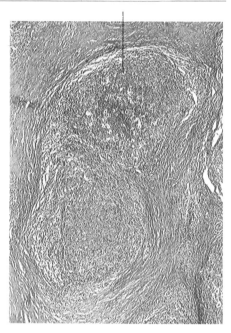

Fig. 11.12. Hodgkin's disease, nodular sclerosis; H & E, 100×.

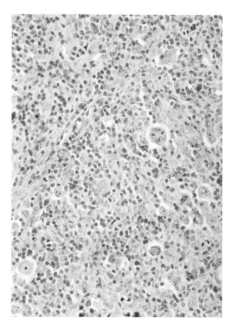

Fig. 11.13. Hodgkin's disease, mixed form; Giemsa stain, 200×.

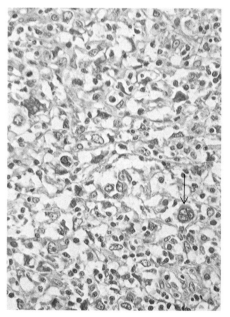

Fig. 11.14. Hodgkin's disease, reticular form; H & E, 200×.

Hodgkin's Disease (Lymphogranulomatosis)

Hodgkin's disease (malignant lymphoma of Hodgkin, Figs. 11.11–11.15) *is the most frequent of all malignant diseases of lymph nodes* (50% of primary lymph node tumors). *It has a proliferative, granulomatous type of growth that possesses specific tissue characteristics.* The typical histological appearance shows the following: destruction of the normal structure of lymph nodes by granulation tissue comprised of atypical reticulum cells (eventually epithelioid cells), lymphocytes, eosinophilic granulocytes, Hodgkin and Reed-Sternberg giant cells (Fig. 11.15). The characteristic cell type of the disease is the Hodgkin cell which arises either from reticulum cells or lymphoblasts (× and → in Fig. 11.15). Hodgkin cells have a striking, pale, vesicular nucleus with a distinct nuclear membrane surrounded by a narrow margin of poorly defined, basophilic cytoplasm (Giemsa stain). From these cells are derived the multinucleated Reed-Sternberg cells. Their nuclei are likewise vesicular and partially overlap and they have abundant cytoplasm (Fig. 11.15 → 2). As a result of Luke's studies (see Kaplan, 1972) different forms of Hodgkin's disease each with a different prognosis are recognized:

1. **Lymphocytic predominance** (diffuse or nodular): previously called paragranuloma. Figure 11.11 shows the predominance of lymphocytes whereas only a few atypical reticulum cells and Hodgkin cells (→) are seen.

Eosinophilic leukocytes for the most part are lacking. Mostly affects young men (30–40 years). Good prognosis (50–60% live longer than 6 years). Transition to mixed form or reticular forms is possible.

2. **Nodular sclerotic form:** a special form that seldom changes to another type of Hodgkin's disease. Figure 11.12 shows the typical findings. The lymph nodes are traversed by broad bands of collagenous connective tissue (doubly refractive in polarized light) having a ring-like arrangement. The granulation tissue consists chiefly of lymphocytes, solitary atypical reticulum cells and so-called "lacunar cells" (histiocytes with finely granular cytoplasm) which appear as small, round clear cells, (→) in Figure 11.12. Chiefly affects young women. Sixty per cent live longer than 6 years.

3. **Mixed form** (Fig. 11.13): There are typical granulomatous tissue as described above and atypical reticulum cells, lymphocytes, eosinophilic leukocytes, Reed-Sternberg giant cells and Hodgkin cells. Survival rate: 25% live longer than 6 years. Occurs about equally in men and women.

4. **Lymphocytic depletion:**
a) **Diffuse fibrosis:** Collagenous scar tissue with little granulomatous tissue. Scanty lymphocytes, abundant atypical reticulum cells and Reed-Sternberg giant cells.

b) **Reticular form** (Hodgkin sarcoma): Figure 11.14 shows that the cellular growth consists chiefly of reticulum cells and Hodgkin cells especially Reed-Sternberg giant cells (→) while lymphocytes are almost completely lacking. Hematogenous metastases. Both sexes are equally affected. Course: only 20% live longer than 2 years.

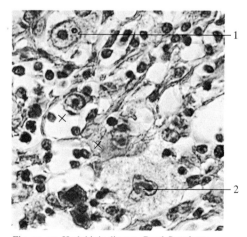

Fig. 11.15. Hodgkin's disease, Reed-Sternberg giant cells; Giemsa stain, 400×.

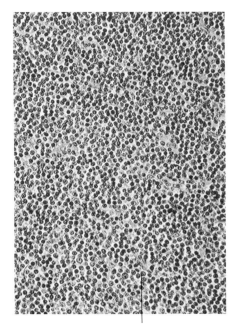

Fig. 11.16. Chronic lymphatic leukemia; H & E, 300×.

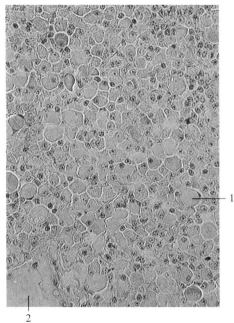

Fig. 11.17. Immunocytoma; H & E, 300×.

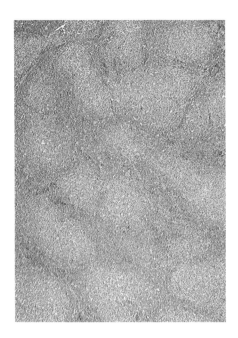

Fig. 11.18. Brill-Symmers disease; Giemsa stain, 40×.

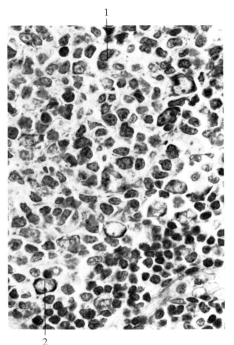

Fig. 11.19. Brill-Symmers disease; Giemsa stain, 500×. (Stein).

Non-Hodgkin Lymphomas

Malignant lymphoma (non-Hodgkin lymphoma, see Fig. 11.1. p. 232). By the coordinated use of subtle investigative techniques (Giemsa stain, electronmicroscopy) and recent advances in immunology and of retrospective clinical studies, it has been possible to devise a prognostically significant classification of malignant lymphomas (Lennert et al, 1975). Unfortunately there is still no uniformly agreed on nomenclature. As of today we distinguish between *lymphomas with low grade malignancy* (average course between 5–15 years; chronic lymphatic leukemia, immunocytoma, lymphocytic lymphosarcoma, Brill-Symmers disease) and *lymphomas with higher grade malignancy* (course up to 3 years: immunoblastic sarcoma, lymphoblastic lymphosarcoma).

Chronic lymphatic leukemia (CLL., Fig. 11.16) may occur with an aleukemic (so-called lymphadenosis) subleukemic or leukemic blood picture. Histologically (Fig. 11.16) there is characteristically diffuse proliferation of typical lymphocytes with only a few lymphoblasts ($\rightarrow$). Lymph node sinuses are mostly preserved. Splenic follicles and hepatic periportal fields are infiltrated with leukemic cells. Bone marrow is also involved.

Most frequent of all leukemias. Age 60–70 years. $\male : \female = 2:1$. Course 3–10 years. Immunoglobulin (IgM) can be detected in the tissue.

Immunocytoma *(lymphocytoid-plasma cell immunocytoma* Fig. 11.17). These cases were formerly called *Waldenstrom's macroglobulinemia,* which showed a somewhat different tissue pattern (lymphocytoid plasma cells, mast cells, protein lakes) and a constant increase of blood IgM. Figure 11.17 shows the typical increase of plasma cells containing cytoplasmic Russel bodies ($\rightarrow$ 1, storage of secreted immunoglobulin). In addition there are lymphoid elements that resemble in part lymphoid plasma cells. Immunoblasts are also seen, similar to those shown in Figure 11.21. At $\rightarrow$ 2 there is a portion of a protein lake. IgM and IgG can be detected in tissue but not always in blood.

Higher age groups: men attacked more frequently than women. Longer course. Corticoid therapy.

Giant follicular lymphoma (synonyms—germinoblastoma, **Brill-Symmers disease,** giant follicular lymphoblastoma, Figs. 11.18 and 11.19). Figure 11.18 shows the lymph nodes to contain numerous pale germinal centers which for the most part are smaller than in nonspecific lymphadenitis. With higher magnification (Fig. 11.19) it is possible to identify the cells in the germinal centers: germinocytes with oval nuclei ($\rightarrow$ 1) and germinoblasts with marginal nucleoli and basophilic cytoplasm ($\rightarrow$ 2). Absent are macrophages containing nuclear debris such as are seen in nonspecific lymphadenitis.

Age: 20–30 years and 60 years. Men are chiefly affected. 60% live longer than 5 years. Fifty per cent of cases progress to sarcoma (germinoblastic sarcoma). Tissue IgM or IgG increased.

Lymphocytic lymphosarcoma (well-differentiated or small cell lymphosarcoma): diffuse proliferation of lymphocyte-like cells but having paler nuclei than lymphocytes, appearing more square than round and without distinct cytoplasm. According to Lennert, these should be considered as germinocytes (diffuse germinocytoma). May have leukemic manifestations. Occurs at all ages. Prognosis variable (months–years). Tissue IgM present.

Lymphoblastic lymphosarcoma (Fig. 11.20): the best known representative of this group is the *Burkitt tumor* (see p. 288) which occurs mostly in central Africa but has been observed also in other places. There is proliferation of large lymphoblasts derived from B-lymphocytes, with round nuclei, 1–2 nucleoli and basophilic cytoplasm. Numerous histiocytes containing nuclear debris ($\rightarrow$) are very characteristic.

Children are chiefly affected. $\male : \female = 3:1$. Epstein-Barr virus or its genome is present as it is in nasopharyngeal carcinomas in Chinese.

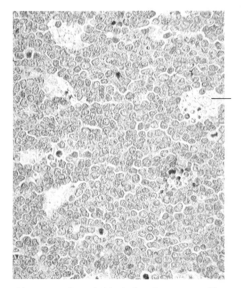

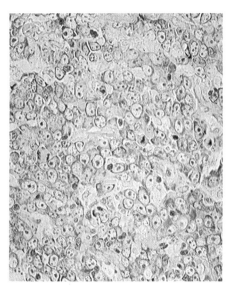

Fig. 11.20. Lymphoblastic lymphosarcoma; Giemsa stain, 300×.

Fig. 11.21. Immunoblastic sarcoma; Giemsa stain, 400×.

Immunoblastic sarcoma (histiocytic lymphoma, formerly reticulum cell sarcoma). Figure 11.21 shows diffuse proliferation of large cells with basophilic cytoplasm and round or ovoid nuclei with a distinct nuclear membrane and a large nucleolus. With electromicroscopy the cytoplasm is seen to be rich in polysomes and ribosomes. The network of reticulin fibers, which were formerly considered typical of reticulum cell sarcoma, are often conspicuous. IgM can almost always be demonstrated in the tumor tissue. Age 60–70 years. Course: $1/2$–1 year.

Immunological Considerations.

As shown on p. 243 there are B- and T-cell regions in lymph nodes. The immunological response of an organism can involve **B-cells** (-bone marrow lymphocytes) with stimulation of lymph nodes (Fig. 11.23): enlargement and loosening of nuclear chromatin, increase in the width of the cytoplasm with abundant rough endoplasmic reticulum and microvilli on the cell membrane), or **immunoblasts** (increase of all organelles, above all, ribosomes) or differentiation to **plasma cells** (formation of humoral antibody-immunoglobulin). Simultaneously cells increase by mitosis.

If the **T-cell system** (thymus-dependent lymphocytes) is stimulated the same cellular processes result (stimulated lymphocytes, immunoblasts). Further differentiation, however, leads to production of lymphocytes designated as "killer lymphocytes" since they have the capability of recognizing foreign cells not belonging to the organism and destroying them with lymphotoxin (e.g., destruction of tumor cells). In autoimmune diseases also there may be destruction of body specific cells. Morphologically killer lymphocytes cannot be differentiated from resting lymphocytes that have not yet come into contact with the antigen, so-called "memory cells". Memory cells have at one time already come in contact with antigen, have produced antibodies and possess an immunological memory for the specific antigen so that on further contact they again produce antibody. Current opinion is that antigen is first taken up by macrophages and further processed by them and that a specific immunological message is transferred to lymphocytes. Figure 11.22 shows that specific antigen receptors (immunoglobulin) are located on the surface of lymphocytes, which thus can bind antigen (sheep erythrocytes in figure) by immunoadherence.

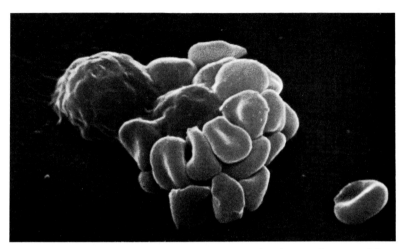

Fig. 11.22. Antigen binding by lymphocytes (mouse): scanning electron microscopy. Adsorption of antigen by immunoadherence (sheep erythrocytes) to a lymphocyte with an antigen specific surface; immunoglobulin receptor (rosette test of Biozzi). 4700× (Brücher, Gudat & Villiger).

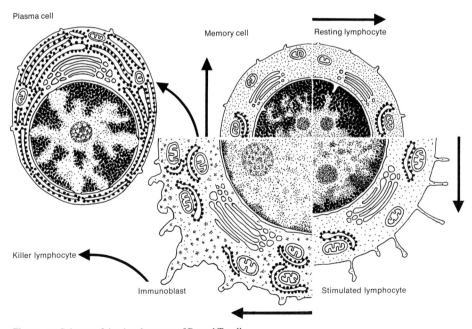

Plasma cell

Memory cell

Resting lymphocyte

Killer lymphocyte

Immunoblast

Stimulated lymphocyte

Fig. 11.23. Schema of the development of B- and T-cells.

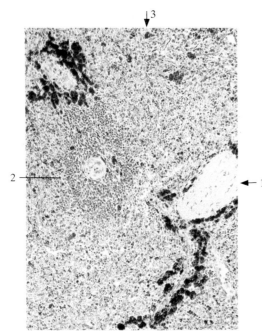

Fig. 11.24. Hemosiderin in the spleen; Berlin blue reaction, 100×.

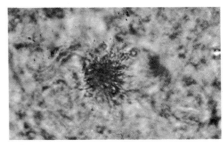

Fig.11.25. Hematoidin crystals in a splenic infarct; H & E, 380×.

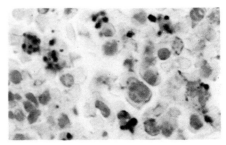

Fig.11.26. Formalin pigment in the spleen; Nuclear fast red 950×.

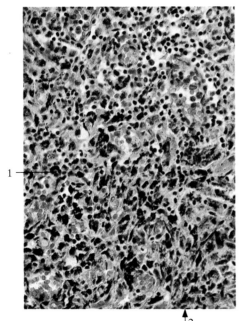

Fig. 11.27. Anthracosis of lymph nodes; H & E, 300×.

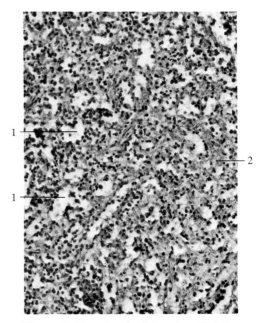

Fig. 11.28. Fibroadenosis of the spleen; H & E, 180×.

Spleen

Pathological changes occurring in the spleen are considered with respect to the trabecular architecture, the sinuses of the red pulp and the white pulp. Special attention should be paid to: blood content, the fibrous framework, the number of cells and any foreign deposits.

Siderosis of spleen (Fig. 11.24). In increased erythrocytic destruction (hemolytic anemia, repeated blood transfusions) and after large parenteral iron supplements, iron pigment is stored in the reticulum cells of the spleen (see p. 18). Histologically, low-power examination of sections stained with Berlin blue shows foci of greenish blue, layered masses in the red pulp and trabeculae ($\rightarrow$ 1), ($\rightarrow$ 2: follicles). High power shows that the siderin, which is stained blue by the Berlin blue reaction, lies within the cytoplasm of reticulum cells. To see this clearly, look for a part of the section in which the pigment is not so thick and where individual cells can be recognized ($\rightarrow$ 3).

Hematoidin crystals in a splenic infarct (Fig. 11.25). These consist of crystals of bilirubin in the form of red or orange needles or rhomboid plates. When blood is broken down and not removed by cellular resorption, for example, as may occur in the center of a hematoma or splenic infarct, iron-free pigment is formed from the hemoglobin freed from the erythrocytes (compare p. 9).

Formalin pigment (Fig. 11.26) is an artifact. The dark brown, granular, doubly refractile deposits are grouped together. They arise from the reaction of formaldehyde with unbound hemoglobin (probably protoporphyrin). The pigment gives a positive benzidine test and is soluble in weak acid.

Macroscopic: With formalin fixation, the blood appears brown or brownish black.

Anthracosis of lymph node (Fig. 11.27): Inhaled carbon pigment leaves the lung by way of the lymph channels and travels to the hilar lymph nodes, whence it can be carried even farther to the para-aortic lymph nodes. Rupture of markedly anthracotic lymph nodes into blood vessels in the hilus of the lung can result in spread via the blood stream and thus give rise to so-called pigment metastases in various organs.

In the hilar lymph nodes, the granular carbon pigment is first phagocytized by the sinus histiocytes. With further accumulation, pigment is also found in histiocytes in the cortical and medullary pulp, especially around the lymphoid follicles. Higher magnification shows the carbon granules to be in individual histiocyte cells and to surround and compress the nucleus ($\rightarrow$ 1). Progressive atrophy of lymphoid tissue occurs, and finally fibrosis of the node. Figure 11.27 shows the atrophy of the lymphocytes $\rightarrow$ 2.

Macroscopic: Early, there is diffuse or mottled gray discoloration of the lymph nodes; later, they are homogeneous black (the cut surface is moist in contrast to silicosis).

Fibroadenosis of spleen (Fig. 11.28): This term is used to describe chronic congestive induration of the spleen in portal hypertension; for example, in cirrhosis of the liver. Following dilatation of the sinus from acute congestion, hyperplasia of reticulum cells and reticular fibers develops between the sinusoids and increases with the duration of the stasis. Collagenization of the reticular fibrils ensues. The sinusoids, which are largely free of erythrocytes in the illustration ($\rightarrow$ 1), become surrounded by thick, rigid walls ($\rightarrow$ 2). Simultaneously, the white pulp atrophies.

Macroscopic: Marked splenic enlargement. The spleen frequently weighs more than 500 Gm. The splenic capsule is thickened by fibrosis and often hyalinized. The spleen has a tough, elastic consistency. The cut surface is dark red. After hemorrhage, for example from esophageal varices, the organ is light red, firm but elastic.

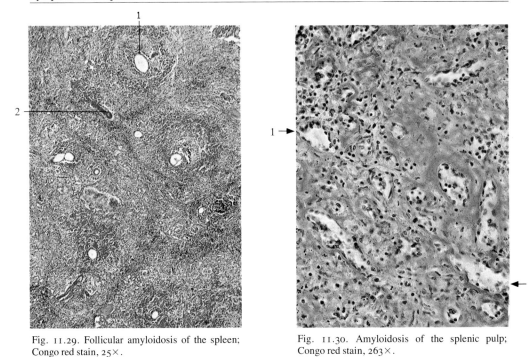

Fig. 11.29. Follicular amyloidosis of the spleen; Congo red stain, 25×.

Fig. 11.30. Amyloidosis of the splenic pulp; Congo red stain, 263×.

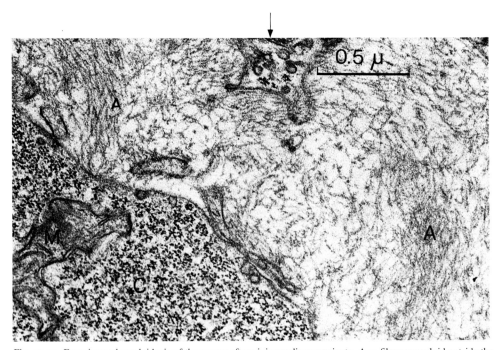

Fig. 11.31. Experimental amyloidosis of the mouse after giving sodium caseinate. A = fibrous amyloid outside the cytoplasm (C) of a reticulum cell of the spleen. In the cytoplasm, there are numerous aggregates of ribosomes (polysomes), an indication of high protein synthesis. M = fusion of mitochondria (giant mitochondria), → part of a neighboring cell, 49,000×. (Caesar).

Amyloidosis

Amyloid is a glassy, translucent, homogeneous substance of firm consistency which stains red with eosin and positively with Congo red (see p. 11). The composition of amyloid is 90% protein (by amino acid analysis this is immunoglobulin). Amyloid fibrils consist of variable fragments of light chain molecules of antibody and 1% carbohydrates (chondroitin sulfate and neuraminic acid). The binding of Congo red probably takes place with the carbohydrate component of amyloid in which a distance of 10 Å of the reactive groups of the stain is required (similar to cellulose, Puchtler *et al.*, 1965). The fact that after staining with Congo red the amyloid is doubly refractile is proof of direct deposition of the stain on the amyloid fiber. Electron microscopically, amyloid shows fibers about 80 Å (50–150 Å) thick (Figs. 11.31; 11.32), which, with the usual techniques, show no internal structure (Caesar, 1961). However, with special techniques, it has now been observed that these fibers consist of 2 fibrils, each 25 Å in diameter, forming a double helix with a space 25 Å between them. The two fibrillar strands are wound around each other, producing a transverse striation with 40 Å periodicity (Boeré *et al.*, 1965). According to Benditt and co-workers, 1966, there is a globular subunit 30–37 Å in diameter. Amyloid is formed by mesenchymal cells (reticulum cells, endothelial cells, Cohen and co-workers, 1965) in which the high content of ribosomes speaks for marked protein synthesis (Schneider, 1964, see Fig. 11.31). Cohen *et al.* also have seen amyloid fibrils in the cytoplasm of cells and concluded that the fibrils are formed intracellularly or from phagocytosed circulating immunoglobulins. One hypothesis states that light chains are taken up by the cells and after partial proteolysis are secreted as amyloid fibrils. However, there are also cases of amyloidosis in which the amyloid contains little or no immunoglobulin (Glenner *et al.*, 1974).

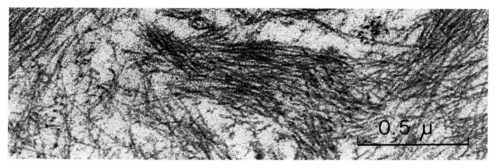

Fig. 11.32. Amyloid fibers without distinct internal structures, experimental amyloidosis in a mouse, 63,000× (Caesar).

Several types of amyloidosis are recognized morphologically: 1. **Typical amyloidosis:** Spleen, kidney, liver, adrenal, intestinal mucosa (rectal biopsy for confirmation of diagnosis). 2. **Atypical amyloidosis:** any organ in addition to those mentioned above may be affected. *Amyloidosis in the aged* particularly involves the heart; 3% of cases over 70 years. 3. **Tumor forming amyloidosis:** nodules of amyloid infiltrated by plasma cells may occur, e.g., in the tongue. Tumor-like deposits may also occur in pancreatic islets and in C-cell thyroid tumors (calcitonin producing cells). *Etiological classification:* 1. **Primary hereditary amyloidosis,** e.g., familial Mediterranean fever (typical amyloidosis), neuropathic amyloidosis (atypical amyloidosis). 2. **Secondary acquired amyloidosis:** (typical amyloidosis) in chronic inflammation (tuberculosis is present in 50% of cases of amyloidosis, osteomyelitis 12%, chronic lung infection 10%, other chronic infections 12% (hyperimmunization). In primary chronic polyarthritis 20% of cases show amyloidosis. *Experimental:* repeated doses of foreign protein.

Follicular amyloidosis (Fig. 11.29). Low magnification of a section stained with Congo red demonstrates the red-colored follicles which are seen as red circles or little disks sometimes with a central artery (→ 1). → 2 amyloid in an artery in the pulp. The follicles contain no lymphocytes, the pulp is poor in cells.

Macroscopic: Multiple small glassy nodules = Sago spleen.

Pulp amyloidosis (Fig. 11.30): Low magnification shows red homogeneous tissue and focal round pale areas corresponding to the follicles. Higher magnification shows the amyloid lying between dilated sinuses lined by large endothelial cells (→ 1).

Macroscopic: Enlarged, firm spleen of wooden consistency and lardaceous glassy cut surfaces.

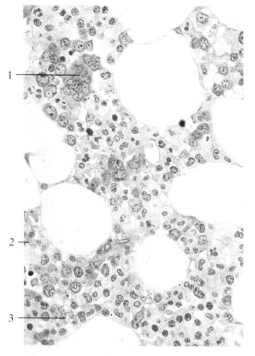

Fig. 12.1. Normal bone marrow; Giemsa stain, 320×.

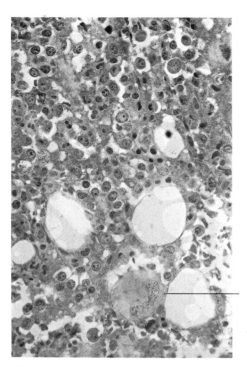

Fig. 12.2. Polycythemia vera; Ladewig stain, 320×.

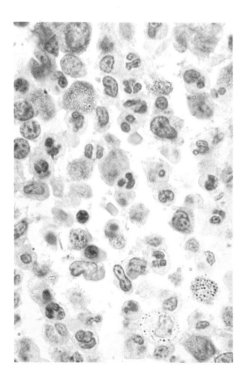

Fig. 12.3. Chronic myelocytic leukemia (mature cell); Giemsa stain, 600×.

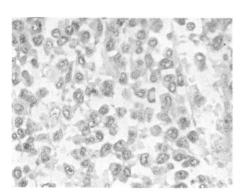

Fig. 12.4. Acute myelocytic leukemia (immature cell); Giemsa stain, 320×.

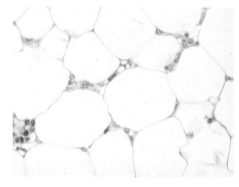

Fig. 12.5. Aplasia of bone marrow; Ladewig stain, 200×.

12. Blood–Bone Marrow

Definitive diagnosis of diseases of the blood depends on examination of a peripheral blood smear and a bone marrow biopsy. With the introduction of bone marrow biopsy and the use of pathological-anatomical methods of investigation (paraffin embedding, histological staining, histochemical reactions and electronmicroscopy) the pathologist is frequently confronted with the collection and interpretation of hematological data. A bone marrow biopsy (pelvic crest) has distinct advantages over a bone marrow smear but does not replace it. The cells can be studied as a tissue rather than as isolated cells and in relation to the other components of the bone marrow, e.g., bone trabeculae, osteoblasts, osteoclasts and blood vessels. A biopsy rather than a smear is especially advantageous in evaluating a *cellularly depleted* bone marrow with replacement by fat cells (e.g., *bone marrow aplasia*, Fig. 12.5) or by fibrous tissue (in *osteomyelofibrosis*). The greatest difficulty of bone marrow biopsy heretofore has been the difficulty of cytomorphological cell differentiation in paraffin sections over 5 μ thick. This difficulty has now been overcome by the introduction of other embedding materials. Today with material embedded in methacrylate it is possible to prepare semithin sections of 0.1–2 μ thickness with which the routine staining (H & E, Giemsa, Ladewig, Gomori) or histochemical (PAS, Berlin blue) procedures can be carried out without disturbance of cellular and nuclear relationships.

Normal bone marrow (Fig. 12.1) is cellular and very variegated in its composition. In semithin sections it is possible to differentiate the first stages of myelopoiesis. Especially clearly shown are the multinucleated megakaryocytes ($\rightarrow$ 1), the dark blue erythrocytes ($\rightarrow$ 2) and the granules of the eosinophiles ($\rightarrow$ 3). Large fat cells are present in the marrow (optically empty spaces).

In **polycythemia vera** (Fig. 12.2) *the blood forming elements are increased and in addition there is polyglobulinemia, leukocytosis and thrombocytosis.* An increase in megakaryocytes ($\rightarrow$) which lie chiefly in the marrow sinuses is very characteristic.

Polycythemia commonly occurs between 50 and 60 years of age and after a long course progresses to osteosclerosis or chronic myelocytic leukemia (about 10% of cases). Pure erythropoietic hyperplasia, in which the peripheral erythrocyte count may be over 10 million/cubic mm, is referred to as *polyglobulinemia*. In addition to the *idiopathic form* there is *secondary polycythemia* resulting from other causes (chronic lung diseases, hypernephroma [due to increased production or erythropoietin]).

Leukemia (or leukosis) *is a neoplastic disease in which the blood-forming cells of the hemopoietic system show abnormal, autonomous proliferation that may develop either quickly or slowly.* Any series of the hematopoietic system may be involved *(myelocytic, lymphocytic, monocytic, erythrocytic, megakaryocytic or plasma cell leukemias).* Depending on the maturity of the cells and the duration of the disease we distinguish *chronic* (mature cells) and *acute* (immature cells) *leukemias.* Chronic leukemias as a rule are accompanied by the appearance of the abnormal cells in peripheral blood, so that there may be a leukocytosis of 500,000 to 1,000,000 cells. In acute leukemias the leukocyte count more often may be normal or even subnormal *(aleukemic leukemia).* As a consequence of the increased number of leukemic cells the appearance of the bone marrow is altered by displacement of normal cells leading to reduced erythropoiesis ($\rightarrow$ anemia) and thrombocytopoiesis ($\rightarrow$ thrombocytopenia $\rightarrow$ hemorrhagic diathesis). Figure 12.6 and Table 12.1 set forth the different sorts of leukemia with the frequency of their occurrence, and their macroscopic and histologic features.

In **chronic myelogenous leukemia** (Fig. 12.3) semithin sections stained with Giemsa have a variegated and richly cellular appearance. Besides mature polymorphonuclear granulocytes there are immature cells, especially pro- and metamyelocytes. In **acute myelocytic leukemia,** by contrast, the cellular picture is monotonous. Chiefly there are paramyeloblasts (Fig. 12.4). Smears of peripheral blood usually show segmented leukocytes as well as paramyeloblasts, but no intermediate forms *(leukemic hiatus).*

We are indebted to Dr. Mobius of Freiburg for the semithin sections.

Leukemias

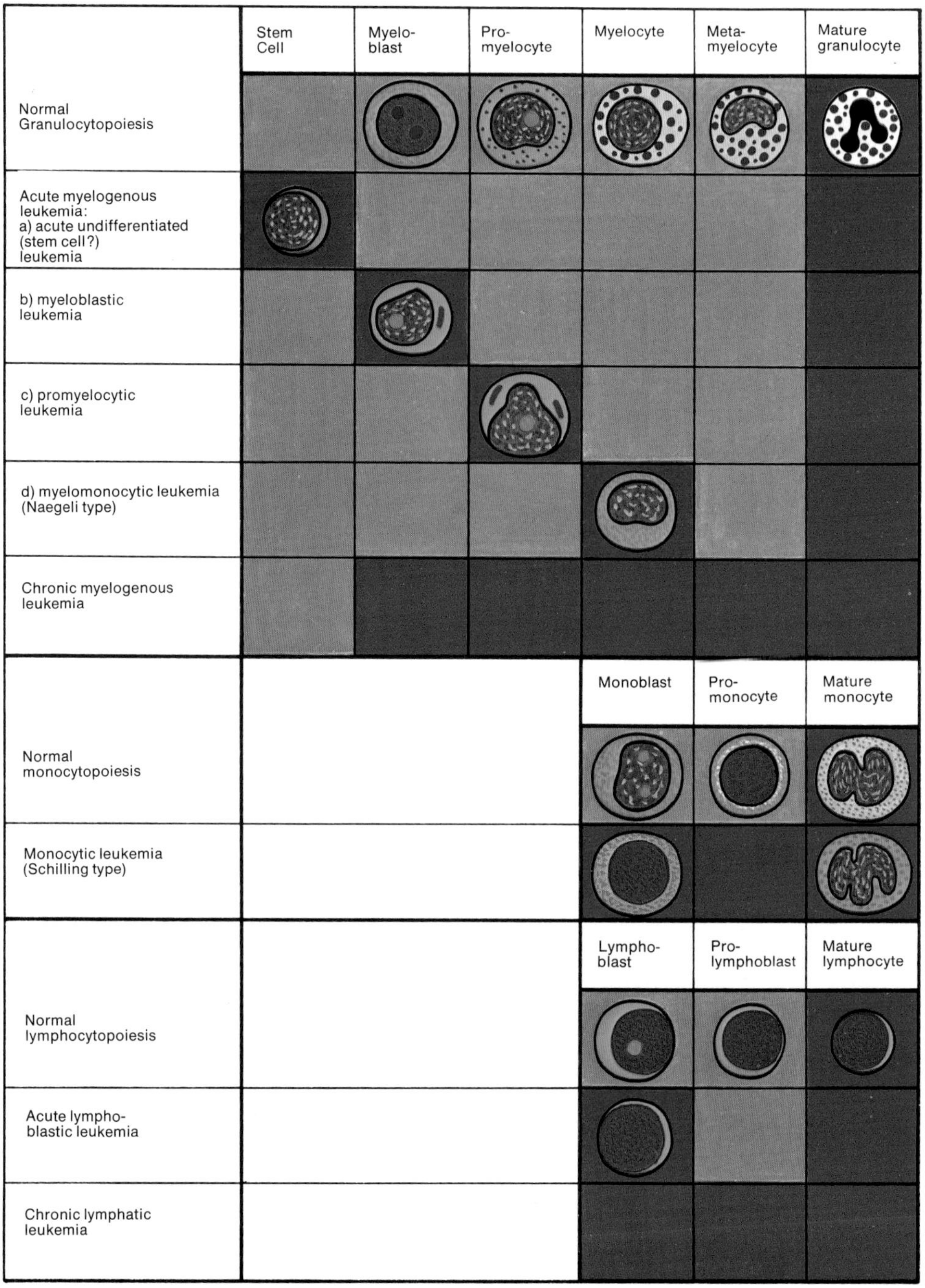

	Stem Cell	Myelo-blast	Pro-myelocyte	Myelocyte	Meta-myelocyte	Mature granulocyte
Normal Granulocytopoiesis						
Acute myelogenous leukemia: a) acute undifferentiated (stem cell?) leukemia						
b) myeloblastic leukemia						
c) promyelocytic leukemia						
d) myelomonocytic leukemia (Naegeli type)						
Chronic myelogenous leukemia						

	Monoblast	Pro-monocyte	Mature monocyte
Normal monocytopoiesis			
Monocytic leukemia (Schilling type)			

	Lympho-blast	Pro-lymphoblast	Mature lymphocyte
Normal lymphocytopoiesis			
Acute lympho-blastic leukemia			
Chronic lymphatic leukemia			

Fig. 12.6. Schematic diagram of the leukemias. Orange: bone marrow, Red: peripheral blood.

Table 12.1. Outline of morphological, hematological and clinical findings in leukemias

Type of Leukemia	PAS	Esterase	Peroxidase	Alkaline Phosphatase	Liver Infiltrate	Liver Hepato-megaly	Bone marrow — color	Lymphodenopathy	Splenomegaly	Gingivitis	Age range	Sex distribution
Acute myelocytic leukemia												
a) acute undifferentiated leukemia	−	−	−	+	diffuse	+	gray-red	+	+++	(+)		
b) myeloblastic leukemia	(+)	+	(+)	+	diffuse	+	gray-red	+	+++	(+)		
c) promyelocytic leukemia	+	+	+++	+	diffuse	+	gray-red	+	+++	+	15–20 years	60% ♂
d) myelomonocytic leukemia	+	+++	+	+	diffuse	+	gray-red	(+)	+++	+,++		
Chronic myelogenous leukemia	(+)	−	+	−	diffuse	+	pyoid	+	+	(+)	50–65 years	
Monocytic leukemia	+	+++	+	+	diffuse often lacking	(+)	gray-red	(+)	(+)	+++		
Acute lymphoblastic leukemia	+++	−	−	+	portal	++	gray	+++	+	−	5–15 years	
Chronic lymphatic leukemia	+	−	−	+	portal	++	gray	++++	+	−	45–50 years	70% ♂

Pathology of Erythropoiesis

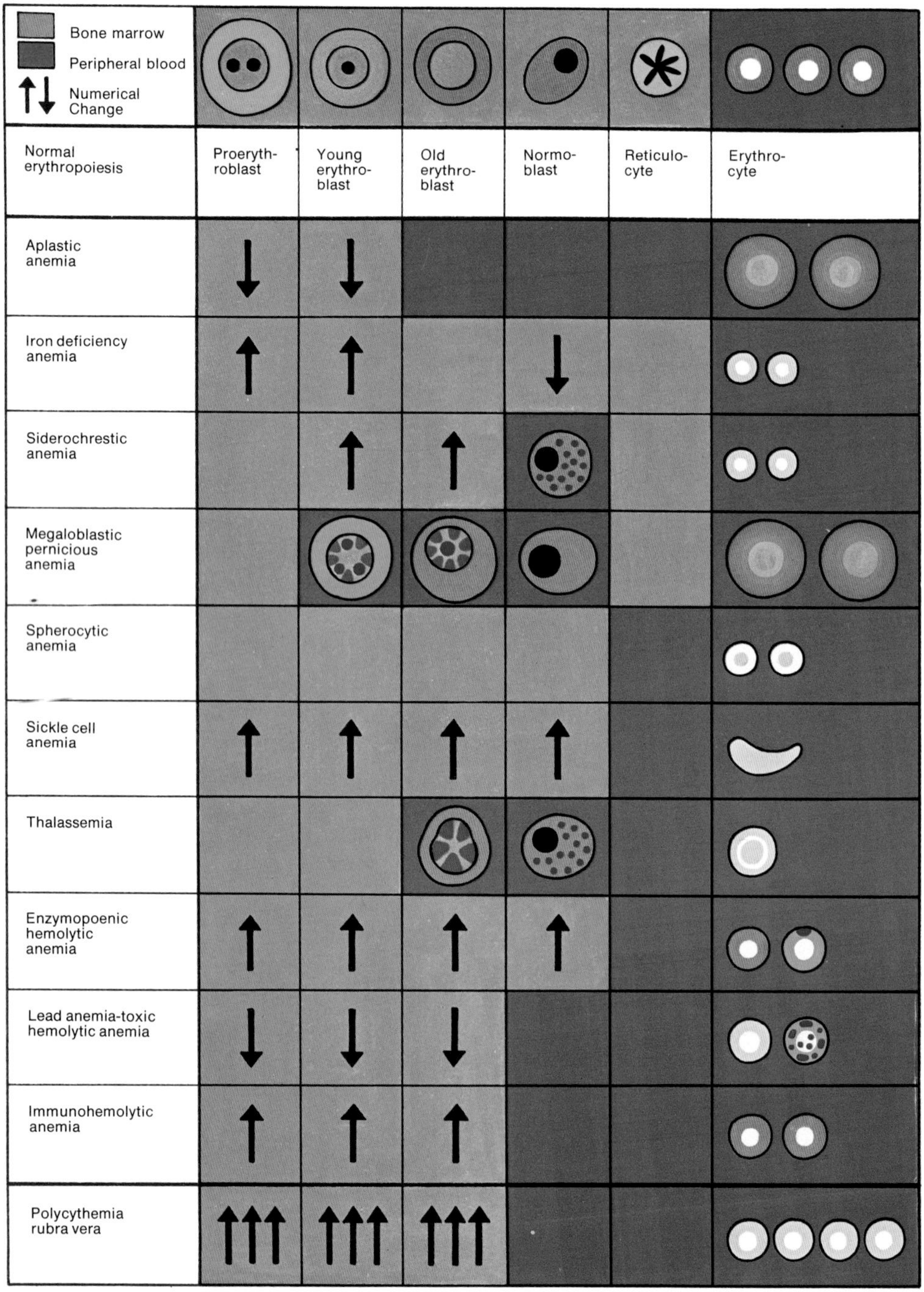

	Proeryth-roblast	Young erythro-blast	Old erythro-blast	Normo-blast	Reticulo-cyte	Erythro-cyte
Normal erythropoiesis						
Aplastic anemia	↓	↓				
Iron deficiency anemia	↑	↑		↓		
Siderochrestic anemia		↑	↑			
Megaloblastic pernicious anemia						
Spherocytic anemia						
Sickle cell anemia	↑	↑	↑	↑		
Thalassemia						
Enzymopoenic hemolytic anemia	↑	↑	↑	↑		
Lead anemia-toxic hemolytic anemia	↓	↓	↓			
Immunohemolytic anemia	↑	↑	↑			
Polycythemia rubra vera	↑↑↑	↑↑↑	↑↑↑			

Legend: Bone marrow / Peripheral blood / Numerical Change ↑↓

Fig. 12.7. Schematic diagram of disturbances of erythropoiesis.

Table 12.2. Disturbances of hemopoiesis in different anemias.

Legend: ↗ Cause ⇗ Consequence

Cause / Consequence	DNA synthesis (Proerythroblast)	Mitoses (Young erythroblast)	Heme-synthesis (Old erythroblast)	Hb synthesis (Normoblast)	Iron deposit (Reticulocyte)	Glycolysis (Erythrocyte)	Membrane function (Erythrocyte)
Normal Erythropoiesis							
Aplastic anemia		⇗					
Iron deficiency anemia				⇗	↗		
Siderochrestic anemia			⇗		⇗		
Megaloblastic pernicious anemia	⇗						
Spherocytic anemia							↗
Sickle cell anemia						↗	⇗
Thalassemia				↗	⇗		⇗
Enzyme deficient hemolytic anemia				⇗			⇗
Lead anemia toxic hemolytic anemia			↗		⇗	⇗	⇗
Immunohemolytic anemia							⇗
Polycythemia rubra vera	↗	↗					

Pathology of Erythropoiesis (Fig. 12.7 and Table 12.2)

Anemias are usually divided according to the following characteristics: a) changes in *size*. Normal erythrocytic volume at mid-cross section = $84-95\mu^3$ macrocytes: $> 100\mu^3$, microcytes $< 80\mu^3$. b) Changes in *shape*: poikilocytosis = morphologic changes of erythrocytes, anisocytosis = variations of size. c) Changes in *hemoglobulin content* (=Hb): monochromatic = normal Hb content, hypochromatic, hyperchromatic = lowered or raised Hb content, anisochromatic = varying Hb content, polychromasia = immature bluish erythrocytes, see p. 249.

Myelophthisic Anemias

Anemias due to disturbances of blood formation—*osteomyelosclerotic anemias:* replacement of blood forming bone marrow by fibrous bone formation in the mature spongiosa; hardly any extramedullary blood formation. *Aplastic anemia* (Fig. 12.5 panmyelophthisis, erythroblastophthesis). Toxic bone marrow injury by gold, benzol or irradiation. Often, however, the cause is unknown. Bone marrow (=BM): hypoplastic with increased number of fat cells. Erythroblastopenia. Early forms of the red and white cell series are reduced. Blood: macrocytic hyperchromatic, anisopoikilocytic anemia, reticulocytopenia. Erythroblasts can occur.
Anemias of disturbed maturation. Nephrogenic, e.g., in uremia: no erythroprotein production and no Hb synthesis. Hepatogenic, e.g., cirrhosis: disturbed vitamin B_{12} function (B_{12} antibodies?). Toxic: blast cell injury by chloramphenicol, lead, benzol, etc.

Metabolic Anemias

Iron deficiency anemias (Fig. 12.7). Iron deficiency due to chronic bleeding. Disturbance of resorption (e.g., sprue). Disturbance of nutrition (e.g., goat's milk). As a result of the iron deficiency a smaller amount of Hb is manufactured. BM: hyperplastic (of all erythropoietic elements). Sideroblastopenia. Normal granulocytopoiesis and thrombopoiesis. Blood: microcytic, hypochromatic, anisopoikilocytic anemia. Reticulocyte count: mostly normal.

Sideroblastic anemia (Fig. 12.7). *Hereditary sideroblastic anemia.* Results from disturbance of heme formation (hereditary X-chromosome?). Less iron formation in Hb. Diffuse sideroblastosis in BM (= normoblasts with iron granules) and hypochromatic erythrocytes in spite of raised serum iron. BM: hyperplastic erythrocytopoiesis with sideroblastosis. Blood: microcytic, hypochromic anemia with sideroblastosis. Mostly reticulocytopenia. *Acquired form:* Vitamin B_6-sensitive anemia, lead anemia, toxic drug induced anemia.

Macrocytic, hyperchromic deficiency anemias. *Megaloblastic pernicious anemia* (= Addison's disease) *with neurologic symptoms* (Fig. 12.7). Vitamin B_{12} (= extrinsic factor) is reabsorbed in the ileum by intrinsic factor (produced by gastric parietal cells). Vitamin B_{12} catalyzed step wise during DNA synthesis. Because of antibody production against the gastric mucosa or against the intrinsic factor, Vitamin B_{12} deficiency develops. As a result of the disturbance of erythrocyte maturation megaloblasts and giant myelocytes appear in the BM with thrombocytopoiesis. BM: hyperplastic, megaloblastic with giant forms in erythro- and granulocyte series. Blood: macrocytic, hyperchromic, anisopoikilocytic anemia with megaloblasts and megalocytes. The enlarged nuclei of these cells show a loose chromatin network and clumping of chromatin. Reticulocytopenia. Hypersegmented granulocytes. *Megaloblastic pernicious anemia without neurological symptoms.* Caused by folic acid deficiency due to faulty nutrition, folic acid antagonists (tumor retarding agents) or antiepileptic agents. Vitamin B_{12} also catalyzes folic acid production during DNA synthesis. BM and blood are similar to Addisonian anemia.

Hemolytic Anemias

Corpuscular hemolytic anemias. *Spherocytic anemia (hereditary spherocytosis, Minkowski-Chaufford,* Fig. 12.7). There is an inherited autosomal defect of the erythrocyte membrane which causes sodium uptake and spheroidal erythrocytes. Increased destruction of erythrocytes results. BM: hemolytic crises start with an aplastic phase with reticulocytopenia and giant forms of mature erythroblasts. Regeneration is ushered in with reticulocytosis. Blood: microcytic, normo-polychromic anemia with spherical erythrocytes (= microspherocytosis). *Reticulocytosis.* In a hemolytic crisis there is an outpouring of erythroblasts. *Eliptocytosis (ovulocytic anemia).* An inherited abnormality of erythrocyte shape without clinical significance.

Sickle cell anemia (Fig. 12.7). An inherited hemoglobinopathy with Hb-S and allemorphic genes which cause sickle-shaped erythrocytes in an hypoxic environment (chiefly in the negro race: increased resistance to malaria!) BM: increased erythropoiesis. Blood: sickle-shaped erythrocytes in hemolytic crises. Reticulocytosis.

Thalassemia (Mediterranean anemia, Fig. 12.7). Inherited hemoglobinopathy with diminished formation of a specific globulin chain and substitution of increased numbers of pathological globulin chains. Iron is absorbed from normoblasts, but can not be incorporated in the abnormal Hb (= sideroblastic anemia). BM: increased erythropoiesis. Shift to the left. Blood (in thalassemia major): hypopolychromic, microcytic, anisocytic, poikilocytic anemia with target cells. Reticulocytosis. Outpouring of paraerythroblasts (= atypical chromatin precursor). *Anemias resulting from unstable hemoglobin.* Inborn hemoglobulinopathies (e.g., Hb Zürich) in which Heinz bodies form after taking certain drugs. *Paroxysmal nocturnal hemoglobulinuria.* Due to defective erythrocyte membrane which results in nocturnal hemolysis of erythrocytes oversensitive to acidity. BM: increased erythropoiesis. Blood: macrocytic, polychromic anemia with reticulocytosis, lymphocytosis and leukopenia. *Enzymatic hemolytic anemias* (Fig. 12.7) enzyme defect of aerobic glycolysis shortens the life span of the erythrocytes. Following use of certain drugs or beans (favism) hemolysis may develop. BM: hyperplastic erythropoiesis. Blood: normochromic anemia with reticulocytosis and Heinz bodies.

Extracorpuscular anemias. *Parasitic hemolytic anemias:* malarial plasmodia and *Bartonella bacilliformis* (= Oraya fever) attack and destroy erythrocytes. *Toxic hemolytic anemias.* Phenacetin and sulfonamides cause formation of sulf-Hb and later precipitation of globulin (morphological equivalent = Heinz body). Plant poisons (male fern, fungi). Snake toxins (= lecithinases), toxins of hemolytic streptococci and illuminating gas damage the erythrocyte membrane. Nitrous oxide gas, arsenic, H_2S and lead arrest synthesis of heme. Lead blocks formation of δ aminolevulinic acid (= ALA) by blocking ALS synthesis; blocks iron formation in protoporphyrin and thus heme synthesis by interfering with heme synthetase. Iron production in erythrocytes is defective. Blood in lead anemia: outpouring of erythroblasts and normoblasts. Reticulocytosis. Basophilic spotting of erythrocytes. Hypochromatic, polychromic anemia. Hypoplastic BM.

Physical hemolytic anemias. Thermal hemolysis in burns, mechanical hemolytic anemias: march hemoglobulinuria: anemia due to defective heart valves; microangiopathic anemias. *Immunohemolytic anemias* (Fig. 12.7). Autoimmune hemolytic anemias: caused by release of antibodies (=AB) against erythrocytes of the same body, e.g., warm AB (=IgG); cold AB against foreign erythrocytes of the same sort (ABO, Rhesus), e.g., hemolytic disease of the newborn. Transfusion hemolysis: BM: hyperplastic erythropoiesis.

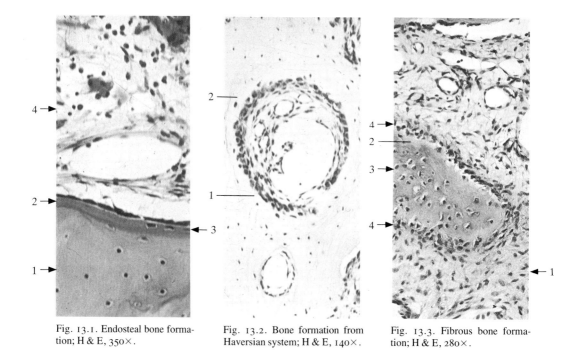

Fig. 13.1. Endosteal bone formation; H & E, 350×.

Fig. 13.2. Bone formation from Haversian system; H & E, 140×.

Fig. 13.3. Fibrous bone formation; H & E, 280×.

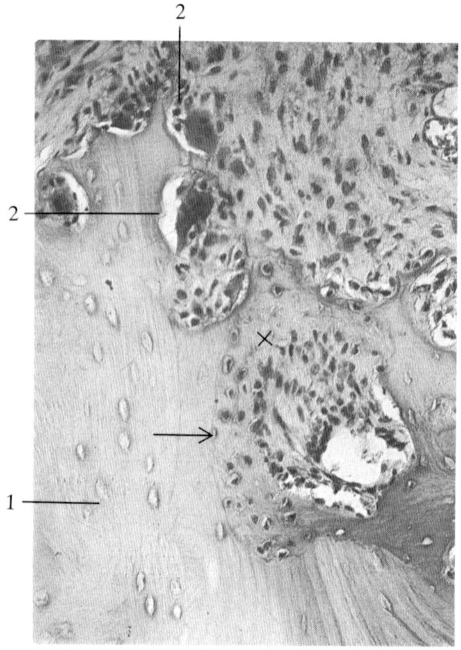

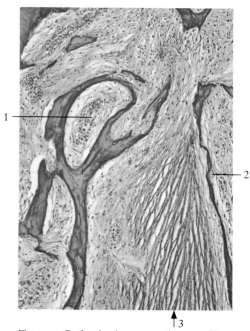

Fig. 13.4. Smooth resorption and formation of lacunae in bone; H & E, 250×.

Fig. 13.5. Perforating bone resorption; van Gieson stain, 80×.

13. Bones–Joints

Microscopic study of bone sections necessitates knowledge of the *type of bony tissue* being examined (whether compact bone with Haversian systems or spongy bone without Haversian systems). The *quantitative relation between cancelous part and marrow space* must be evaluated (e.g., in the rarefaction due to osteoporosis) as well as the *types of cells appearing in the marrow spaces* (active hematopoietic, fatty or fibrous marrow, inflammatory infiltrates, etc.). It is important to see if the osteocytes in the *trabeculae* are stained (in bone necrosis the nuclei do not stain. Care must be exercised, however, for severe decalcification causes negative nuclear staining). The number of osteoblasts, the width of the osteoid margins, the degree of calcification of newly formed bone and the number of osteoclasts serve as an *indication of bone formation or resorption*.

In order to simplify the study of the various bone diseases, they will be considered only from the point of view of general pathology. Thus, the reaction of bony tissue to the stimulus of disease will be considered in terms either of *bone formation* or of *bone resorption*.

New bone is formed from connective tissue cells which, because of chemical or physical stimuli, differentiate to form osteoblasts. During this process of differentiation, the nuclei and nucleoli enlarge, the rough endoplasmic reticulum increases and the increased RNA causes increased basophilia. The *osteoblasts* fulfill three basic functions: 1. formation of mucopolysaccharide (MPS)-protein complexes, 2. synthesis of collagen fibers, 3. participation in mineralization. The acid and neutral mucopolysaccharides act as ion exchangers. They concentrate calcium and phosphate and are destroyed by enzymatic action after mineralization.

With the light microscope, the following sites of bone formation can be differentiated: 1. *Periosteal bone formation* (proceeding from osteoblasts in the periosteum). This occurs in pathological situations, e. g., ossifying periostitis, chronic osteomyelitis, formation of a fracture callus. 2. *Endosteal bone formation* (proceeding from endosteal osteoblasts). This also is seen in pathological situations, e. g., formation of a fracture callus, chronic osteomyelitis (Fig. 13.1). This type of bone formation often leads to gradual substitution of bone (Fig. 13.4). Thus, there may be simultaneous bone resorption by cells with a single nucleus as well as formation of new bone. This occurs, for example, in osteitis deformans of Paget (simultaneous action of osteoclasts and osteoblasts). 3. New bone formation from the *Haversian systems* (see Fig. 13.2). In this case, the formation of new bone is accomplished by cells derived by differentiation from perivascular connective tissue cells. 4. Finally, *osteocytes* from the interlamellar osseous tissue can form bone (mostly when there is bone substitution and, therefore, accompanying bone resorption). In these various ways new bone is built like a shell around existing lamellar bone. However, new bone may also form without contact with bone previously formed in connective tissue, mostly in the bone marrow, (fibrous bone formation: no Haversian canals). Such fibrous bone can later convert to lamellar bone with Haversian canals.

Figure 13.1 shows **endosteal new bone formation.** Below, there is mineralization of bone ($\rightarrow$ 1) which is lying on a narrow zone of newly formed osteoid ($\rightarrow$ 2). Osteoid contains collagen fibers, MPS-protein complexes, but not hydroxyapatite, although there are large amounts of calcium (attached by ion binding to the acid MPS). Osteoid is formed by osteoblasts which can be seen as a single layer of cells with one nucleus ($\rightarrow$ 3). Above this is the loose connective tissue of the marrow cavity ($\rightarrow$ 4). Figure 13.2 shows **new bone formation in the region of a Haversian canal.** Osteoblasts are forming an edge of bone in the periphery of the perivascular connective tissue ($\rightarrow$ 1). The boundary between new and old bone is marked by a cement line ($\rightarrow$ 2). **Fibrous bone** (Fig. 13.3). In the midst of the richly cellular collagenous connective tissue ($\rightarrow$ 1), fibroblasts differentiate to osteoblasts which become mineralized (nonmineralized intercellular substance: $\rightarrow$ 2; mineralized intercellular substance: $\rightarrow$ 3). The resulting bone trabeculae are again surrounded by osteoblasts ($\rightarrow$ 4). By special staining, it is possible to show that the collagen fibers in the surrounding connective tissue are continuous with those in the bone trabeculae.

Bone resorption results from the action of mononucleated or multinucleated connective tissue cells (osteoblasts). These cells are concerned with demineralization, enzymatic resorption of collagen (collagenase) and splitting of the MPS-protein complex (lysosomal enzymes). The most important morphological forms are 1. *smooth resorption* (often in company with slow substitution), this is the commonest form of bone resorption by cells with a single nucleus. 2. *Lacunar resorption* by multinucleated osteoclasts. These arise by fusion of cells with a single nucleus and can convert back to uninuclear cells. During the process of bone resorption, the osteoclasts develop numerous microvilli (electron microscopy) on the outer cell membrane (this is morphological evidence of the increased work of resorption). 3. *Perforating resorption ("tunneling")*, which results from the action of cells of the Haversian system with one nucleus. This leads to excavations or lacunae in the bone trabeculae. Occurrence: e.g., in osteomyelitis and brown tumors.

Continued on page 259.

Healing of Fractures

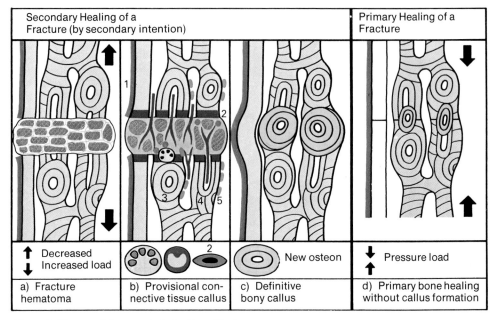

Fig. 13.6. Diagram of the stages in the healing of fractures.

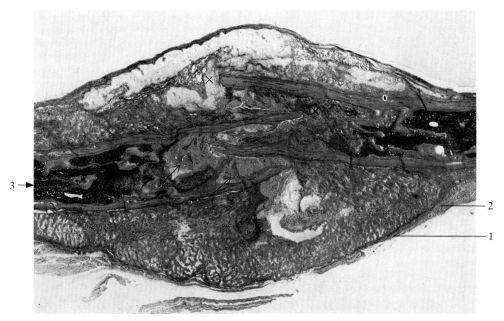

Fig. 13.7. Rib fracture with definitive callus; H & E, 7×.

Figure 13.4 shows **slow substitution** with smooth resorption and lacunar formation. In the lower left part of the picture there is necrotic bone (→ 1: empty spaces left by bone cells). At →, the old bone has been resorbed in layer fashion. In all probability, the resorption has been accomplished by the same uninucleated cells that are forming new bone at X. Bone resorption by osteoclasts (→ 2) leads to formation of lacunae (Howslip's lacunae) in resorbed bone.

Perforating resorption (Fig. 13.5) "tunnels" the bone trabeculae. Connective tissue cells with a single nucleus from the Haversian canals resorb the bone (→ 1). This process of resorption leaves only narrow strips of spongy trabecular (→ 2), until, finally, these also are resorbed and only poorly cellular connective tissue remains behind (→ 3).

The *regulation of bone resorption and bone formation* is accomplished under both normal and pathological circumstances by physical forces (chiefly effective locally) and chemical agents (generalized effect). For example, the operation of the piezoelectric effect, in which electric currents are formed that apparently change the cell performance (the exact mechanism of translation of electric current into the chemical "language" of the cell is still unknown). The action of parathyroid hormone is an example of a chemical agent which, along with other influences (kidney), has an effect on the cells of the skeletal system (this has been demonstrated in organ cultures) and in all probability stimulates bone resorption.

Bone Fracture

A fracture is a complete or partial break in the continuity of a bone. It sets in motion a series of regular tissue reactions, which lead to restoration of continuity. The results of these tissue reactions are depicted schematically in Figure 13.6. First, a **hematoma** forms between the two ends. As early as the second day, capillary loops and fibroblasts (granulation tissue) begin to grow into the hematoma. Starting points for formation of new tissue are (refer to the number in the second column of Fig. 13.6): 1. the periosteum, 2. the endosteum, i.e., osteoblasts, 3. the Haversian canals, 4. blood vessels in the marrow cavity, 5. blood vessels in the subcutaneous tissues and muscle. This leads to subsequent formation of a **provisional callus of connective tissue.** At the end of the first week, however, this already shows signs of being converted to a **provisional bony callus.** First, the immature connective tissue cells put down ground substance and collagen fibers. The fibroblasts develop into osteoblasts and produce osteoid, which is the organic matrix of bone. As a result of certain chemical reactions, calcium and phosphate from a supersaturated solution from which the mineralizing substance (secondary calcium phosphate hydroxyapatite) precipitates. This process constitutes the genesis of so-called *fibrous bone,* which by repeated remodeling by the action of osteoblasts and osteoclasts will give rise to *compact bone.* This, in turn, forms the **definitive callus.** Fracture healing may be regarded as the prototype of all healing processes in bony tissue.

Figure 13.7 (scanning lens view) shows a **rib fracture** with definitive callus formation. The fractured ends (×) are not well aligned, possibly because of the shearing forces of the respiratory or other movements. Such shearing forces produce cartilage formation (→) in the provisional callus. The healing process in the ribs (and cheek bone) is thus atypical, since the formation of the cartilaginous callus continues to progress. The fractured ends are surrounded not only by cartilaginous tissue but also by immature connective tissue and newly formed bone (→ 1) covered by periosteum (→ 2). Typical hematopoietic marrow can be seen at a distance from the fracture (→ 3).

The following *complications* of fracture or its delayed healing may occur: 1. *Fat embolism* (especially after fractures of long bones). 2. *Infection* of the reparative hematoma (osteomyelitis, especially after compound fractures). 3. Insufficient callus formation interposition of soft tissues *(pseudarthrosis).* 4. *Hyperactive callus formation* (exuberant callus causing pressure on soft tissues, nerves, etc.). 5. Formation of a *cartilaginous callus* (due to the development of shearing forces, leading to delayed healing of the fracture).

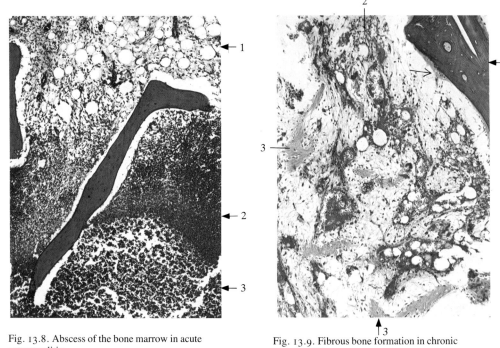

Fig. 13.8. Abscess of the bone marrow in acute osteomyelitis; H & E, 60×.

Fig. 13.9. Fibrous bone formation in chronic osteomyelitis; H & E, 95×.

Disorders in development of growing bones

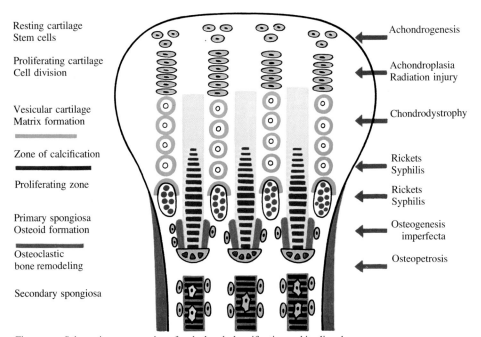

Resting cartilage
Stem cells

Proliferating cartilage
Cell division

Vesicular cartilage
Matrix formation

Zone of calcification

Proliferating zone

Primary spongiosa
Osteoid formation

Osteoclastic
bone remodeling

Secondary spongiosa

Achondrogenesis

Achondroplasia
Radiation injury

Chondrodystrophy

Rickets
Syphilis

Rickets
Syphilis

Osteogenesis
     imperfecta

Osteopetrosis

Fig. 13.10. Schematic representation of endochondral ossification and its disorders.

Inflammation of Bones

As in other organs, inflammations of bones can be either *nonspecific* (acute osteomyelitis, chronic osteomyelitis) or *specific* (e.g., tuberculosis, actinomycosis, syphilis). Whereas nonspecific inflammations seem to have a predilection for *metaphysis or diaphysis,* specific inflammations (especially *tuberculosis*) preferentially affect the *epiphysis*. The regional bony structures are destroyed in the course of inflammation (loss of osteocytes, resorption by osteoclasts and blood vessels). The pieces of dead bone are partly sequestered. In addition, new tissue grows (from the periosteum) around the dead bone (*sequestrum* of osteomyelitis). As is to be expected, all types of inflammatory cells are found in the bone itself.

A *nonspecific osteomyelitis* has been chosen as an example of a bone inflammation. Such an osteomyelitis can arise at a site of injury (e.g., in fractures or in otitis media) or it can be hematogenous (e.g., in septicemia). Figure 13.8 shows a **marrow abscess** in an acute osteomyelitis of hematogenous origin. In the upper part of the picture there is fat marrow that has been infiltrated with granulocytes ($\rightarrow$ 1). At $\rightarrow$ 2 is seen the necrotic wall containing granulocytes and fibrin. In the lower portion of the picture ($\rightarrow$ 3) there is destruction of tissue and numerous polymorphonuclear leukocytes (abscess). Because of the necrosis, the bone trabeculae have lost their supporting matrix and are themselves necrotic. A sequestrum of bone is formed (a piece of dead bone). In more advanced stages of osteomyelitis (**chronic osteomyelitis,** Fig. 13.9), there are dead bone trabeculae ($\rightarrow$ 1) which can be seen in the picture to be overlaid with newly formed bone ($\rightarrow$), thus forming a case for the dead bone. The marrow space shows fibrosis (loose collagenous tissue) and a perivascular inflammatory infiltrate of lymphocytes and plasma cells ($\rightarrow$ 2). Beneath this, there is fibrous bone formation ($\rightarrow$ 3).

Disorders in Development of Bones

Osteodystrophies are in some ways comparable to metabolic disturbances in other organs. One way to consider them is in terms of *growing* and *grown or adult bones.* Figure 13.10 is a **schematic representation of endochondral ossification and the possible causes of its disturbed development.** At the left are represented the various zones which normally make up the zone of ossification: Quiescent or resting cartilage, cartilage columns and the provisional zone of calcification, osteoid formation, bone remodeling into compact lamellar bone.

Disturbances can occur at any step of this complex process. *Defective or absent growth of columnar cartilage* gives rise to a disease entity known as *chondrodystrophy* (p. 263). In *rickets,* the process of *calcification in the zone of provisional calcification may be deficient* (see p. 263). Deficient *osteoid formation* leads to *osteogenesis imperfecta* (see p. 263). In compact bones, the disorder may be in the zone of remodeling as in *osteopetrosis.*

In most cases of disordered development, the changes are not restricted to endochondral ossification alone but also involve other aspects of bone formation (hatched areas in Table 13.1).

Table 13.1. Diagram of the different disturbances in ossification in the osteodystrophies

	Chondro-dystrophy	Rickets	Syphilitic Osteochondritis	Osteogenesis Imperfecta	Osteopetrosis
I. *Compensatory Bone Formation* 1. Enchondral O. a) epiphyseal O.					
b) metaphyseal O.					
2. Perichondral O.					
II. *Periosteal bone formation*					

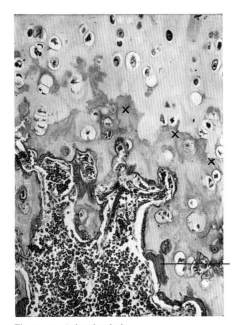

Fig. 13.11. Achondroplasia;
H & E, 110×.

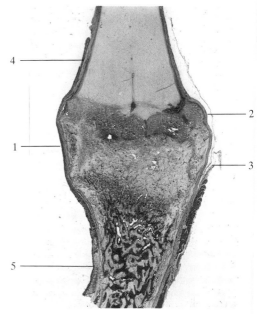

Fig. 13.12. Rickets;
H & E, 5×.

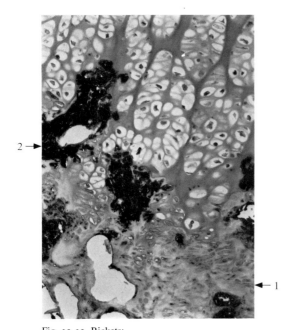

Fig. 13.13. Rickets;
Azan stain, 110×.

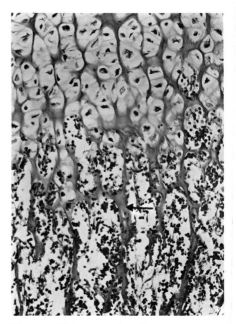

Fig. 13.14. Osteogenesis imperfecta;
H & E, 110×.

Inflammatory Diseases of Joints

The nonspecific inflammatory joint diseases may be subdivided into:
1. *Suppurative inflammations of joints;*
2. *Rheumatic inflammations of joints*
   a) joint inflammation in rheumatic fever,
   b) chronic arthritis (arthritis deformans, osteoarthritis),
   c) ankylosing spondylitis;
3. *Rheumatoid arthritis.* (The clinical picture resembles that of rheumatic fever with its involvement of joints. The causes, however, are different; e.g., dysentery, tuberculosis, ulcerative colitis, etc.)
4. *Degenerative joint disease* (osteoarthritis, see p. 271).

In *active (febrile) rheumatic fever,* true Aschoff nodules may occur in the loose connective tissues of the joint capsule (compare with heart, pp. 49, 217). *Young individuals* are most commonly affected. In most instances, antistreptolysin and antistaphylolysin titers are often markedly elevated. The joint lesions ultimately regress completely.

Chronic arthritis (see Figs. 13.22–13.24) has the morphological appearance of a nonspecific chronic inflammation. *The small joints* (fingers, toes) are preferentially affected. *Older individuals* are afflicted more frequently than young persons. Very frequently results of the latex-fixation and Waaler-Rose tests are positive. Ankylosing of joints occurs as a result of the severe destructive changes.

Ankylosing spondylitis (Bechterew's disease) begins with scanty inflammation infiltration of lymphocytes into the capsule and ligaments of the *small vertebral joints.* The prominent feature of this disease is the excessive bone formation which leads to ankylosis of the vertebral column.

Chronic arthritis (rheumatoid arthritis) can serve as an example of inflammatory joint disease. Compare the schematic drawings in Fig. 13.23 a. The disease begins with inflammation of the joint capsule, as has been shown recently by study of biopsies of the capsule. There is exudation in the joint space of blood plasma and emigration of cells (granulocytes with cytoplasmic inclusion bodies containing rheumatoid factor, synovial cells, lymphocytes, plasma cells). the synovial cells covering the joint capsule are focally destroyed and the foci covered with fibrin. In other places the synovial cells proliferate (→ 1). The synovial connective tissue is densely infiltrated with plasma cells and lymphocytes (→ 2), which often form small lymph follicles. Occasional foci of fibrinoid may be seen.

Chronic arthritis (destruction of cartilage by granulation tissue), 13.23b. The stage of exudation may lead to a stage of proliferative inflammation. Richly vascularized connective tissue called a panus (→) from the synovium or the subarticular bone marrow may grow into the joint cartilage (→ 2) and destroy it on both the joint and bone surfaces.

Chronic arthritis (fibrous ankylosis), Fig. 13.24. The final phase of fibrous ankylosis develops when granulation tissue proliferating from both joint surfaces meets. The subarticular portions of the bone are still intact (→ 1). Only small portions of the joint cartilage are still visible and they show secondary degenerative changes. Solitary slit-like spaces remain from the former joint space (→) within the picture. The articulations of the bones are fused by connective tissue (→ 2).

Macroscopic: White, fibrous cartilaginous deposits (panus), ulceration of cartilage and ankylosis.
NOTE: 1. Subcutaneous periarticular rheumatoid nodules (see p. 217) have diagnostic significance (excision, histopathological examination). 2. The following complications may occur: a) amyloidosis (in about 20%), b) panarteritis nodosa (in about 25%, muscle or liver biopsy may be indicated as diagnostic measure).

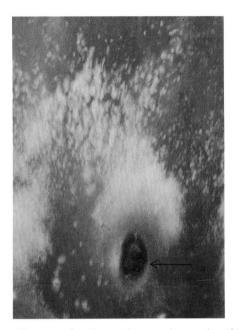

Fig. 13.25. Granular proteinaceous degeneration of joint cartilage; eosin stain, photographed under fluorescent light, 625×.

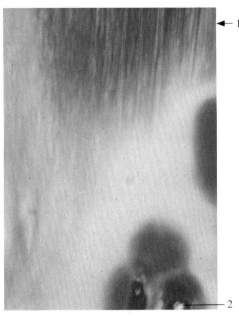

Fig. 13.26. Unmasking of collagen fibers in joint cartilage;
toluidine blue stain, 625×.

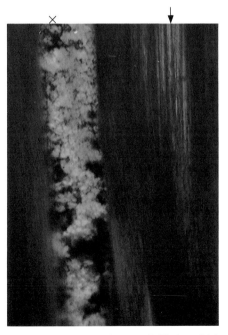

Fig. 13.27. Cyst formation and fibrillation of joint cartilage;
toluidine blue stain, 625×.

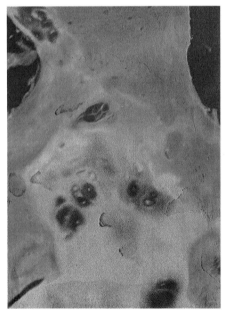

Fig. 13.28. Bone formation in a joint cartilage in arthritis deformans;
acridin orange stain, fluorescent light, 400×.

Degenerative Joint Disease (Osteoarthritis)

In contrast to inflammatory joint diseases, the degenerative joint disorders (e.g., *arthritis deformans, spondylosis deformans*) always begin in the joint cartilage itself. The first detectable change is mucoid or **granular proteinaceous degeneration of the joint cartilage.** Figure 13.25 shows a section through such a joint cartilage. In the lower part of the picture there is a preserved cartilage cell (→) surrounded by numerous yellow granules having a fan-shaped arrangement. These consist of protein or mucopolysaccharides, as can be demonstrated by histochemical techniques. These changes are interpreted as a process of disintegration in which the refractive index of the ground substance is altered, and the normally invisible collagen fibers of the hyalin joint cartilage become visible (→ 1 in Fig. 13.26).

Unmasking of collagen fibers in the joint cartilage (Fig. 13.26). This section shows that the cartilage cells (→ 2) in the vicinity of the unmasked fibers (→ 1) are still intact. Once these cells are destroyed, the lesion is described as **fibrillation** of the cartilage (Fig. 13.27), such as is frequently seen in rib cartilage. The portions of cartilage affected in this manner frequently develop **cysts** and in such regions cells are no longer demonstrable. Only denuded fibers (→) and elongated, cystic spaces (×) remain. Bone may arise in these cysts as a result of proliferative budding of granulation tissue. Figure 13.28 is stained with acridin orange and photographed under fluorescent light to show cancellous bone (green) within bright yellow cartilaginous ground substance (cartilage cells are stained red).

In summary, it is the destruction of cartilaginous tissue which is responsible for the loss of the shearing strength of the hyalin cartilage, and the increasing transfer of pressure is to the bone (Fig. 13.29), since it can no longer be transformed into thrust. The effect of this pressure is to stimulate **new bone formation** (Fig. 13.28). This leads to overgrowth of subchondral cancellous bone (Fig. 13.29), ossification in the joint cartilage itself, and marginal bony outgrowths which finally give the afflicted joint its characteristic structure (so-called lipping of the joint).

Macroscopic: The cartilage is ulcerated and there is marginal enlargement and beading (e.g., spondylosis deformans).

Early phase

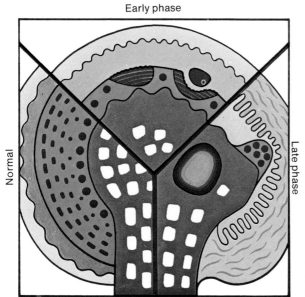

Normal

Late phase

Results of chronic changes in joints in arthritis deformans
1. Normal joint
2. Early phase
   fibrillation of joint cartilage, osteochondritis dissecans and subchondral spongiosa hypertrophy
3. Late phase
   hyperplastic fibrosis of joint capsule, subchondral involuted cysts and capsular regeneration

Fig. 13.29. Diagram of the development of the bony changes resulting from degenerative injury of the joint cartilage.

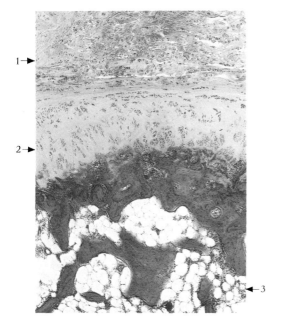

Fig.13.30. Cartilaginous exostosis;
H & E, 36×.

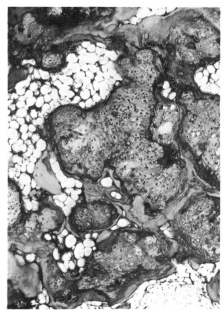

Fig.13.31. Enchondroma;
H & E, 41×.

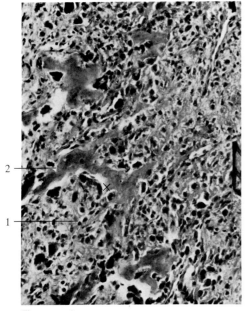

Fig.13.32. Osteosarcoma;
H & E, 102×.

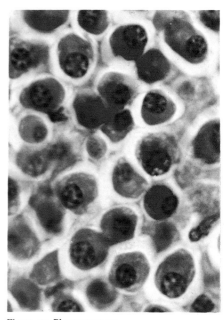

Fig.13.33. Plasmacytoma;
H & E, 1,200×.

Tumors of Bones

Osteochondroma (osteocartilaginous exostosis. Fig. 13.30). *Cartilaginous exostoses are considered to be developmental abnormalities, some representing multiple hereditary lesions, others a benign tumor, i. e., osteochondroma.* Their structure consists of a sparsely cellular cartilaginous cap covering hyperplastic cortical bone and is reminiscent of normal bone growth by enchondral ossification. At the top of the picture there is a layer of periosteal connective tissue (→ 1). Beneath this is a layer of cartilage with groups of small chondrocytes with single nuclei (→ 2), suggesting columns of cartilage, which becomes part of the newly formed thick cortical and spongy bone below. The cancellous bone contains fat tissue and a single focus of hematopoiesis (→ 3).

Enchondroma (Fig. 13.31). *Chondromas, confined chiefly to the hands and feet, occur as either ecchondromas (periosteal chondroma) in epiphyseal regions or as solitary enchondromas of bone marrow.* Histologically, masses of hyaline cartilage of varying shapes can be seen, which, in this particular instance, have developed in the fatty marrow (enchondroma). The cartilaginous tissue has an abundance of uniformly sized cartilage cells with single nuclei that lie in well-defined blue staining ground substance. The cartilage cells are more numerous and arranged less regularly than in normal cartilage. There are no mitoses. Along the edges of the blue staining cartilaginous ground substance (acid mucopolysaccharides) may be seen newly formed bone tissue that stains red (enchondral ossification). Enchondromas of fingers and toes are benign. Those in long bones have a poorer prognosis (chiefly malignant transformation). Chondromas of the pelvis are always malignant.

Osteosarcoma (Fig. 13.32). Osteogenic sarcomas have a varied morphological appearance. They destroy the normal bone tissue but, at the same time, promote development of pathologic bone from connective tissue and cartilage (Albertini, 1955). Characteristically they show a checkerboard histological structure with sarcomatous stroma, islands of hyaline cartilage (neoplastic cartilage), calcification, mucoid material, fibrous bone (neoplastic bone), collections of giant cells and neoplastic osteoid. The neoplastic osteoid and bone are formed from the sarcomatous connective tissue stroma. The formation of osteoid distinguishes osteosarcoma from chondrosarcoma. The osteoplastic variety of osteosarcoma contains numerous pleomorphic spindle cells, whereas the osteolytic variety contains many giant cells and thus may closely resemble a giant cell tumor of bone (see p. 266). Figure 13.32 reveals polymorphocellular tumor tissue containing cartilage-like structures with a homogeneous ground substance (neoplastic cartilage). Atypical cartilage cells with darkly stained nuclei can be seen embedded in homogeneous ground substance (→ 1). In some places (→ 2), structures are found that are reminiscent of uncalcified bony trabeculae (neoplastic bone). Beneath is a layer of uncalcified osteoid (×). There are, however, some totally undifferentiated portions which have the appearance of polymorphocellular sarcoma.

Clinical: Although osteochondrosarcomas are seen particularly in children, they also occur in somewhat older age groups (peak incidence at 10–20 years). Sites of predilection are metaphyses of the femur (distal) and tibia (proximal). Radiologically, osteosarcomas show spicules; the osteolytic form has a mouse-eaten appearance. In order to make a histological diagnosis of bone tumors, it is essential to know the clinical and x-ray findings.

Plasmacytoma or Multiple Myeloma (Fig. 13.33) *is a circumscribed or diffusely growing tumor of bone marrow which destroys the bone. There is an accompanying increase of immune globulins in the blood plasma* (chiefly IgG, IgA; less often IgD or IgE, so-called monoclonal immunoglobulin; part heavy (H) or light (L) chain or L and H antibodies). The kidneys frequently excrete a pathological protein (Bence Jones protein, light chain protein), which is reabsorbed and produces hyalin droplet degeneration in the tubular epithelium (compare p. 160). The disease is also frequently associated with paraamyloidosis. A smear or section of the bone marrow reveals the characteristic atypical plasma cells with eccentrically placed nuclei and pronounced wheel-spoke arrangement of the chromatin. The cytoplasm is eosinophilic.

Macroscopic: Focal lesions in the cranial tables (x-ray!) and focal or diffuse lesions in the spinal column, sternum, pelvis, etc., with concomitant osteolysis. Red or grayish red, gelatinous nodular lesions.

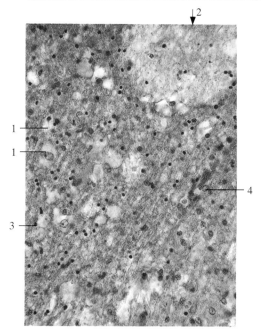

Fig. 14.1. Focal area of recent encephalomalacia or softening of the brain;
pallid area (honeycomb area);
H & E, 248×.

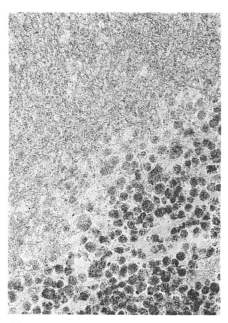

Fig. 14.2. Center of an area of encephalomalacia with granular, fat-containing phagocytic cells (gitter cells or compound granular corpuscles);
Sudan stain, 250×.

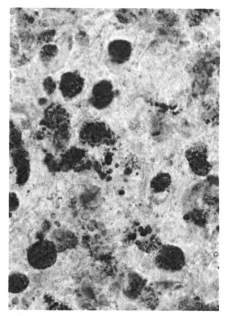

Fig. 14.3. Granular fatty cells;
scarlet red-hematoxylin, 512×.

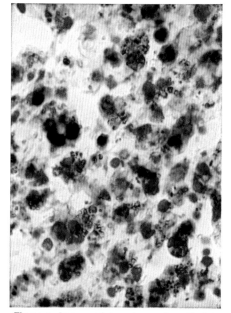

Fig. 14.4. Iron-containing phagocytic cells (pigmented granular cells) in encephalomalacia;
Berlin blue reaction, 800×.

14. Brain–Spinal Cord

Histological examination of the brain and spinal cord should start with an investigation of the condition of the meninges (cellularity, vascular changes, unusual deposits). The substance of the brain and spinal cord is composed of *neurons with their cytoplasmic processes* (dendrites and axis cylinders or axons surrounded by a myelin sheath – special stains must be used to demonstrate them), *neuroglia (astrocytes* with relatively large round nuclei and cytoplasm which is seen well only with special stains, *oligodendroglia* with small round nuclei, and *microglia* with small fusiform nuclei) and *blood vessels.* Both the intact and injured portions of the tissue must be examined (e.g., areas of softening, foci or demyelinization). Perivascular or tissue infiltrates and the types of cells that compose them should be noted.

Encephalomalacia

This is due to **necrosis** of the brain substance followed by *liquefaction* and *secondary cavitation* (cyst formation) resulting either from occlusion of a nutrient artery (arteriosclerosis, thrombosis, embolization) of from generalized hypoxia. The process has several stages. 1. The stage of *cortical pallor* with ischemic changes in the neurons (shrinkage of both the cell body and nucleus with loss of Nissl substance). There may also be interstitial edema with fiber and nuclear degeneration (so-called honeycomb appearance) and, finally complete *necrosis* with loss of nuclei. 2. The stage of *softening with granular fatty cells,* also called gitter cells or compound granular corpuscles (stage of resorption). 3. The stage of *cyst formation and glial scarring* (end stage).

Figure 14.1, which shows **focal, recent brain softening,** will serve as an example of the *first stage* (cortical pallor). There is conspicuous edema between fibers and focally around cells (→ 1), and degeneration of the myelin sheaths, resulting in their complete dissolution (→ 2). The oligodendrocytes have a shrunken appearance (→ 3). The nuclei of the macroglia stain weakly (beginning of karyolysis, → 4). In the upper portion of the picture (→ 2) there is a pale red focus in which the process is further advanced. Nuclei are almost totally lacking, the myelin sheaths dissolved.

Macroscopic: The brain tissue is of slightly soft consistency, and the gray substance is pallid.

The *second stage* (stage of *focal softening*) is characterized by resorption of the destroyed myelin substance (lipids). Figure 14.2 shows the center of an area of **brain softening.** Even with the unaided eye, fat stains show a red lesion that stains with Sudan, as well as a loosening of the tissues, which is discernible in the bluish red brain substance. Examination of the lesion with medium high power reveals numerous round cells, the cytoplasm of which is filled with red sudanophilic granules. High power clearly shows (Fig. 14.3) these **granular fatty cells** with their eccentrically located nuclei (they are either phagocytic microglial cells or histiocytes derived from the sheaths of blood vessels). In paraffin sections, the fat droplets are dissolved and the cytoplasm has a vacuolated appearance. In many cases, bleeding into the tissues has occurred in addition to the softening (*hemorrhagic softening*, frequently seen with emboli). The extravasated erythrocytes and hemoglobin are also taken up by phagocytes and stored as hemosiderin. Such phagocytic cells are called **pigmented granular cells** (Fig. 14.4), since the cytoplasm contains brown hemosiderin granules (iron-reaction positive). In addition, granular fatty cells as well as extra-cellular deposits of brown pigment can be seen (*hematoidin* = iron-free hemoglobin, see also pp. 9, 245).

Macroscopic: There is softening and liquefaction of brain tissue. In cases of hemorrhagic softening, there are punctate hemorrhages which show a brown discoloration when the lesion is a little older. In unstained fresh microscopic preparations, numerous granular fatty cells may be seen (granular cytoplasm with glassy granules).

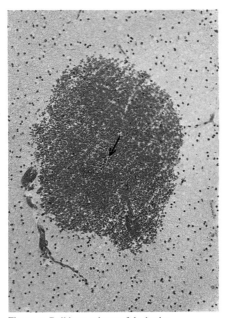

Fig. 14.5. Ball hemorrhage of the brain;
H & E, 120×.

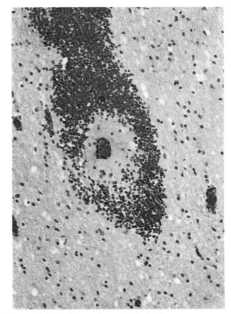

Fig. 14.6. Ring hemorrhage of the brain;
H & E, 175×.

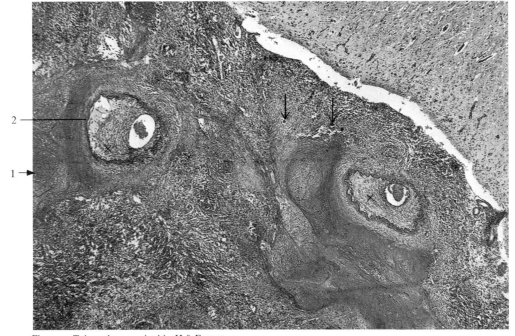

Fig. 14.7. Tuberculous meningitis; H & E, 33×.

Ball and ring hemorrhages of the brain (Figs. 14.5, 14.6). *These hemorrhages are due to circulatory disturbances accompanied by necrosis of the vessel wall. Ball hemorrhages* are spherical lesions composed of compactly arranged extravasated erythrocytes, in the center of which can be seen a venule with a necrotic wall (→ in Fig. 14.6). In **ring hemorrhages,** the center of the lesion is occupied by a vessel that is completely plugged with erythrocytes. This is surrounded by a ring of necrotic brain tissue (in this case, homogeneous myelin sheaths and an occasional cell with an intact nucleus). The outer zone consists of a ring of erythroctyes.

Macroscopic: Punctate hemorrhages, which cannot be wiped away, are present on the cut surfaces of the brain. They are common in hypertension, air embolism, stroke and hemorrhagic encephalitis.

Tuberculous meningitis (Fig. 14.7). *Tuberculous inflammation of the meninges is hematogenous in origin, affects the base of the brain and occurs chiefly in children.* In the acute exudative stage there is a rich fibrinous and protein-rich exudate containing polymorphonuclear leukocytes that is especially prominent around blood vessels. Caseation sets in rapidly in the vicinity of the vessels. Figure 14.7 shows the perivascular necrosis and network of fibrin (→) and the dense cellular infiltration (mainly lymphocytes) of the neighboring tissues. In some areas, the necrosis is already delineated by epithelioid cells. Solitary Langhans giant cells (→ within the picture) are also seen *(subacute proliferative stage).* Of great importance is the fact that the caseation also affects arteries, causing partial or complete necrosis of the vessel walls (→ 2). In addition, if the caseation involves the adventitia, an arteritis develops, which, by a process of inward extension, causes marked endarteritis obliterans (×) with intimal proliferation and marked reduction of the lumen. For this reason, secondary foci of encephalomalacia may be seen in the healing stages of tuberculous meningitis. Thus it is especially important to diagnose tuberculous meningitis early. Caution: since it is rare today, typical cases may not be diagnosed.

Macroscopic: Acute: Gray, gelatinous exudate covers the base of the brain. *Subacute-subchronic:* Small yellow or grayish white, translucent nodules. In the *end stage,* there is connective tissue proliferation with grayish white thickening of the meninges.

Purulent meningitis (Fig. 14.8). *This inflammation of the leptomeninges arises either from blood-borne infection, from direct spread from suppurative infection of adjacent tissues or from penetrating wounds.* Microscopic examination with low power reveals a dense cellular exudate in the leptomeninges. Higher magnification shows that the exudate consists of densely packed polymorphonuclear leukocytes intermingled with fibrin strands. Frequently, the inflammation extends into the cortex (→) along blood vessels (meningoencephalitis).

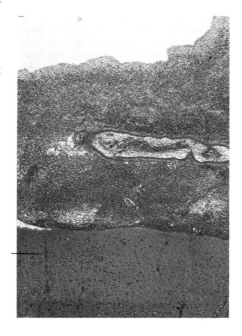

Fig. 14.8. Purulent meningitis; H & E, 38×.

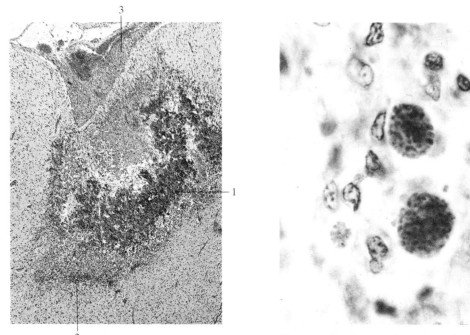

Fig. 14.9. Encephalitis caused by toxoplasmosis; H & E, 10×.

Fig. 14.10. Pseudocysts of toxoplasmosis in the brain;
thionine stain, 1,400×.

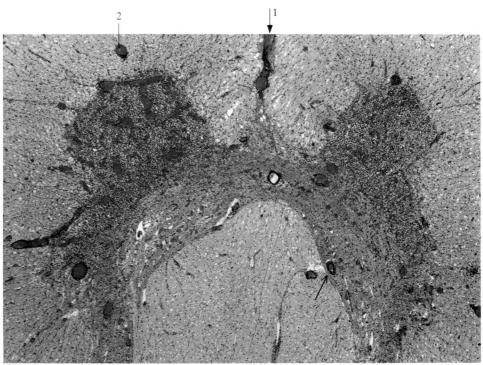

Fig. 14.11. Poliomyelitis; H & E, 51×.

Encephalitis in toxoplasmosis (Fig. 14.9). *This is a granulomatous, necrotizing and calcifying encephalitis caused by Toxoplasma gondii (a protozoon) and occurring chiefly in neonates.* Examination of the specimen with a scanning lens discloses conspicuous cellular nodules and blue-stained calcified foci in the cortex and white matter. Sometimes there are larger necrotic lesions. Closer inspection shows that the cellular nodules are granulomas consisting of lymphocytes, plasma cells, histiocytes and glial cells. Figure 14.9 shows such a cortical lesion with a calcified central zone of necrosis (stained violet blue, → 1) surrounded by a cellular infiltrate (→ 2), consisting largely of lymphocytes and histiocytes. The arachnoid (→ 3) is also infiltrated by lymphocytes.

With oil immersion, **pseudocysts** can often be seen in the granulomas (Fig. 14.10) consisting of intracellular colonies of the causative organisms. The infected cells are round and the cytoplasm is filled with bow-shaped toxoplasma containing small, oval inner bodies. There are histiocytes in the surrounding tissues. Toxoplasmosis in adults causes lymphadenopathy with small foci of epitheloid cells (see p. 235).

Macroscopic: Brown or yellow nodular lesions are seen on the cut surface of the brain.

Poliomyelitis (Figs. 14.11, 14.12). *This viral infection affects the motor neurons of the anterior horn of the spinal cord, causing cell destruction and resorption.* Examination of the section with the scanning lens shows dense cellular infiltration of the anterior horns. At the bottom of Figure 14.11 is the anterior median fissure in which may be seen the lymphocytic infiltration of the leptomeninges (→ 1). The central canal is clearly visible. Dilated vessels (→) in the white matter are also surrounded by mantels of round cells (→ 2). The posterior horns are uninvolved.

Under **higher magnification** (Fig. 14.12), leukocytes and proliferated glial cells are seen to have replaced the phagocytosed necrotic cells *(neuronophagia)*. In places, the shadowy outlines of nerve cells may be seen in the middle of the exudate (→ 1: phagocytosed neuron, → 2: shrunken neuron).

Macroscopic: The anterior horns are deformed.

Typhus fever encephalitis (Fig. 14.13). *This results from systemic infection with Rickettsia prowazekii and is characterized by a nodular form of panencephalitis.* The section shows the olive of the medulla oblongata with two cellular nodules of proliferating microglial cells. These glial cell nodules are situated perivascularly (reaction to rickettsial toxin). The neurons are unchanged. The nodules are not specific for typhus fever and may occur in other sorts of encephalitis.

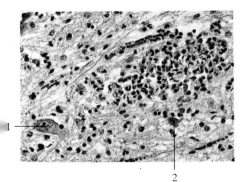

Fig. 14.12. Poliomyelitis;
H & E, 227×.

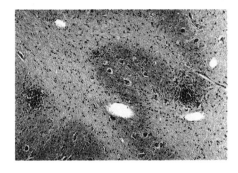

Fig. 14.13. Typhus fever encephalitis;
H & E, 60×.

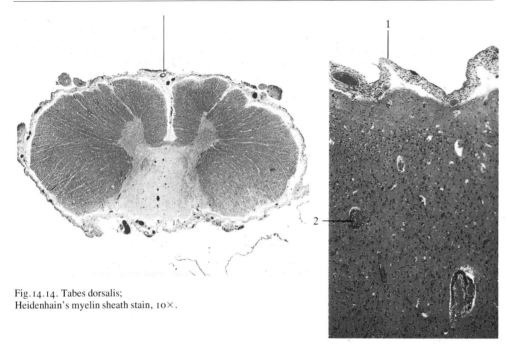

Fig. 14.14. Tabes dorsalis;
Heidenhain's myelin sheath stain, 10×.

Fig. 14.15. General paresis;
H & E, 60×.

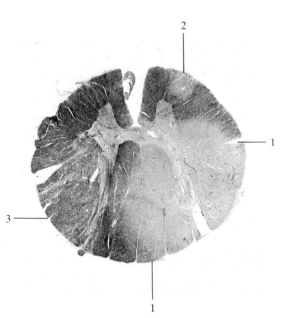

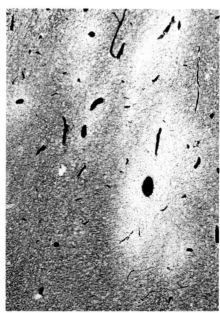

Fig. 14.16. Multiple sclerosis;
Sudan stain, 5×.

Fig. 14.17. Multiple sclerosis;
myelin stain, 60×.

Tabes dorsalis (Fig. 14.14). *In the tertiary stage of syphilis, a chronic, slowly progressive meningitis may develop, with injury of the dorsal roots of the spinal cord and secondary degeneration of posterior columns.* The histological appearance in sections stained for myelin is very typical. With the histological section oriented according to the deeply indented anterior longitudinal fissure (→), the lack of myelin stain in the region of the posterior columns and dorsal roots is immediately apparent. The gray matter (neurons and unmyelinated fibers of the anterior gray horns) is of almost identical hue. Under higher magnification, individual preserved myelin sheaths or sheaths with clumped degenerated myelin may still be recognized. In the florid stages, sections stained for fat show tissue disintegration and granular fatty cells. The meninges are fibrotic and thickened and infiltrated by lymphocytes.

Macroscopic: The meninges are opaque, especially in the thoracic region, and the spinal cord is shrunken and the posterior columns are discolored gray.

General paresis, also called general paralysis of the insane or dementia paralytica (Fig. 14.15). This is a *chronic syphilitic encephalitis with frontal lobe atrophy and deposits of iron in the brain tissue.* In contrast to *luetic meningoencephalitis,* in which there is a predilection for the base of the brain with secondary progression of the inflammation along vascular channels to the cortex, *paresis* affects primarily the *frontal lobes* (insular cortex and temporal lobes) and encephalitis is more marked than is meningitis. The leptomeninges (→ 1) are thickened by fibrosis and sparsely infiltrated by lymphocytes and plasma cells. The most conspicuous feature is in the cortex, where the adventitia of the small vessels is infiltrated by lymphocytes and plasma cells (→ 2) which, even under low-power magnification, may be seen as bluish cuffs. In addition, there is a diffuse increase of microglial cells which contain cytoplasmic hemosiderin, as do the macrophages derived from the perivascular tissues.

Macroscopic: Atrophy of the convolutions of the frontal lobe with opaque, thickened, meninges.

Multiple sclerosis (Figs. 14.16, 14.17). *A chronic, progressive, focally disseminated, demyelinating disease of the brain and spinal cord of unknown etiology.* Myelin stain or Sudan stain (Fig. 14.17) demonstrates the demyelinated lesions clearly. A cross section of the spinal cord shows a well-demarcated, pale round lesion located mostly in the vicinity of the dorsal roots (between → 1 in Fig. 14.16). However, there are isolated smaller lesions (→ 2) that are not restricted to anatomically distinct fiber tracts (compare this to the picture of tabes dorsalis, Fig. 14.14). The spreading of the demyelinating process has been compared to an ink stain on a blotter. An early stage may also be seen in Figure 14.16, in which there is resorption of the myelin substance by granular fatty cells (→ 3). Even under low power, the light red stain of the neutral fats stored in macrophages is conspicuous, and under higher power these prove to be typical granular fatty cells (p. 274).

The **myelin stain** (Fig. 14.17) shows that the demyelinating process proceeds from the vessels, but nevertheless does not correspond to the area of distribution of the vessel.

Axons are preserved. A glial scar forms secondarily, consisting of a network of glial fiber and slightly increased numbers of glial cells (sclerosis). The myelin stain colors the erythrocytes in the vessels a deep blue.

Macroscopic: Old lesions appear gray, more recent lesions are salmon colored. Pathogenesis: It is now thought to be either a virus infection (slow virus) or an aggressive disease (IgG increased in spinal fluid). Slow virus = viral infection of long duration; occurs in sheep in England, so-called "scrapie" disease (chronic pruritis). Newborns in New Guinea with the disease (Kuru) show a paralysis agitans (Field, 1969). Genetic factors play a role (familial incidence).

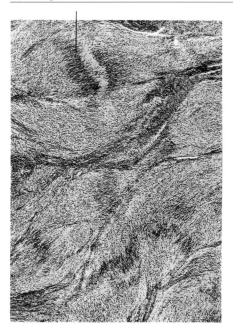

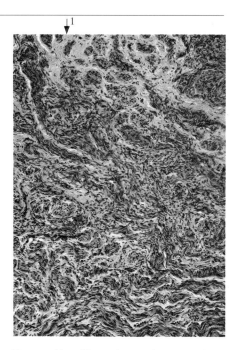

Fig. 14.18. Neurinoma;
van Gieson, 47×.

Fig. 14.19 Neurofibroma (amputation neuroma);
H & E, 90×.

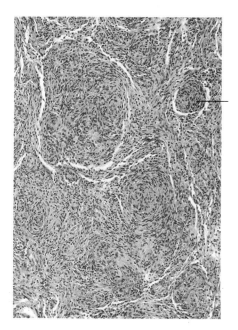

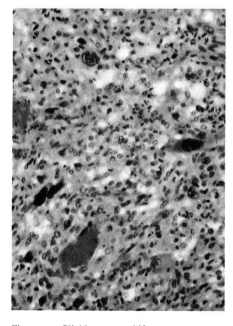

Fig. 14.20. Meningioma;
van Gieson, 180×.

Fig. 14.21. Glioblastoma multiforme;
H & E, 190×.

Tumors of Nerve Tissues

The **neurinomas** (Fig. 14.18) present a typical histological picture, even when examined only with a scanning lens. There are densely packed spindle-shaped cells and fibers arranged in wide bands. The nuclei are pointed and have an orderly, rhythmic arrangement (so-called palisading of the nuclei: →). Medium magnification of a van Gieson preparation reveals the yellow, drawn-out cytoplasm of the cells which form a syncytium. These cells are derived from the Schwann cells of the nerve sheath ("schwannoma").

Macroscopic: Round, discrete tumors, e.g., in the pontine-cerebellar angle.

Neurofibromas (Fig. 14.19) may be solitary or multiple and frequently are generalized (as part of *von Recklinghausen's neurofibromatosis)*. It is only the large amount of collagenous fibrous tissue that distinguishes them from the neurinomas. The tumors are essentially fibromas, infiltrated by nerve fibers and proliferated Schwann cells. The bundles of nerve fibers (van Gieson yellow) are divided and pressed apart by the proliferating connective tissue (→ 1: van Gieson: red). Figure 14.22 shows a so-called *amputation neuroma,* i.e., a club-shaped proliferation of nerve fibers (→ 2) and connective tissue following injury or severance of a nerve. Such a lesion is probably not a true neoplastic condition; rather, it appears to be compensatory regeneration.

Meningioma (Fig. 14.20). *Grossly, most meningiomas are spherical tumors situated on the dura and compressing the brain. They derive from the arachnoid fibroblast.* The typical structures can be best located under low magnification. There are spindle-shaped cells in an onion-skin arrangement (→ 1), in the center of which there are hyalin or calcified nodules (necrotic cells) arranged concentrically – the so-called *dural psammoma body* (→2). Scattered between these foci, there are solid portions containing great numbers of ovoid cells (→ 3) surrounded by collagenous fibrous tissue. Should proliferation of connective tissue predominate, the tumor will resemble a fibroma histologically.

Glioblastoma multiforme (Fig. 14.21). the glioblastoma multiforme is the most common malignant brain tumor of adults. Histologically, the tumor is highly cellular with focal areas of necrosis and hemorrhage and has invaded normal brain. A prominent feature is the marked variation of the cells, which have pleomorphic cytoplasm and bizarre, hyperchromatic and pleomorphic nuclei, and frequently are arranged in perivascular fashion. Scattered throughout the tissue there are small round cells. It is not possible to identify any of these cells specifically as either glial cells or astrocytes.

Macroscopic: Variegated cut surface with a mixture of red hemorrhagic portions, yellow areas of necrosis and gray tumor tissue. Frequently, the surrounding brain tissue is edematous (yellowish gray, gelatinous).

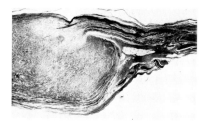

Fig. 14.22. Club-shaped amputation neuroma of a nerve (right); myelin stain, 10× (Noetzel).

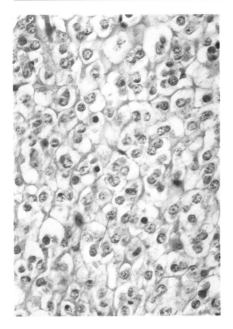

Fig. 14.23. Oligodendroglioma; H & E, 320×.

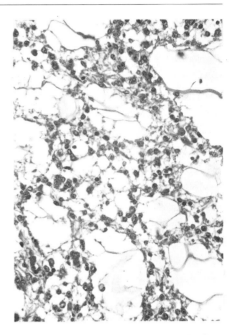

Fig. 14.24. Fibrillary astrocytoma; H & E, 180×.

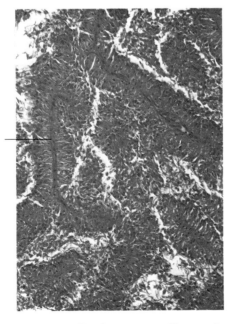

Fig. 14.25. Ependymoma; van Gieson stain, 180×.

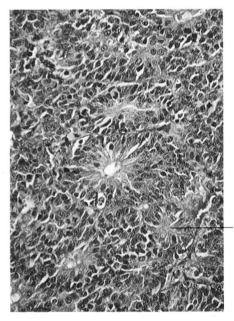

Fig. 14.26. Medulloblastoma; cresyl violet stain, 150×.

Oligodendroglioma (Fig. 14.23). This is a slowly growing brain tumor which occurs chiefly in the cerebrum. The figure shows that it is composed of relatively uniform cells having round nuclei with compact chromatin structure and optically empty cytoplasm. The cell borders are distinct and resemble those of plants (compare hypernephroma of the kidney). The tumor is poor in blood vessels. Capillaries in the neighborhood of the tumor are frequently calcified (X-ray!)

Mostly 30–50 year olds. $\male : \female = 3:7$.

Fibrillary astrocytoma (Fig. 14.24). In adults it occurs in the cerebrum; in children, in the cerebellum or pons. It has an invasive growth pattern and macroscopically is poorly demarcated (surgery!). There are two types: a) protoplasmic astrocytoma with plump astrocytes, i.e., large round cells with homogenous, eosinophilic cytoplasm and eccentrically situated nuclei. These occur only in the cerebrum; b) fibrillary astrocytoma (Fig. 14.24) composed of bipolar fibrillary astrocytes with round only moderately polymorphic nuclei. The fibrillary processes of the cells intermingle, forming a loose network. $\male : \female = 3:2$.

Ependymoma (Fig. 14.25): Ependymomas arise from the ependymal cells in the ventricles and accordingly occur in the region of the cerebral ventricles (30% of cases, especially young persons), the fourth ventricle (45% of cases) or in the spinal cord (25% of cases). They grow expansively and also into the ventricle and frequently recur. Histologically they have a rosette-like pattern: at the center there is a capillary (→) to the adventitia of which is attached the stretched out cytoplasm of the ependymal cells. The nuclei lie in the periphery at the opposite end of the cells thus forming a nucleus free halo around the central blood vessel.

Medulloblastoma (Fig. 14.26): this is the most common brain tumor in childhood (6–14 years) and arises in the cerebellar vermis or cerebellar hemispheres. It is an embryonal tumor and in this respect is similar to embryonal renal tumors. Histologically there are oval, carrot-shaped nuclei which often form pseudorosettes (→) or show a palisade arrangement. If the tumor grows in the fourth ventricle obstructive hydrocephalus may develop. Metastases may occur within the ventricular system or diffusely in the leptomeninges.

Spongioblastoma also occurs at a young age, especially in girls. These tumors occur in the optic nerves, pons, cerebellum or hypothalamus. Elongated tumor cells are arranged in fibrous tufts or whorls and produce an abundance of glial fibers. Mostly the tumors are well defined but because of their deep location are difficult to approach surgically.

Brain tumors occupy a special position among malignant tumors because they do not metastasize outside the brain and cerebral symptoms predominate (no cachexia). The commonest intracranial tumor is meningioma (15–20% of all brain tumors); then follow glioblastoma multiforme with 12%, oligodendroglioma, spongioblastoma and astrocytoma with 6–8% and ependymoma and medulloblastoma with 4%.

Table 15.1 Differences of behavior of benign and malignant tumors

Characteristics	Benign Tumors	Malignant Tumors
Clinical Findings		
1. Sex	Not significant	Not significant
2. Age	Chiefly in young persons	Chiefly in older persons
3. Location of tumor	Both benign & malignant tumors occur in all organs. Tumor characteristics determined by localization: a histologically benign tumor can have a malignant behavior because of its location (e.g., in the brain).	
4. Clinical symptoms	Rather slight, nonspecific (many exceptions, e.g., endocrine tumors).	Marked, often detected first in advanced stages
5. Duration of illness	Long (years or decades)	Rather short (months)
6. Specific cell function	Chiefly normal	Mostly lacking
7. Growth	Expanding, displacing	Infiltrating, invasive
8. Metastases	Lacking	Common
9. Recurrence	Can occur	Common
Pathological Findings		
10. Organ changes	Pressure atrophy	Destruction
11. Tumor capsule	Present	Lacking
12. Consistency	Variable	Mostly soft
13. Cut surface	Uniform	Variegated (red hemorrhages, yellow necrosis)
14. Tissue type (resembles parent tissue)	Homologous, mature	Heterologous, immature
15. Cellularity	Often poorly cellular	Richly cellular
16. Cell size and shape	Regular, isomorphous	Irregular, polymorphous
17. Cell atypia	Lacking	Common
18. Mitoses: number and type	Rare, typical	Common, atypical
19. Chromatin	Regular division	Irregular: partly dense, partly vesicular
20. Chromosomes (DNA content)	Euploid	Chiefly aneuploid with chromosomal aberrations
21. Nucleolus	Similar to parent cells	Distinctly large, often prominent
22. Nucleus/cytoplasm ratio	Normal	Displacement in favor of of nucleus
23. Cytoplasmic staining	Normal	Often increased by DNA, slightly basophilic
24. Enzyme content of cells	Normal	Often deficient

15. Tumors

Tumors (synonyms: neoplasm, new growth, blastoma) *are abnormal tissue masses, which arise by autonomous, progressive and excessive proliferation of the body's own cells.*

For useful **diagnosis** and **classification** of a tumor it is necessary to consider several individual factors, especially the morphology (microscopic structure) and the histogenesis (recognition of the parent tissue from which the tumor arises). It is desirable not only to make an *accurate diagnosis* of a tumor but also to give an opinion of the *prognosis* and of the *appropriate therapy*. The most important consideration in classifying a tumor, without doubt, is its *biological behavior*. It should be borne in mind, however, that the terms *benign* and *malignant* are man-made concepts and do not describe any innate natural phenomena of the tumor. There are tumors that are truly benign (e.g., cutaneous warts) and others of which there is no question of their malignancy (e.g., malignant melanoma). For *locally malignant tumors* that have a locally destructive growth pattern and recur but do not metastasize the term *"semi-malignant"* is used. Basal cell carcinoma (basaloma, cylindroma), carcinoid and salivary gland tumors belong to this group. In the current WHO nomenclature basaloma and cylindroma are considered as basal cell carcinoma or as adenoidcystic carcinoma and so unequivocally counted among malignant tumors. Carcinoids behave differently depending upon their location: carcinoids of the appendix are often benign; carcinoids of the ileum may metastasize to the liver. Today salivary gland tumors are placed with pleomorphic adenomas, since they recur only after incomplete surgical removal.

The diagnostic assessment of a tumor demands the collection and evaluation of numerous individual pieces of clinical and pathological information. Thus it must be remembered that the final diagnosis of any pathologist is the result of his experience and that he predicts the possible final outcome of the disease from the static appearance of the fixed tissue submitted to him. The most important pieces of information are summarized in Table 15.1. In practice one is always faced with the question, *is the tumor still benign or already malignant?* We know that a malignant tumor (e.g., a carcinoma) does not arise directly from a normal cell but is rather the end stage of a series of changes that may progress from the normal cell through regenerative changes and benign tumors to malignant tumors. This course is considered as *progressive*. Thus it is possible that a tissue sample may be of a transitional phase or intermediate stage of a tumor and the question of its behavior cannot be definitely settled. Such cases are called *borderline* tumors.

In recent years it has been observed repeatedly that the *prognosis of a tumor*—measured in terms of 5- or 10-year survival—depends upon certain well-established pathological-anatomical facts which are taken into account either by the **TNM system** or by tumor grading. In the **TNM system** (T-tumor, N-node, M-metastasis) the macroscopic findings such as tumor size, its localization, spread, involvement of lymph nodes and the presence of distant hematogenous metastases, are taken into account. At present there is a TNM coding for each organ. In **tumor grading** the prognosis of a tumor is estimated from its histological structure and degree of differentiation, well-differentiated tumors as a rule having a better prognosis than undifferentiated tumors (see salivary gland tumors).

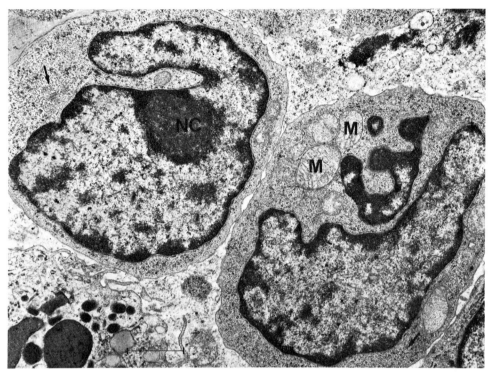

Fig. 15.1. *Burkitt tumor* (Burkitt, 1958). *Malignant lymphoma* occurring chiefly in the jaws of children. It consists of lymphoblasts with scanty cytoplasmic margins and distinctly polymorphous nuclei, irregular, clump-like divisions of heterochromatin and large nucleolus (NC). The cytoplasm is rich in free ribosomes and polysomes but poor in mitochondria (M). 10,000× (Bernhard).

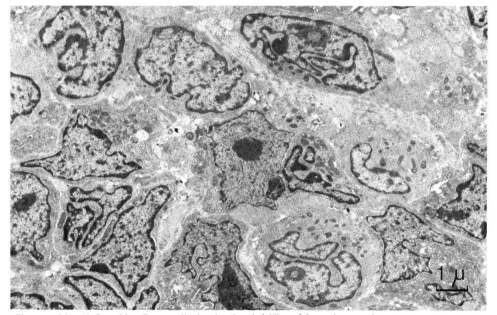

Fig. 15.2. Mycosis fungoides. Tumor cells showing deep infolding of the nuclear membrane. 5000×.

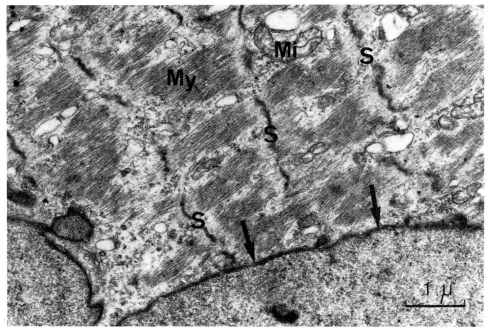

Fig. 15.3. Section of a rhabdomyosarcoma cell. Myofilaments (My) are clearly shown and have a sarcoma-like arrangement (S). Mi = mitochondria. The arrow points to the nuclear membrane. 12,000×.

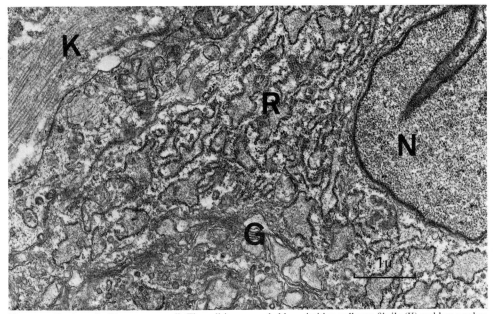

Fig. 15.4. Section of a fibrosarcoma cell. The cell is surrounded by primitive collagen fibrils (K) and has a valve-like nucleus (N) and well-developed rough ER (R) and Golgi apparatus (G). 12,000×.

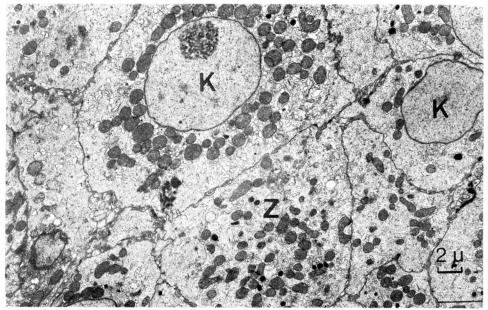

Fig. 15.5. Section of a moderately fast growing Morris hepatoma. The cytoarchitecture of the tumor cells for the most part resembles that of normal hepatocytes. The orderly lobular pattern is lacking. Z = cytoplasm, K = nucleus. Note the large nucleolus, 7500×.

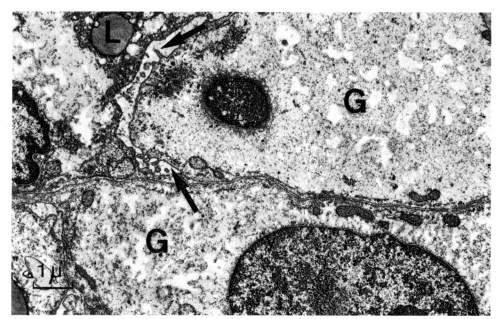

Fig.15.6. Section of a clear cell from a hypernephroma (renal clear cell carcinoma). The cytoplasm contains large amounts of glycogen (G) and lipid droplets (L). The arrow points to brushlike differentiation of the cell surface. 10,500× (Kistler).

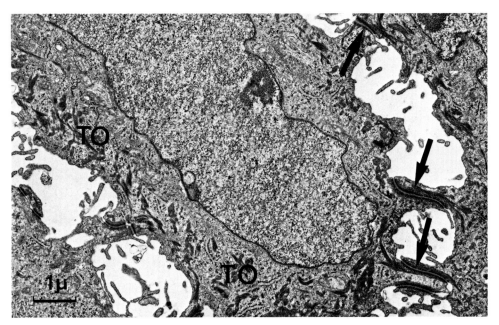

Fig. 15.7. Section of a tumor cell from a squamous cell carcinoma of the bronchus. The typical intercellular bridges are clearly seen with their desmosome-like structures (→), which are characteristic of squamous epithelium. The cytoplasm is rich in tonofibrils (TO). 12,000 (Kistler).

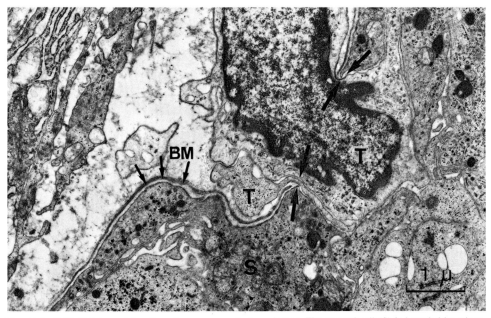

Fig. 15.8. Epithelial-stromal junction of a mammary duct carcinoma. The stromal cell (S) is bounded by a basement membrane (BM). Tumor cells (T) penetrate the stroma through a break in the basement membrane (→). 15,000×. (Ozello and Sanpitak).

Tumors—Electron Microscopy

There is no one specific ultramicroscopic feature by which a cancer cell can be invariably recognized. There are, however, certain recognizable morphological changes that differentiate a normal cell from a tumor cell.

In animals oncologic viruses can be detected in certain tumors, for example, breast carcinoma, leukemia and other tumors. In man viruses have been identified only in certain papillomas and cutaneous warts. It is true, nonetheless, that similar particles have been observed in human leukemia cells and a few other cancer cells, but such particles have not been proven to be viruses despite their morphological similarities.

Electron microscopic evaluation of the **nuclear membrane** is of the utmost importance. Marked infolding of the nuclear membrane is typical of certain tumor cells, e.g., mycosis fungoides cells (Fig. 15.2) or Reed-Sternberg cells in Hodgkin's disease, although the change usually can only be identified with certainty in semi-thin sections (thickness less than 1μ).

The **cytoplasm** also shows ultrastructural alterations. Certain tumors, such as oncocytoma, show pathological changes of *mitochondrial* DNA. The cells are filled with plump functionally defective mitochondria (histologically oxyphilic, pale, granular cytoplasm). Tumors of a high grade of malignancy by comparison are mostly *poor in mitochondria* or show *dystrophic giant mitochondria* indicating mitochondrial antibodies (Thomas et al, 1977). The *endoplasmic reticulum* is likewise an indication of the degree of differentiation of a tumor. The cells of a benign tumor (adenoma) or of a well-differentiated liver cell carcinoma (Fig. 15.5), for example, may indicate the degree of functional activity of the protein system. Consequently these cells contain well-developed endoplasmic reticulum. In a rapidly growing malignant hepatoma, on the other hand, the tumor cells lose their *metabolic capability:* smooth endoplasmic reticulum is absent. Differentiation is poor and the amount of endoplastic reticulum and membranes decrease in sarcoma cells.

Study of the ultrastructure of tumors can contribute to the *differential diagnosis* and histogenetic differentiation and especially to their classification. *Desmosome-like intercellular bridges* are typical of a squamous cell carcinoma (Fig. 15.7) The carcinoma cells are recognizable because of the *microvillus-like differentiation of the margins of the cell membrane* which derives from the lumen or from holes in the covering cells (glands, respiratory tract, mesothelium). The recognition of *intracytoplasmic granules* with a zigzag internal structure suggests a melanoma. In spindle cell sarcomas an accurate histogenetic classification is often possible only after electronmicroscopic investigation. The presence of a *sarcomatous arrangement of myofilaments* suggests a rhabdomyosarcoma (Fig. 15.3); of heavy *bundles of filaments*, a leiomyosarcoma.

Electron microscopy, especially in regard to the *tumor-stroma relationship,* can also give information about the *spread of a tumor*. In these cases the ultrastructural findings (e.g., the basement membrane, Fig. 15.8) contribute to better demarcation of the invasive stages of precancer and of early cancer changes.

Benign Epithelial Tumors

Benign epithelial tumors can arise from a mucous membrane (*fibro-epithelial exophytic growth* = papilloma or polyp) or from a solid, parenchymatous organ (*endophytic growth* = adenoma).

Chronic irritation or inflammation can cause circumscribed thickening of a mucous membrane. In **leukoplakia** (Fig. 15.9a) there is acanthotic thickening of the epithelium with superficial parakeratotic cornification (cornified lamellae containing nuclei) and an inflammatory infiltrate in the depths of the stroma. Leukoplakias of oral mucous membrane, lip, tongue, larynx and of the urinary bladder are considered precancerous lesions. In contrast, simple hyperkeratosis *(leukoplakic thickening)* of the esophagus or uterine cervix is harmless.

Papillomas (Fig. 15.9c) are benign, broad based, epithelial new growths which develop on squamous or transitional epithelial surfaces. They occur in the urinary bladder, skin, or oral cavity and as villous polyps in the colon where they are demarcated by the muscularis mucosae. Invasion is a sign of malignant transformation (Fig. 15.9f).

Polyps (Fig. 15.9d) are benign epithelial new growths with a narrow base and a long stalk. The surface is covered by glandular epithelium. Example: adenomatous polyp of the colon.

Pseudopolyps (Fig. 15.9b) arise by expansion of a submucosal tumor. Example: submucous or subcutaneously situated lipoma.

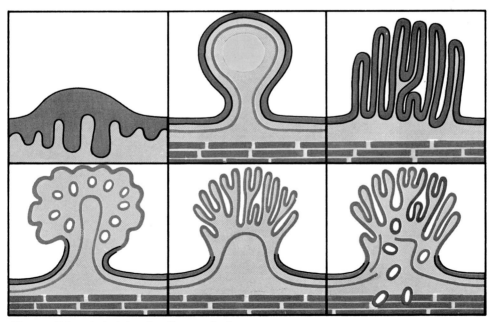

Fig. 15.9. Schematic depiction of papillomas and polyps.

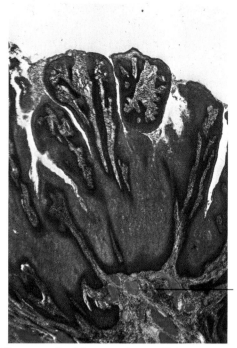

Fig. 15.10. Condyloma acuminatum; H & E, 20×.

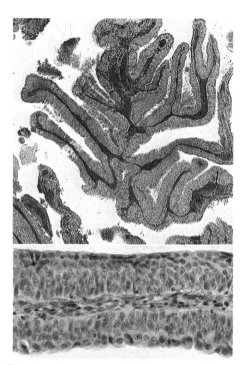

Fig. 15.11. Low power and high power magnification of a papilloma of the urinary bladder; H & E, 30× & 150×.

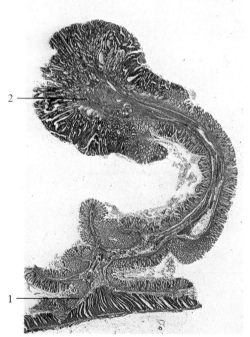

Fig. 15.12. Adenomatous polyp of the rectum; H & E, 8×.

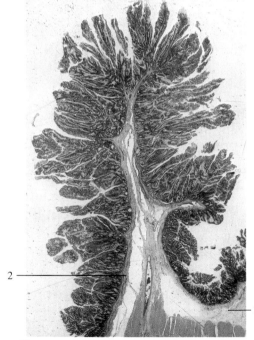

Fig. 15.13. Villous (papillary) polyp of the rectum; H & E, 6×.

Papilloma–Polyp

Condyloma acuminatum (Fig. 15.10). *A benign, broad-based fibro-epithelial new growth, chiefly occurring in the perianal and periurethral regions, or on the penis or external female genitalia.* Histologically the lesion consists of a papilloma resting on a broad base of connective tissue and covered on the surface by a thickened layer of squamous epithelium (stratum spinosum shows many mitoses). The basal stroma is inflamed and vascular.

Condyloma acuminatum is a virus caused hyperplasia of mucous membrane induced by chronic irritation—usually as an accompaniment of some other disease (e.g., gonorrhea). The lesion tends to recur but not to become malignant. It must be differentiated from syphilitic *condylomata*.

Urinary bladder papilloma (Fig. 15.11) *is a* **histologically** *benign, exophytic growing, fibroepithelial tumor of the upper urinary passages and bladder which, however, frequently recurs and shows malignant transformation. It is therefore* **clinically** *considered at least an obligate precancerous lesion or even a well-differentiated transitional cell carcinoma (Grade 1).* Low magnification (Fig. 15.11, above) shows the many layered transitional epithelium. It is a papilloma with a broad cellular layer (more than 7 cell layers), cell atypia (distinctly large cells and nuclei) as well as mitoses which are signs of marked proliferation or malignant transformation, although signs of invasive growth in the material examined may be entirely lacking.

Papillomas of the urinary bladder commonly develop in men 60 to 70 years old. Recurrences occur in about 70% of cases and are seldom as low grade as the primary tumor. In 10% of papillomas the evidences of invasive growth are present from the first. Proliferating mucous membrane showing all the cytological criteria of malignancy, but with an intact basement membrane is designated *carcinoma-in-situ* and often is flat and spreading.

Polyps of the Colon (Figs. 15.12, 15.13)

Polyps of the gastrointestinal tract are benign exophytic new growths occurring chiefly in the colon and infrequently in the gastric mucosa and small intestine. Both clinically and pathologically the following types are recognized: 1. Solitary *retention polyps*. These usually develop in children under 6 years, are localized in the rectum and are benign. 2. Solitary *adenomatous polyps* (Fig. 15.12) occur in adults and very rarely become malignant. 3. Large (over 3 cm diameter), solitary, *villous, rectal polyps* by contrast commonly become carcinomas. 4. *Polyposis coli* shows many mucosal polyps that are of adenomatous type histologically, but develop at an earlier age (young men under 36 years of age). 5. In *polyposis intestini (Peutz-Jeghers syndrome)* benign polyps with long stalks develop in the gastrointestinal tract accompanied by prominent, fleck-like melanin pigmentation of the lips and oral mucous membranes. Polyps also occur in the *Gardner* and *Cronkhite-Canada* syndromes.

Figures 15.12 and 15.13 show the prognostically important differences in structure between an adenomatous and a villous polyp of the rectum. An *adenomatous rectal polyp* has a narrow site of attachment (→ 1), a long, thin stalk and a thick, knob-like head. The stroma arises from the muscularis mucosa, submucosa and blood vessels. Near the surface (→ 2) there are collections of erythrocytes and macrophages containing hemosiderin (sign of bleeding). The superficial layer is made up partly of pale mucous containing epithelium and partly of dark regenerating and hyperplastic epithelium. A *villous rectal polyp* (Fig. 15.13) on the other hand has a broad-based papillary structure and the pattern of the superficial epithelium has changed to a hyperplastic adenomatous one. The tumor-free submucosa (→ 1) and the intact muscularis mucosa exclude malignancy in this case.

295

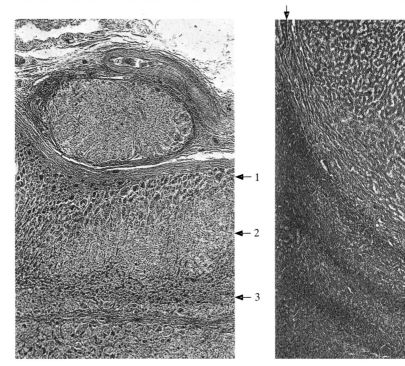

Fig. 15.14. Adrenal cortical adenoma; H & E, 35×.

Fig. 15.15. Benign liver cell adenoma; H & E, 36×.

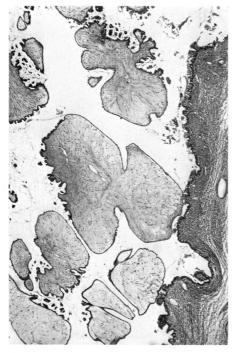

Fig. 15.16. Papillary serous cystadenoma of ovary; H & E, 30×.

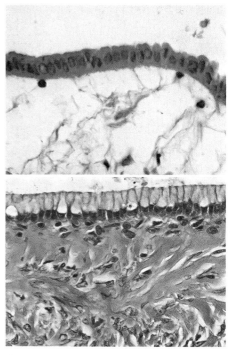

Fig. 15.17. Above: serous cystadenoma, Below: pseudomucinous cystadenoma of ovary; H & E, 250×.

Adenoma–Cystoma

An **adenoma of the adrenal cortex** (Fig. 15.14) *is a well circumscribed, encapsulated, benign neoplasm arising from the adrenal cortex.* Since these and similar tumors—especially those found in other endocrine organs—are an expression of marked hormonal demand, they are sometimes spoken of as adaptation hyperplasia. This means that—at least at the beginning—both growth and function are under hormonal control. The figure shows an adenoma lying in the capsule of the adrenal and isolated from the underlying adrenal which shows the normal cortical layers (lower half of figure): *zona glomerulosa* (→1), *zona fasciculata* (→2) and *zona reticularis* (→3).

Adrenal cortical adenomas are frequently multiple in patients with hypertension *(nodular hyperplasia of adrenal cortex).* They also occur as true autonomous adenomas and can be hormonally silent or active (Conn or Cushing syndromes). These adenomas are especially rich in lipids (yellow cut surface).

Hepatoma (Fig. 15.15) *is a benign new growth arising from proliferating hepatocytes.* Histologically it is a circumscribed but not encapsulated nodule (→) composed of cells having a trabecular arrangement. Under high magnification the tumor is seen not to be bounded by normal liver cells. The adjacent tissue at the periphery shows pressure atrophy and is bloody.

Hepatomas develop with special frequency in cirrhosis of the liver and in the advanced stages of the disease cannot be differentiated from *regenerative nodules.* Isolated hepatomas develop in normal liver but only occasionally and are thought to be tumor-like malformations *(hamartomas).* Well-circumscribed *benign cholangiomas* are also regarded as hamartomas. They consist of proliferating glandulo-alveolar bile duct epithelium supported by fibrous stroma.

Cystadenoma, (cystic adenoma, cystoma) (Figs. 15.16, 15.17). Cystadenomas occur chiefly in the ovary and rarely in other organs (e.g., pancreas). They consist of *single or multilocular cysts* lined by flattened or papillary, simple or pseudomucinous epithelium and contain thin, yellow usually mucinous fluid. On the basis of these features there are *uni- or multilocular, simple or papillary, serous or pseudomucinous cystadenomas.* This classification has both prognostic and therapeutic significance. **Serous ovarian cystadenomas** develop in both ovaries in about 50% of cases and tend to have the same percentage of malignant transformation. By contrast, **pseudomucinous cystadenomas** are solitary and only occasionally show malignant change (less than 5% of cases). They may rupture and cause **pseudomyxoma peritonei** (rupture → mucinous and tumor adhesions develop in the peritoneum → implantation metastases → further mucin production and spread of intraperitoneal adhesions, especially of the small intestines).

Serous papillary **cystadenoma of the ovary** (Figs. 15.16, 15.17 above) consists of a cyst lined with cuboidal epithelium. In the cavity of the cyst there are papillary structures (→) having a loosely arranged fibrous stroma and a superficial layer of epithelium. Higher magnification (Fig. 15.17 above) reveals cuboidal cells with eosinophilic cytoplasm and centrally situated nuclei. Commonly there are small concentrically layered calcium deposits in the stroma (psammoma bodies).

Pseudomucinous cystadenoma of the ovary (Fig. 15.17 below) consists of a single layer of cylindrical epithelium with basally placed nuclei and apical cytoplasmic mucous vacuoles. These cells resemble the goblet cells of large bowel mucosa. The cysts contain PAS positive mucus *(pseudomucin* because it is not dissolved by acetic acid).

Ovarian cysts are derived from germinal ovarian epithelium. Differentiation between benign and malignant cysts is often very difficult. In such *borderline tumors* there is often beginning invasion of stroma by clumps of cells showing glandular differentiation.

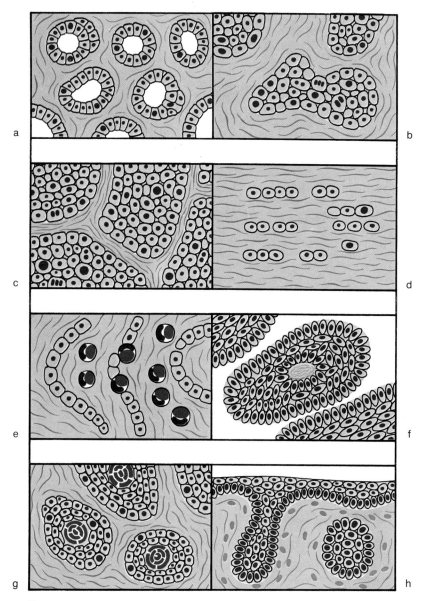

Fig. 15.18. Schematic representation of carcinomas; a) gland-forming carcinoma (adeno-carcinoma), b) solid carcinoma, c) medullary carcinoma, d) scirrhus carcinoma, e) signet ring cell carcinoma, f) transitional cell carcinoma, g) squamous cell carcinoma, and h) basal cell carcinoma.

Carcinoma—Malignant Epithelial Tumor

Carcinomas *are epithelial tumors which both clinically and pathologically show signs of malignancy.* They are classified according to the parent tissue from which they come (e.g., hepatocellular carcinoma) or according to their cellular and tissue differentiation (e.g., squamous carcinoma or signet ring cell carcinoma).

Carcinomas which arise from a glandular parenchymatous organ are called **adenocarcinomas.** Such tumors may show advanced **glandular differentiation,** e.g., follicular, alveolar, cystic or cystic papillary structures (Fig. 15.18a).

Undifferentiated adenocarcinomas are classified on the basis of their tumor cells stroma proportions:

1. In **solid carcinoma simplex** (Fig. 15.18b) tumor cells and stroma are present in about the same proportion (1:1 ratio). Figure 15.19 shows small carcinoma deposits comprised of 10–20 tumor cells and surrounding collagenous connective tissue stroma. Mitoses and cellular atypia are common, in contrast to carcinoid.

2. **Medullary carcinoma** (Fig. 15.18c) typically shows a predominance of the tumor component and only scanty stroma. Figure 15.20 is a completely undifferentiated carcinoma traversed only by occasional septa of breast connective tissue.

3. In **scirrhus carcinoma** (Fig. 15.18d) the collagenous connective tissue stroma clearly predominates. Enclosed in the stroma are single tumor cells or small strands and clusters of tumor cells *(tumor cells in goose step).* These neoplasms have an especially firm, compact consistency and were formerly called *linitis plastica.* All three types of tumor are especially common in stomach and breast.

Signet ring cell carcinoma (Fig. 15.18e) shows a special sort of cell differentiation. The cells are round and the cytoplasm contains a large PAS positive vacuole of mucin which pushes the nucleus to the periphery of the cell (Fig. 15.25). Signet ring cells are observed in mucinous carcinoma of the breast and in early carcinoma of the stomach.

Among carcinomas of surface epithelium are **transitional cell carcinoma** (Fig. 15.18f: urinary bladder and passages) and **squamous epithelial carcinoma** (squamous carcinoma, Fig. 15.18g) which can arise either from normal pavement epithelium or by squamous metaplasia. Malignant epithelial tumors developing from basal cells are called *basal cell carcinoma* (Fig. 15.18h, see skin tumors).

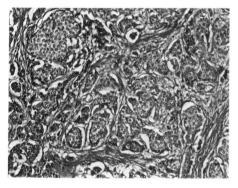

Fig. 15.19 Solid carcinoma simplex of the breast; H & E, 80×.

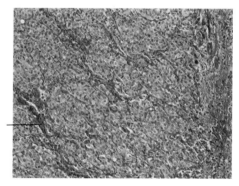

Fig. 15.20. Medullary carcinoma of the breast; H & E, 80×.

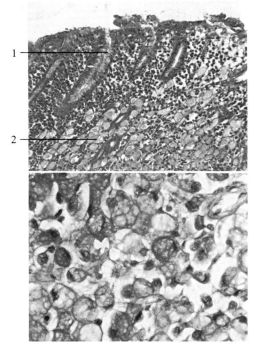

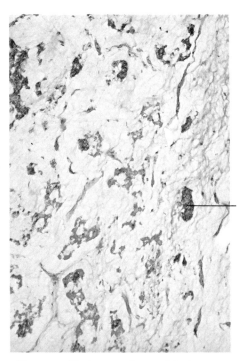

Fig. 15.21. Above: early carcinoma of the stomach; H & E, 80×. Below: signet ring cells; PAS stain, 320×.

Fig. 15.22. Mucinous carcinoma of the breast: H & E, 100×.

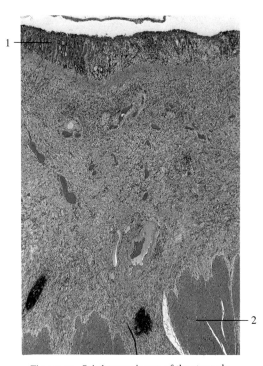

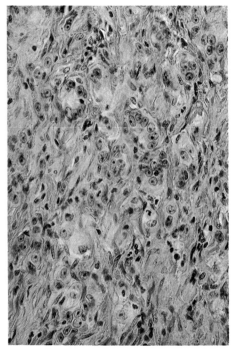

Fig. 15.23. Scirrhus carcinoma of the stomach; H & E, 30×.

Fig. 15.24. Scirrhus carcinoma of the stomach; van Gieson stain, 320×.

Early Carcinoma–Mucinous Carcinoma–Scirrhus Carcinoma

Early carcinoma of the stomach (carcinoma-in-situ, Fig. 15.21) *is an invasive proliferating epithelial tumor, limited to the mucosa and frequently taking the form of a signet ring cell carcinoma.* The mucosa is still preserved so that tumor invasion is easily overlooked. In Figure 15.21 (above), the superficial epithelium and the foveolae gastricae (→ 1) can be seen. The stroma contains small groups of somewhat clear cells (→ 2), which under higher magnification and especially with PAS staining (Fig. 15.21) can be identified as signet ring cells.

The introduction of gastroscopy and gastric biopsy has led to the recognition of this type of tumor which is considered by most authors to be an early form of gastric carcinoma. Treatment at this stage of the tumor results in a 5-year survival rate of more than 90%. Histologically it is possible to differentiate M-type early carcinoma (tumor limited to the mucosa) and SM-type early carcinoma which has already broken through the muscularis mucosa. The prognosis for SM type, however, is quite good. Signet ring cell carcinoma and early carcinoma are not necessarily synonomous designations. Signet ring cell carcinoma may show markedly invasive growth and produce distant metastases. On the other hand, early carcinoma may also take the form of an adenocarcinoma.

Mucinous or **colloid carcinoma** (Fig. 15.22) *manifests itself morphologically by marked mucin production.* The large, clear, slightly basophilic and finely thready masses of mucin may easily be confused with edematous stroma. They contain small groups of carcinoma cells (→) which have a signet ring cell appearance when they contain intracytoplasmic mucin.

Signet ring cell carcinomas occur in the gastrointestinal tract, ovary and especially frequently in the breast. Breast carcinomas showing signet ring cells have a better prognosis than do other infiltrating carcinomas, although they become very large.

Scirrhus carcinoma (Figs. 15.23, 15.24) *has an especially rich fibrous stroma in which are isolated tumor cells.* Low power magnification (Fig. 15.23) reveals marked thickening of the stomach wall. At the top there is a dark band of still preserved mucosa (→ 1) and below remnants of the invaded muscularis propria (→ 2). In between lies the submucosa beneath the large infiltrating tumor. Higher magnification (Fig. 15.24) shows small masses of carcinoma cells with large nuclei and particularly prominent nucleoli. The carcinoma cells are surrounded by collagen fibers (stain red with van Gieson) and fibroblasts (smaller, elongated nuclei). Especially fibrous, scirrhus mammary carcinomas may present diagnostic difficulties. Frequently there are a marked inflammatory reaction and increased vascularization. Such carcinomas are designated *granulomatous carcinomas* and not infrequently are misdiagnosed as granulation tissue.

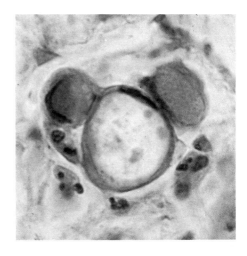

Fig. 15.25. Signet ring cell; H & E, 900×.

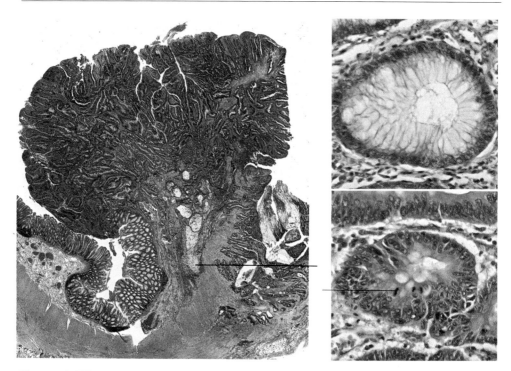

Fig. 15.26. Villous rectal polyp showing malignant change in the base; H & E, 8×.

Fig. 15.27. Above: normal crypt in the large bowel, Below: gland in adenocarcinoma,; H & E, 200×.

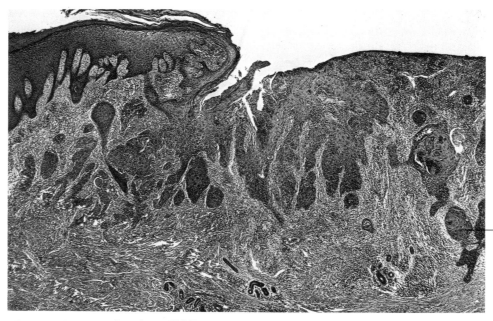

Fig. 15.28. Squamous cell carcinoma; H & E, 30×.

Large Intestine Tumors–Squamous Cell Carcinoma

Malignant change in a polyp of the large intestine (Figs. 15.26, 15.27). Carcinoma of the large intestine frequently arises at the base of a villous polyp. Figure 15.26 shows a broad based polyp the superficial portion of which has a papillary structure. The tumor is essentially darker staining (increased basophilia) than the adjacent normal tissue which contains goblet cells. *Breeching of the muscularis mucosa and invasion of the submucosa by the tumor are the histological signs of malignant transformation.* In our case the invasion extends into the base of the polyp, i.e, the intestinal wall already contains strands of carcinoma (→). The differences in structure between a normal crypt of the large intestine and a glandular carcinoma are shown in Figure 15.27. The upper picture shows a **normal, large intestinal crypt** with its round lumen. The goblet cells have typical basally placed nuclei and large mucin containing cytoplasmic vacuoles. The **gland in the carcinomatous tissue** (Fig. 15.27, below) has irregularly shaped nuclei. The cells are stained more deeply, the nuclei vary in size, are hyperchromatic and no longer uniformly situated at the base of the cells. Mitoses are common (→).

Squamous cell carcinoma (Figs. 15.28, 15.29) *is a malignant tumor that shows invasive growth and occasionally differentiated prickle cells (intercellular bridges) and evidence of cornification.* Low magnification (Fig. 15.28) shows the predominance of invasive growth. Elongated, pointed epithelial pegs infiltrate the corium. In the deeper parts of the section there are islands of detached carcinoma cells (→) surrounded by inflamed stroma. On the left hand side of the figure there is some still intact epidermis showing hyperplastic thickening.

High magnification (Fig. 15.29) shows the very pale prickle cells (→ 1). The pattern of the tumor at the periphery, i.e., the carcinoma cells nearest the stroma, suggests basal cell differentiation. Cornification is typical of squamous cell carcinoma: small spheres consisting of concentric lamellae of cornification (→ 2) are enclosed in the tumor tissue. They usually lack a stratum granulosum—indicating orthokeratotic cornification.

Squamous cell carcinomas frequently develop in previously injured skin (sailor's or farmer's skin), the upper digestive tract (lip, oral cavity, tongue, esophagus), the larynx, bronchus and mucosa of the uterine cervix (on the bases of squamous metaplasia). They must be differentiated from *pseudoepitheliomatous hyperplasia* (following chronic irritation), *leukoplakia* and other lesions associated with proliferation of prickle cells (e.g., *keratoacanthoma*).

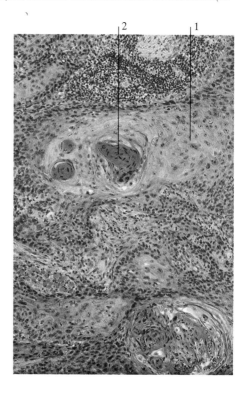

Fig. 15.29. Higher magnification of a squamous cell carcinoma; H & E, 100×.

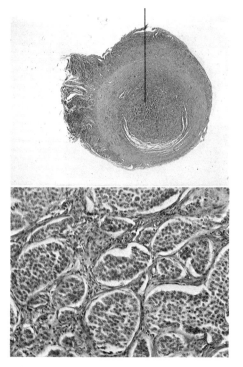

Fig. 15.30. Carcinoid of the appendix. Above: scanning lens, 8×. Below: high magnification; H & E, 100×.

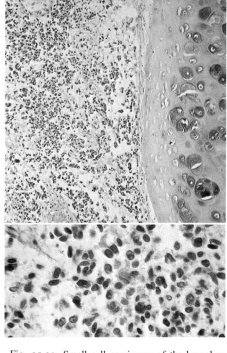

Fig. 15.31. Small cell carcinoma of the bronchus. Above: scanning lens, 80×. Below: high magnification; H & E, 320×.

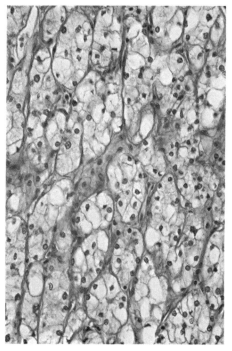

Fig. 15.32. Renal hypernephroma (clear cell adenocarcinoma); H & E, 200×.

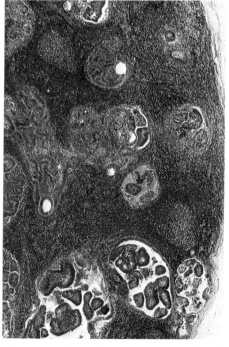

Fig. 15.33. Metastatic carcinoma in a lymph node; H & E, 50×.

Histology of Special Tumors

Carcinoid of the vermiform appendix (Fig. 15.30). The term "carcinoid" arose because of the similarity of this tumor to a true carcinoma. A **carcinoid** *is a solid, infiltrating tumor that arises from the enterochromaffin system and rarely metastasizes (exception carcinoid of the ileum).* Figure 15.30, shows a cross section of an appendix. The lumen is obstructed by a scar. With a scanning lens the diffuse infiltration ($\rightarrow$ 1) of the organ is easily seen. Higher magnification (Fig. 15.30, below) shows the ball-like arrangement of uniform tumor cells. Mitoses are rare.

Carcinoids occur chiefly in the appendix (incidental finding at appendectomy), occasionally in a bronchus or the ileum. They produce serotonin and kallikreinin which are decomposed in the liver. When a metastasis develops in the liver these substances are released into the blood stream and provoke a *carcinoid syndrome.* Carcinoid syndrome may also occur with other tumors, e.g., in bronchial carcinomas (Thomas et al, 1974).

Small cell carcinoma of the bronchus (Fig. 15.31) *is a malignant epithelial tumor composed of lymphocyte-like cells.* Low magnification—adjacent to a still preserved bronchial cartilage—shows tumor invasion. Higher magnification (below) shows a mixture of round (lymphocyte-like) and elongated nuclei (oat cell carcinoma). There is only a sparse stroma.

Bronchial small cell carcinomas are especially malignant tumors, which produce distant metastases very early. Since serotonin granules can be demonstrated electromicroscopically in the cytoplasm, it is thought these tumors are malignant variants of carcinoids.

Renal hypernephroma (adenocarcinoma, clear cell carcinoma, Grawitz tumor, Fig. 15.32) *is a malignant kidney tumor comprised of water clear, plantlike cells with an alveolar or trabecular arrangement, clear, optically empty cytoplasm (glycogen) and round nuclei.* Indications of malignancy in hypernephromas are: size over 3 cm diameter, atypical and polymorphic cells (sarcoma-like growth).

Wilms tumor (adenomyosarcoma, Fig. 15.34) is a special form of malignant kidney tumor that occurs in young children. Histologically it is a mixed tumor with sarcomatous stroma and pseudotubular ($\rightarrow$ 1) as well as pseudoglomerular ($\rightarrow$ 2) structures (see p. 195).

Lymph node metastases (Fig. 15.33). *As a rule the discovery of epithelial tissue in a lymph node indicates metastatic carcinoma.* However, benign ectopic epithelial tissue (e.g., of salivary glands, thyroid or endometrial tissue) does occur occasionally. Figure 15.33 shows a lymph node invaded by small eosinophilic deposits of metastatic carcinoma.

The appearance of lymph node metastasis can have diagnostic (the first clinical manifestation of an occult carcinoma), prognostic (bad sign) and therapeutic significance.

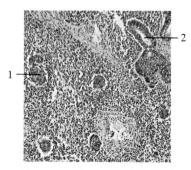

Fig. 15.34. Wilms tumor; H & E, 160×.

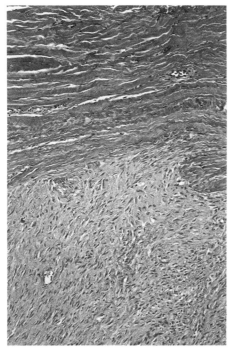

Fig. 15.35. Palmar fibromatosis; H & E, 100×.

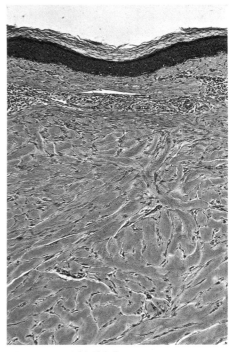

Fig. 15.36. Keloid; H & E, 90×.

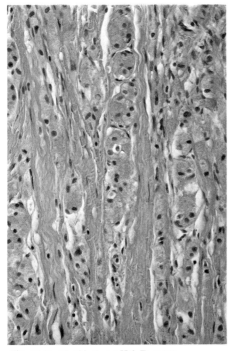

Fig. 15.37. Myoblastoma; H & E, 200×.

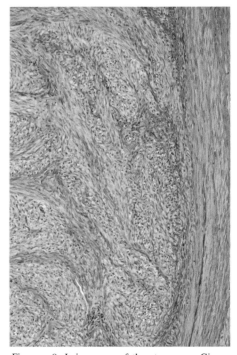

Fig. 15.38. Leiomyoma of the uterus; van Gieson stain, 90×.

Fibroblastoses

Fibroblastoses consist of a diffuse increase in connective tissue comprised of proliferating fibroblasts and newly formed collagen fibers. Fibromatoses may occur at all ages and in every organ. Currently fibromatoses are divided into 12 disease complexes: scar and irradiation fibromatosis, penile, palmar, plantar, abdominal and extra-abdominal fibromatosis, nodular fasciculitis, keloid, fibromatosis coli, nasopharyngeal fibroma and congenital generalized fibromatosis. Fibromatoses show locally invasive growth which can progress over years. Recurrence is common, but metastases are not produced.

Palmar fibromatosis (Dupuytren's contracture, Fig. 15.35) *is a benign fibrosis showing partly diffuse and partly nodular proliferation of the palmar fascia and eventually causes contracture of the finger*. Histologically there is compact, collagen-rich connective tissue (upper half of picture) as well as dense nodules of fibrocytes lying in loosely arranged stroma.

This condition arises chiefly in men 50–60 years of age, develops slowly and in the final stages causes contraction of the palmar fascia.

Keloid (Fig. 15.36) *in most cases is not a true tumor (keloid fibroma) but rather superficial, nodular fibrosis in a scar*. Histologically there is a circumscribed, but not encapsulated, nodule composed of broad glassy, eosinophilic bundles of collagenous tissue, between which the nuclei of a few fibroblasts and inflammatory cells may be seen. Atrophic epidermis (no rete pegs) covers the surface.

Keloids commonly develop in postoperative abdominal scars and in the facial region following trauma. They tend to recur.

Mesenchymal Tumors

Both benign and malignant mesenchymal tumors are encountered. Further separation of these tumors is made from a histogenetic point of view, i.e., taking into consideration the parent tissue from which the tumor arises. *Benign mesenchymal tumors* show a high degree of tissue maturity, slow, expansive growth and lack of metastases. *Malignant mesenchymal tumors* are grouped under the general heading of sarcoma. They may be undifferentiated or show a high degree of cellular and tissue differentiation corresponding to their histogenetic origin (e.g., myo-, lipo- or osteosarcoma).

Myoblastoma (granular cell myoblastoma, Fig. 15.37) *is a benign mesenchymal tumor composed of cells with a strand-like arrangement, central, round nuclei and finely granular cytoplasm. The cytoplasmic granules are PAS positive*.

Myoblastomas are observed in many organs, especially the tongue and larynx. Their pathogenesis is still uncertain. Because they show a marked similarity to Schwann cells electromicroscopically it is thought they are of neurogenic origin.

Leiomyoma (Fig. 15.38) *is a benign tumor of smooth muscle and is particularly common in the myometrium*. Histologically the tumors show an interlacing arrangement of smooth muscle fibers having elongated, cylindrical nuclei with blunt ends and yellow cytoplasm with van Gieson stain. The muscle fibers are separated by a dense collagenous network that stains red with van Gieson.

Leiomyomas grow by expansion and may show hyalinization, calcification and ossification which are signs of regressive changes. Malignant transformation is rare. Retroperitoneal leiomyomas (from blood vessel walls), however, are potentially malignant.

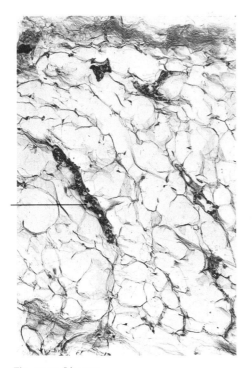

Fig. 15.39. Lipoma:
H & E, 100×.

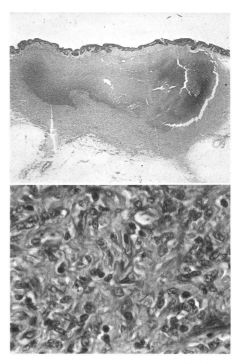

Fig. 15.40. Histiocytoma. Above: scanning lens,
8×. Below: high magnification; H & E, 200×.

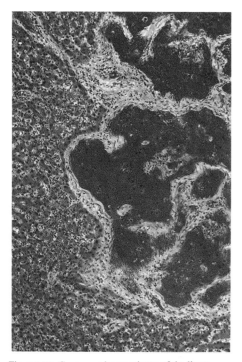

Fig. 15.41. Cavernous hemangioma of the liver;
H & E, 60×.

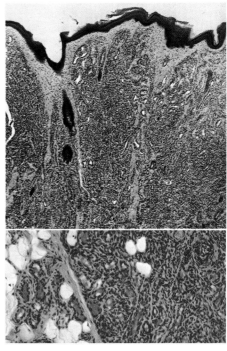

Fig. 15.42. Capillary hemangioma of skin. Above:
scanning lens, 30×. Below: high magnification;
H & E, 60×.

Lipoma–Histiocytoma–Hemangioma

Lipoma (Fig. 15.39). *A benign, lobulated tumor derived from mature fat tissue.* Histologically it is composed of cells that deviate from normal fat cells only in their variation in size. They have distinct cell borders, rounded nuclei situated at the periphery and optically empty cytoplasm; the fat is dissolved by paraffin embedding. A fibrous capsule (Fig. 15.39, above) covers the surface. Many capillaries ($\rightarrow$) are seen lying between the fat cells.

Lipomas develop in subcutaneous fat tissue and occasionally retroperitoneally or in other organs. They grow slowly. *Hibernoma* is a special variant of lipoma that arises from fetal fat cells (small, cuboidal cells with finely vacuolated cytoplasm).

Histiocytoma (Fig. 15.40, sclerosing hemangioma of Wolbach). *This is a circumscribed but not encapsulated tumor located in the subepidermal corium and composed of proliferating histiocytes.* Under low magnification the tumor appears bluish and is covered with intact epidermis. With higher magnification the bizarre nuclei of the histiocytes can be identified and the partly whorled arrangement of the newly formed collagen fibers seen. There are also solitary macrophages containing fat or hemosiderin. The surface epidermis shows in part pseudoepitheliomatous thickening and in part atrophic shrinkage and is separated from the histiocytoma by a narrow band of acellular corium.

Angiomas *are benign vascular tumors that in most cases are hamartomas, i.e., a tumorlike malformation of local tissue.* They may arise from blood vessels *(hemangioma),* from lymph vessels *(lymphangioma)* or from neuromyoepithelial tissue *(angiomyoma* or *glomus tumor).*

Cavernous hemangioma (Fig. 15.41) develops most frequently in the liver. It consists of many large spaces tightly packed with erythrocytes, traversed by connective tissue septa and lined with endothelial cells. The neighboring liver parenchyma may show pressure atrophy.

Capillary hemangioma (Fig. 15.42) is the commonest type of vascular tumor. Under low magnification (Fig. 15.42, above) it appears as an ill defined, lobulated and very cellular new growth, extending from the subepidermal corium to the subcutis. Medium magnification (Fig. 15.42, below) shows fissured or oval spaces bordered by endothelial cells and containing occasional erythrocytes. The newly formed capillaries enclose fat cells. Because this is a tumorlike malformation that develops in the local fat tissue there is no true invasion.

Capillary hemagiomas occur frequently in small children. In the early years they can attain a large size. Later the growth becomes stationary and not infrequently regresses. Hemangiomas also occur as a part of several syndromes (e.g., Hippel-Lindau disease, Sturge-Weber-Krabbe disease) in which retina, skin and central nervous system are affected.

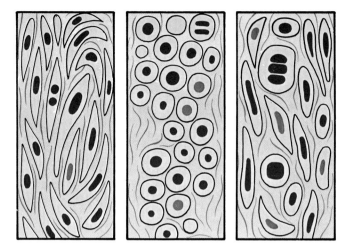

Fig. 15.43. Schematic representation of the sarcomas (morphological classification)
a) spindle cell sarcoma (leiomyosarcoma, fibrosarcoma)
b) round cell sarcoma (lymphosarcoma, immunoblastic sarcoma)
c) polymorphocellular (pleomorphic) sarcoma (rhabdomyosarcoma, liposarcoma, undifferentiated spindle cell sarcoma).

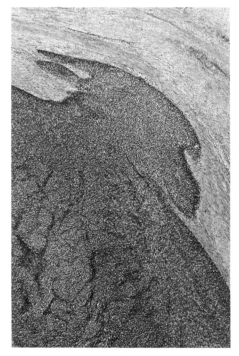

Fig. 15.44. Invasive spindle cell sarcoma;
H & E, 20×.

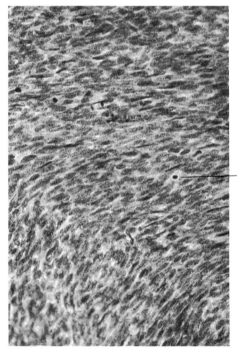

Fig. 15.45. Undifferentiated spindle cell sarcoma;
H & E, 320×.

Sarcoma—Malignant Mesenchymal Tumor

Sarcomas *are malignant tumors of mesenchymal tissues.* They can be classified either according to morphological or histogenetic criteria. For the pathologist a morphological classification has the advantage of simplicity: it separates **round cell, spindle cell** and **polymorphous (pleomorphic) sarcomas** (Fig. 15.43).

It is also known that tumors with similar tissue patterns may have very different prognoses. Thus there are spindle cell sarcomas that metastasize early and are particularly malignant. However, other spindle cell sarcomas are locally invasive and recur but produce distant metastases very late. A histogenetic classification (according to the parent tissue of derivation) allows separation, for example, of a particularly malignant leiomyosarcoma from a so-called fibrosarcoma.

A histological classification gives rise to difficulties in respect of undifferentiated tumors. Histological examination commonly reveals no differences in cell structure or intercellular substances so that it is possible only to make a diagnosis of undifferentiated spindle cell carcinoma (Figs. 15.44, 15.45). In such cases special studies may be helpful, as for example: electronmicroscopy, immunohistology or histochemistry. Electronmicroscopy frequently allows identification of primitive cellular structures such as myofilaments (leiomyosarcoma) or sarcomeres (rhabdomyosarcoma, Fig. 15.3). Myosin in muscle sarcoma cells can be detected immunohistologically by antimyosin serum. These methods, however, are expensive and as a rule require unfixed material (Thomas et al, 1976).

Figures 15.44 and 15.45 show scanning lens and high magnification views of an **undifferentiated spindle cell sarcoma.** The tumor is richly cellular with peg-shaped extensions invading the neighboring eosinophilic connective tissue. The marked basophilia of the tumor is caused by the close proximity of the nuclei. High magnification reveals elongated, parallel lying cells with hyperchromatic nuclei. Mitoses (→) are plentiful. There is no intercellular substance (collagen fibers) between the tumor cells. Poorly differentiated spindle cell sarcomas (few or no collagen fibers between tumor cells) recur (75%) and metastasize (24%) chiefly as collagen forming, so-called fibrosarcomas that have locally invasive growth, recur (40%) but do not metastasize (Stout, 1953).

Pseudosarcoma. Occasionally there are fast growing new growths that morphologically resemble a sarcoma, but—as their later course shows—have a good prognosis. Histologically they correspond to a fibrosarcoma or lymphosarcoma and are grouped together under the general heading of **pseudosarcoma.**

Pseudosarcomatous nodular fasciitis (Fig. 15.46) *is a benign, rapidly developing disease, probably virus induced, that is characterized by sarcoma-like proliferation of fibroblasts in the deeper layers of the subcutaneous fat tissue.* Histologically there is infiltrative growth of fascial fibroblasts (→ 1) with distinctly pleomorphic nuclei and mitoses. In the periphery of the lesion there is inflamed granulation tissue (→ 2). Metastases do not occur.

Pseudosarcomas with a lymphocyte-like pattern are called **pseudolymphomas.** They have been described in many organs chiefly in the gastrointestinal tract. Histologically they resemble a lymphosarcoma. However, their long course over years or decades suggests a benign lesion.

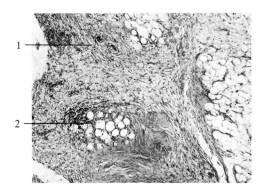

Fig. 15.46. Pseudosarcomatous fasciitis;
H & E, 32×.

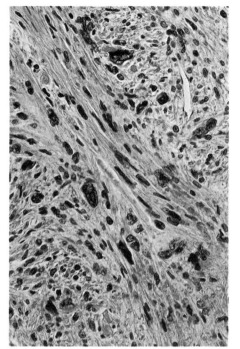

Fig. 15.47. Leiomyosarcoma; H & E, 450×.

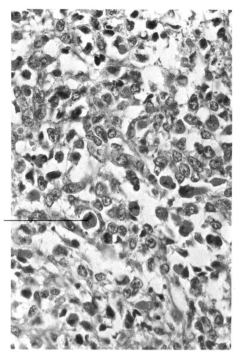

Fig. 15.48. Embryonal rhabdomyosarcoma; H & E, 320×.

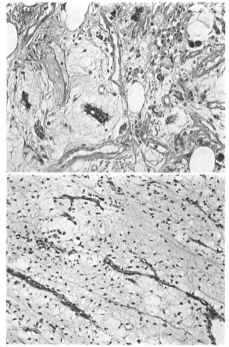

Fig. 15.49. Liposarcoma. Above: pleomorphic cell liposarcoma with lipoblasts, 200×. Below: myxoid liposarcoma; H & E, 80×.

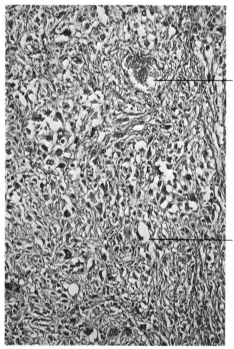

Fig. 15.50. Malignant hemangioendothelioma; H & E, 120×.

Leiomyosarcoma–Liposarcoma–Rhabdomyosarcoma–Malignant Hemangioendothelioma

Leiomyosarcoma (Fig. 15.47) *is a malignant tumor of smooth muscle*. Histologically it is a spindle cell sarcoma with bundles of elongated tumor cells which in the figure are seen partly in longitudinal section (middle of picture) and partly in cross section. The cells have abundant cytoplasm and are very pleomorphic with large, hyperchromatic nuclei. The presence of mitoses is of diagnostic significance since cellular atypia also occurs in degenerative uterine myomas.

Myomas of the uterus seldom undergo malignant change. Leiomyosarcomas are seen especially in the extremities, intestinal and blood vessel walls (retroperitoneal). They produce distant metastases early and thus are particularly malignant, in this respect standing in contrast to well differentiated fibrosarcoma. *Leiomyoblastomas* are benign neoplasms that occur in the gastrointestinal tract as well as the mesentery and retroperitoneal region. They consist of polygonal cells with clear cytoplasm.

Rhabdomyosarcoma (Fig. 15.48) *is a malignant tumor of striped muscle*. In most cases it is a polymorphocellular sarcoma. The recognition of cross striations in the cytoplasm of these tumors is pathognomonic, but they are not often present. Brick red tumor cells with centrally placed, hyperchromatic nuclei (→) are quite typical of **embryonal rhabdomyosarcoma.**

Rhabdomyosarcoma (Fig. 15.48) *belongs to the group of malignant tumors of striated muscle*. A special variant is *sarcoma botryoides* which occurs in the genital tract of young women. The diagnosis of rhabdomyosarcoma in the last analysis can be made only by finding rhabdomyofibrils. Usually these can only be demonstrated by electronmicroscopy as rudimentary sarcomeres (Fig. 15.3). *Rhabdomyomas* are benign, very rare tumors of striated muscle especially of myocardium. The cells have perinuclear glycogen vacuoles, spindle shaped, drawn out nuclei and cytoplasmic cross striations.

Liposarcoma (Fig. 15.49) *is a malignant tumor of fat tissue*. A typical liposarcoma shows large, polymorphous tumor cells (lipoblasts, Fig. 15.49, above) with bizarre, hyperchromatic nuclei and many cytoplasmic vacuoles containing fat. In addition there are large, mature fat cells as well as cells with finely vacuolated cytoplasm (immature or "fetal" fat cells). A **myxoid variant** (Fig. 15.49, below) is a most common liposarcoma. It consists of a myxoid ground substance enclosing star-shaped cells or nuclei. Since mitoses and lipoblasts are rare, a myxoid liposarcoma many times is mistaken for a benign lipoma. All variants of liposarcoma are malignant. In most cases they arise de novo, that is they do not arise as a rule from a preexisting lipoma. Common sites are the gluteal region, thigh, mesentery and retroperitoneum.

Malignant hemangioendothelioma (Fig. 15.50) *is a relatively rare malignant tumor arising from the vascular system*. Histologically is has a polymorphocellular, sarcomatous structure with small slit-like spaces lined by very atypical tumor cells and occasionally containing blood (→). The larger tumor cells often contain phagocytosed erythrocytes (*erythrophagocytosis* occurs commonly in hemangioendotheliomas).

Hemangioendotheliomas occur particularly in the liver (e. g., following chronic arsenic poisoning or storage of thorotrast) and in the thyroid. It is a malignant tumor with a high incidence of metastasis. Together with chorionepithelioma and malignant hepatoma it is the bloodiest of tumors. The malignant counterpart of the lymphatic vascular system is *lymphangiosarcoma* and may give rise to the Stewart-Treves syndrome: sarcoma arising from chronic edema of the arm after total mastectomy and axillary lymph node extirpation for mammary carcinoma.

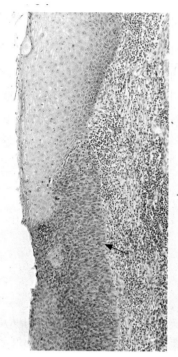
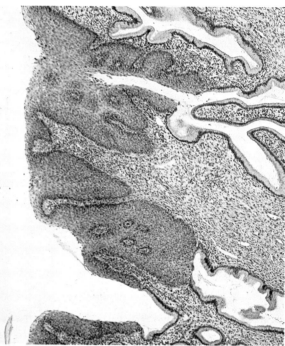

Fig. 15.51. Carcinoma in situ with simple replacement of surface epithelium; H & E, 100×.

Fig. 15.52. Carcinoma in situ with simple replacement of cervical glands; H & E, 80×.

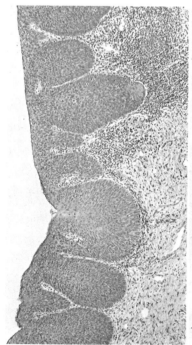
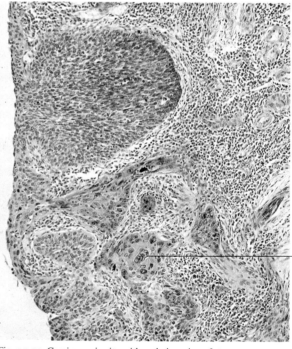

Fig. 15.53. Carcinoma in situ with bulky growth; H & E, 80×.

Fig. 15.54. Carcinoma in situ with early invasion of stroma; H & E, 120×.

Precancerous Lesions–Carcinoma In Situ

Precancerous lesions *are those tissue lesions or disease entities that during their late stages commonly become carcinoma.* If the malignant transformation develops in a relatively short time (less than 5 years) and in a specially high percentage of cases (20–50%), it is called an *obligate precancer*. *Facultative precancer,* on the other hand, changes to cancer after a longer course and in less than 20% of cases.

The term **carcinoma in situ** was first used for the changes in the mucosa of the uterine cervix (Broders, 1932), in which the cytological signs of malignancy were present but the basement membrane was still intact. That is these mucosal alterations that histologically appear to be carcinoma lacked the most important sign of malignancy: invasive growth. At a later date carcinomas in situ were described in other organs. Today we distinguish:
1. **Carcinoma in situ** which develops in the cervix and is clearly precancerous. Untreated, an invasive carcinoma develops in about 60% of cases.
2. **Carcinoma growing in situ** (superficial carcinoma, mucosal carcinoma) is, in contrast, a carcinoma from the beginning. At first it spreads in the mucosa, later—as a rule—breaks through the basement membrane of the mucosa and so becomes an invasive carcinoma (example: surface carcinoma of the colon).
Early carcinoma of the stomach is a special form of carcinoma in situ (see p. 301 and Fig. 15.21, superficial carcinoma, "early cancer"). The tumor cells are located in the mucosal stroma, in SM type even in the submucosa. Even though there is stromal invasion, and thus evidence of invasive carcinoma, it occupies a special position because over 90% of treated patients live more than 5 years.

Additional examples of precancerous tissue changes or diseases: Skin *(Bowen's disease, senile keratosis, lentigo maligna or melanosis circumscripta preblastomatosa of Dubreuilh, intraepidermal epithelioma of Borst-Jadasshon),* vulva *(Bowen's disease, extramammary Paget's disease),* breast *(lobular carcinoma in situ),* uterine cervix *(carcinoma in situ, moderate and marked dysplasia),* endometrium *(adenomatous hyperplasia, carcinoma in situ),* penis *(erythroplasia of Queyrat),* larynx *(proliferative leukoplakia),* colon *(villous polyps, ulcerative colitis),* liver *(cirrhosis)* etc.

Carcinoma in situ (epidermoid carcinoma in situ) of the cervix of the uterus (Figs. 15.51–15.54). *This is a precancerous lesion of the squamous epithelium of the cervix in which the cytological signs of malignancy are present but the basement membrane has not been breeched.* In simple replacement of surface epithelium (Fig. 15.51) there is in addition to the normally layered acidophilic squamous epithelium (upper part of figure) atypical, markedly basophilic epithelium. The normal layering of cells is broken up. The cells have large nuclei and scanty cytoplasm. Mitoses are common. An intact basement membrane (→) separates the carcinoma in situ from the inflamed stroma. Figure 15.52 shows **simple replacement of a cervical gland by carcinoma in situ.** To the right in the figure there are still intact glands with lumens lined by cylindrical epithelium. To the left is the carcinoma in situ which has already filled the necks of the glands and dipped into the stroma, but here also the basement membrane of the surface epithelium as well as of the cervical glands is intact. **Bulky growth** may be a further manifestation of carcinoma in situ (Fig. 15.53). The lesion arches itself against the underlying stroma without infiltrating it. Figure 15.54 shows transformation to an **invasive stage** where besides the bulky growth (left side of figure) there are small markedly acidophilic epithelial pegs showing distinct nuclear pleomorphism (→). Such cases are spoken of as **early infiltration** or **invasion. Net-like infiltration** (interlacing carcinomatous strands in the stroma) is spoken of as **microcarcinoma** when it is not over 5 mm in depth. The *progression of carcinoma* from normal cell to clinically manifest, invasive squamous cell carcinoma is from moderate to marked dysplasia[1] to carcinoma in situ to early infiltration and microcarcinoma.

---

[1]Dysplasia: cells showing dyskeratosis (see p. 213) and disturbed cellular polarity.

Fig. 16.1. Outline of Important Deep Mycoses[1]

Morphology	Mycosis	Fungus	Tissue Reaction	Fungus in Tissue	Si
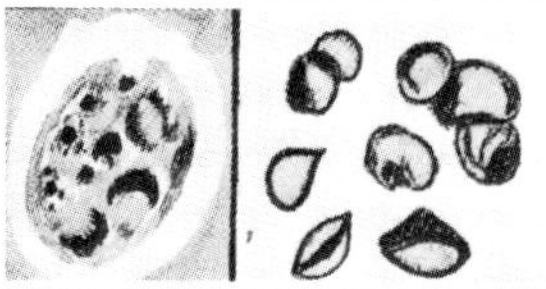	Pneumo-cystosis[2] p. 319	Pneumocystis carinii (Pn. car.)	Interstitial plasma cell infiltrate; lung; occasionally extra pulmonary	Grocott: Round, small; Giemsa: cysts (C) with internal bodies (I)	3 C I
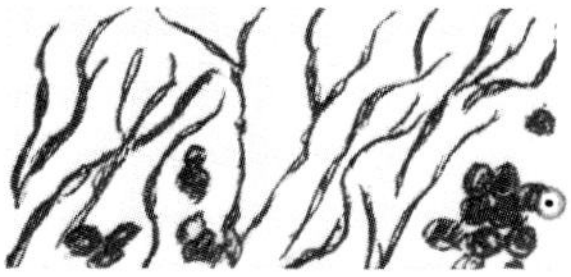	Candidiasis p. 319	Candida albicans, tropic, etc. (Cand. albic.)	Non-specific granulation tissue	Hyphae and small yeast cells	2
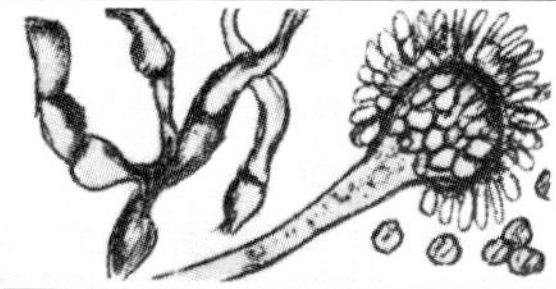	Aspergillosis p. 321	Aspergillus fumigatus	Non-specific; usually granulomas with eosinophils and giant cells	Septated hyphae, conidia "Fruiting bodies"	V
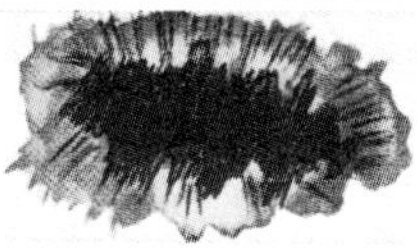	Actino-mycosis[3] p. 321	Mycobacterium actino-mycoses not a fungus	Abscesses with foam cells. Yellow color. Fistulae	Thick bacterial masses; peripherally radiating processes	V
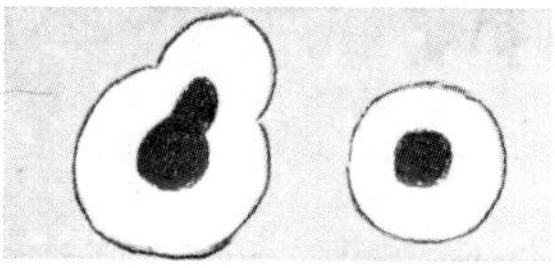	Crypto-coccosis p. 323	Cryptococcus neoformans (Cr. neof.)	Increase in histio-cytes, granulomas	Thick-wall: solitary buds	4
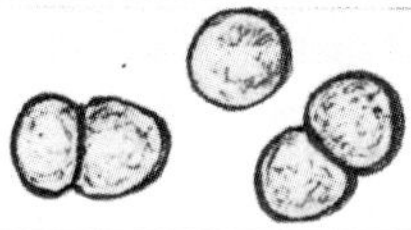	Chromo-mycosis p. 323	Hormo-dendrum and Phialophora	Microabscesses and granulomas of the skin	Brown round sep-tated fungal cells	5
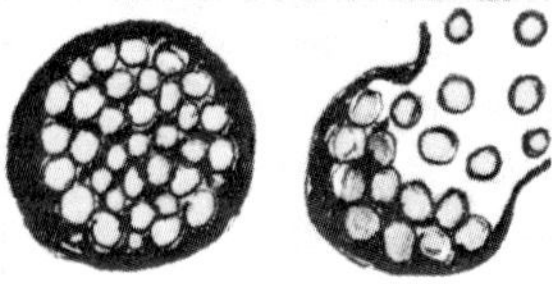	Coccidioido-mycosis p. 323	Coccidioides immitis (Cocc. imm.)	Abscesses, granulomas	Large cysts, Endospores	3
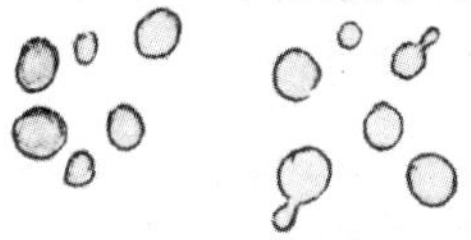	Histo-plasmosis p. 325	Histoplasma capsulatum (H. caps.)	Proliferation of histiocytic tuber-culoid granulomas, calcification	Small round yeast-like fungal cells; intracellular solitary buds	2
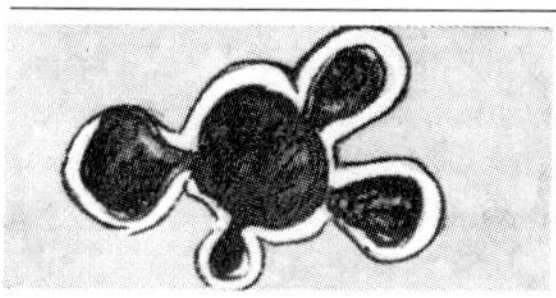	Paracoccidio-idomycosis (South Amer-ican blastomy-cosis) p. 325	Para-coccidioides brasiliensis (Parac. bras.)	Abscesses, granulomas	Yeast-like multiple budding (steering wheel)	5
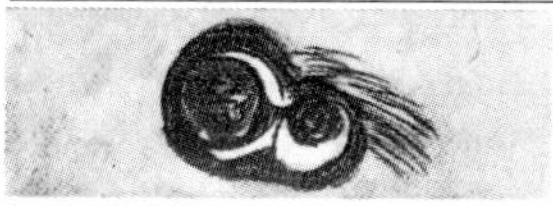	Blastomycosis p. 325	Blastomyces dermatitidis (Blas. derm.)	Abscesses, granulomas	Large yeast-like cells, solitary budding; figure 8 shape	8

[1]Deep mycoses in contrast to superficial mycoses show tissue changes beneath the epidermis and mucosa; often generalized
[2]Fungal nature not proved.
[3]Actinomycetes and nocardes are now considered to be bacteria.

16. Fungi – Protozoa – Parasites

This chapter has been added in order to facilitate a basic knowledge of these important and frequent diseases. Professor Salfeder[1] has kindly provided the following pages, which are written from the viewpoint of a pathologist working in a subtropical or tropical region. Nonetheless, this addition to the book is not without importance for physicians in temperate zones for two chief reasons: On the one hand, we are confronted today with an increasing international commerce, and on the other hand, modern therapeutic agents (cortisone, antibiotics, cytotoxic drugs, etc.) have changed the pattern of infectious diseases, with the result that overwhelming infections (fungi, protozoa, viruses) are common.

The following introduction gives some suggestions for the identification of fungi and parasites (Table 16.1). For ameba, which are easily confused with large tissue cells, the PAS-reaction is recommended. If parasites of small size are found in routine hematoxylin and eosin slides, or Chagas disease, kala-azar or leishmaniasis is suspected, it is helpful to remember that they are negative with the Gram and Grocott stains for fibrin. For the identification of fungi in tissue, the Grocott stain is superior to all other methods. In tissues, dead fungi retain their structural integrity and staining properties for a long time. The mucicarmine stain is recommended for staining the capsule of Cryptococcus in sections. India ink demonstrates the thick capsule of the Cryptococcus very well in smears. The capsule remains colorless, bright and shining. In unstained smears, undesired cell and tissue constituents, especially keratin, can be dissolved with 10% potassium hydroxide (10 min.), which makes the search for infecting organisms easier. Several species are easily identified with the fluorescent antibody technique (Coons and Kaplan).

Table 16.1. Methods Used for Identification of Fungi and Protozoa.

Method	Result	Remarks
Hematoxylin-eosin (H & E)	Blue	Not all fungal elements stain
Fibrin (Weigert)-Gram	Blue	Fungi only partially stained. Protozoa negative
PAS[2])	Red	Cells of small fungi can be overlooked
Gridley[2])	Reddish blue	Stains nearly all fungi
Grocott[2])	Black	Ideal stain, good contrast against light background. Also useful for smears. Note: Coal pigment also stains black, as do erythrocytes and elastic fibers
Mucicarmine[2])	Red	Cryptococcus positive. Excludes other fungi
Polarized light	Shining yellowish blue	Shows double refraction and Maltese crosses of yeast-like fungi in paraffin sections of tissue
Fluorescent antibody	Variable	Fungi of many types positive. Specificity destroyed by cross reactions
Unstained smear	—	Round forms with doubly contoured capsule-suspect fungi
Smear treated for 10 min. with KOH 10%	—	Cell and tissue constitutents better shown
India ink smear	Black	Wide wall of cryptococcus shines forth against dark background
Giemsa, Wright, May-Grünwald Giemsa (smear)	Blue	Stains yeasts and cysts of Pneumocystis carinii positive

[1] Director of the Institute of Anatomic Pathology, University of the Andes, Merida, Venezuela.

[2] Staining of control preparation recommended.

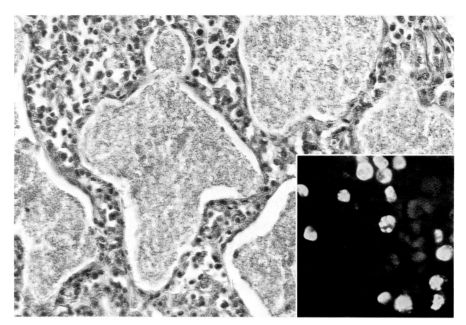

Fig. 16.2. Pneumocystosis with interstitial pneumonia; H & E, 400×.
Inset: Pneumocystis carinii in smear; Rhodamin stain-ultraviolet light, 1050×.

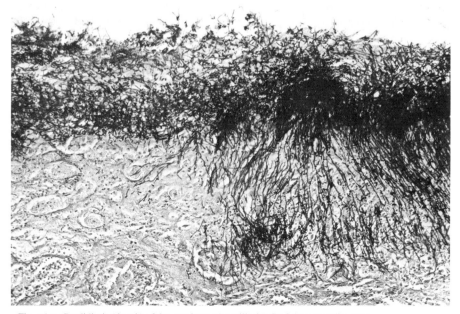

Fig. 16.3. Candidiasis (thrush) of the esophagus (moniliasis); PAS-hematoxylin, 80×.

318

Pneumocystosis with interstitial pneumonia (Figs. 16.2, 16.4). *Pneumocystosis with interstitial pneumonia occurs frequently in prematurely born infants in the 3rd – 6th month of life, but also may occur in older children. When it occurs in adults it is mostly in the end stages of malignant disease (leukemia, sarcoma, carcinoma), particularly after treatment with cytotoxic agents.* **Pneumocystis carinii** is the etiological agent but whether this is a protozoa or a fungus is still debated. Pneumocystis carinii was first seen in Brazil in the lungs of animals (Carini, 1910). Vanek and Jirovec (1952) and Giese (1952) first proved the etiological agent in man over 20 years ago. H & E sections show finely honeycombed granular material in the alveoli (Fig. 16.2). The alveolar lumens are reduced by a thick exudate of alveolar septal cells, lymphocytes, histiocytes and plasma cells. The appearance, indeed, may lead to confusing this form of interstitial pneumonia with atelectasis. The increased cell content of the alveoli and the type of cells should, however, lead to a correct diagnosis. The organisms may be seen in smear preparations stained with Giemsa or Rhodamin in which they appear as cystic forms with internal bodies originating from the honeycombed alveolar contents (see inset in Fig. 16.2). With the Grocott stain, numerous yeast-like bodies 3–4 μ in diameter are seen which are often indented and wrinkled (Fig. 16.4).

Candidiasis *(thrush) of the esophagus* (**candidiasis, moniliasis**) (Figs. 16.3, 16.5). *Various species of* Candida, *but chiefly* Candida albicans, *cause a mycosis that is localized predominantly in the mucous membranes. Spread to the internal organs occurs infrequently (sepsis), mostly in patients with weakened resistance. Macroscopically,* white plaques or membranes are seen on the mucosa of all the upper alimentary and respiratory tracts. *Microscopically,* numerous fungal filaments forming a

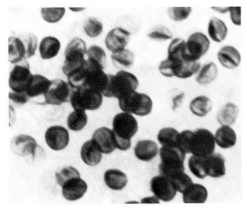

Fig. 16.4. Pneumocystis in a smear; Grocott stain, 1,140×.

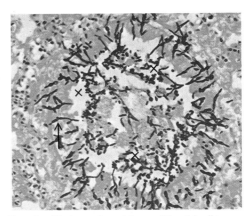

Fig. 16.5. Hyphae and yeast forms of *Candida albicans;* Grocott stain, 400×.

mycelium are seen with H & E, but better with PAS staining (Fig. 16.3). The mycelial filaments penetrate between and into the epithelial cells of the mucous membrane, localizing particularly in the zone between the epithelium and tunica propria (see Fig. 16.3). They penetrate like the roots of a plant into the upper layers of the connective tissue. The tunica propria is infiltrated by lymphocytes. Fig. 16.5 shows the fungal filaments under higher magnification (hyphae, → in the picture). Yeast forms 2–4 μ in diameter are also present (blastospores) which show budding and pseudohyphae formation. If only yeast forms of Candida are present, it may be confused with similar forms of *Histoplasma capsulatum* or small fungus cells of other sorts. The hyphae are thinner than those of aspergillus and some of the phycomycoses.

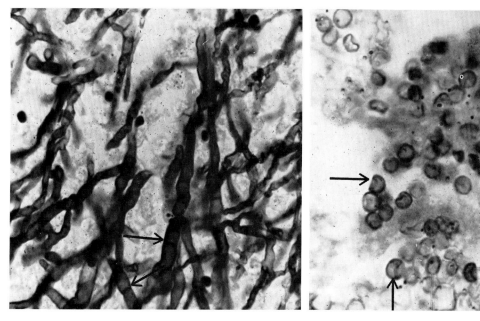

Fig. 16.6. Aspergillus mycelium with hyphae;
Grocott stain, 800×.

Fig. 16.7. Conidia of aspergillus;
Grocott stain, 800×.

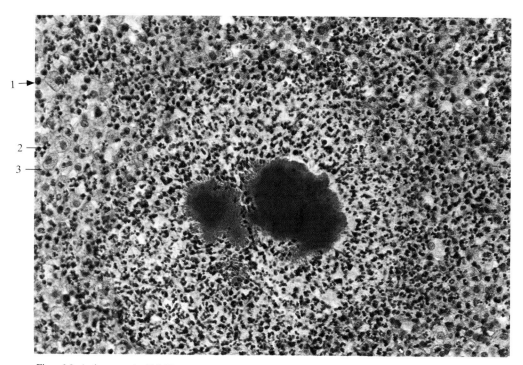

Fig. 16.8. Actinomycosis; H & E, 300×.

Aspergillosis (Figs. 16.6, 16.7, 16.9) *Aspergillus is a fungus of world-wide distribution. The various species produce changes in the lungs and mucous membranes. Less frequently, there is hematogenous spread to other organs. The fungus is a saprophyte-like Candida and the Phycomytes. Aspergillosis occurs frequently in animals, especially birds. The infection is established mostly by inhalation of spores. The mycosis often is seen secondarily in patients whose power of resistance has become greatly reduced (malignant tumors, steroid-antibiotic-cytotoxic treatment or x-irradiation).*

The diagnosis is based upon the demonstration of septate forms (→ in Fig. 16.6) and dichotomous branching of hyphae (Fig. 16.6), which form a network (mycelium). They can penetrate the walls of vessels and other hindrances. In addition, conidia are found (Fig. 16.7). If only conidia are observed in tissues stained with Grocott stain, they can easily be confused with the yeast forms of Candida or Pneumocystis. The conidia are indented and wrinkled (→ in the illustration) similarly to *Pneumocystis carinii* (see p. 319). So-called fruiting bodies (Fig. 16.9) occur in infections with Aspergillus fumigatus, particularly in areas of the body that produce acid (lungs, mucous membranes). The fruiting bodies develop on the end of the hyphae, bear sterigmata and also are known as conidiophores. From the sterigmata, conidia (×) are formed, which then fall from them and lie free in the tissue.

The tissue reaction is predominantly a nonspecific granuloma showing eosinophilic leukocytes and giant cells. Not uncommonly, a tuberculous or bronchiectatic cavity becomes secondarily infected and filled with a so-called fungus ball which may resemble a tumorous mass and for this reason is called an "aspergilloma." Hematogenous spread can lead to involvement of practically all organs (brain, meninges, kidney, spleen, heart, etc.).

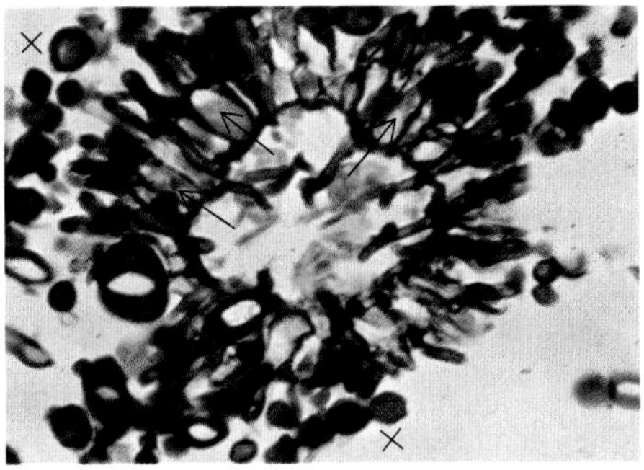

Fig. 16.9. Fruiting body of *Aspergillus fumigatus*; Grocott, 450×.

Actinomycosis *(Mycobacterium actinomyces)* (Fig. 16.8). *In man, the disease is caused chiefly by* Actinomyces israeli, *and in cattle by* Actinomyces bovix *(anaerobic). The portal of entry is usually a break in a mucous membrane (e.g., in the oral cavity, a tooth extraction), the lungs or the gut (appendix). Further spread results from either blood stream invasion (e.g., liver, bone marrow) or lymphatic invasion.*

The bacteria occur in conglomerations and form so-called nodules with characteristic ray-like runners to the periphery. Figure 16.8 shows bacterial masses in the center of an abscess (polymorphonuclear leukocytes and tissue destruction). Granulation tissue containing numerous foam cells (→ 1, → 2, 3) with cytoplasmic fat droplets (foam cells) forms a wall around the abscess. In this way, the abscesses become confluent and form fistulous tracts (especially common, for example, in infections of the mandible). Yellow granules, which contain the nodules, may be demonstrated in the secretion of the fistulas.

Macroscopic: Hard, brawny induration of the skin with numerous fistulas. Sulfur yellow abscess wall (granulation tissue with foam cells).

In the tropics, a **mycetoma** (Madura foot) in the extremities is most frequently due to actinomycosis. The nodules and the tissue reaction in mycetoma have similarities to those in actinomycosis. Various other bacteria and fungi cause indurated swelling and abscesses (Nocardosis, Bothryomycosis). Differential diagnosis is made from cultures since the morphological lesions are very similar.

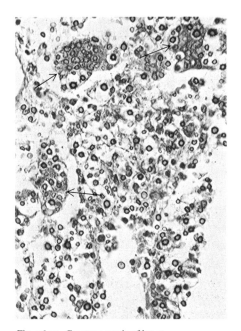

Fig. 16.10. Cryptococcosis of lung: Mucicarmine, 150×.

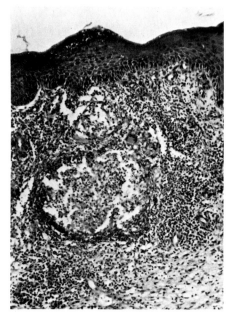

Fig. 16.11. Chromoblastomycosis of skin; H & E, 100×.

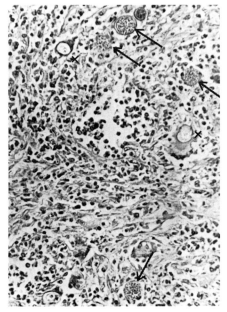

Fig. 16.12. Coccidioidomycosis granuloma of lung, sporocysts (→) with and without (×) endospores; H & E, 140×.

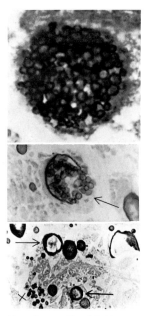

Fig. 16.13. a. Coccidioides sporocyst without membrane H & E, 130×.
b. Endospores released from a spherule; Grocott stain, 100×.
c. Empty fungus spherule and small endospores; Grocott stain, 100×.

Cryptococcosis of the lung (*torulosis, European blastomycosis,* Fig. 16.10). Cryptococcus neoformans (Sanfelice, Busse, Buschke) *has a world-wide distribution. A prime source of infection is the excrement in the nesting places of pigeons. The central nervous system and, above all, the leptomeninges are favored sites for localization of the lesions, although they may occur in any organ. The portal of entry is probably the lungs, where healing results in the development of nodules.*

Figure 16.10 shows many intra- and extracellular cells. The infecting organisms appear as round bodies 4–20 μ in diameter which have a red staining mucous capsule with mucicarmine. In massive infections, the fungi elicit only a marked histiocytic reaction. Chronic granulomatous foci contain only a few fungi. They are usually embedded in dense granulation tissue and, for this reason, often are difficult to discover and easy to confuse with foreign bodies.

Macroscopic: Gelatinous foci which look like a myxomatous tumor when fungal cells are present in the tissues. Often the lesions resemble caseating tuberculosis macroscopically.

Chromoblastomycosis (Chromomycosis) (Figs. 16.11, 16.14). *This fungus has an intrinsic dark brown color, hence the designation. There are five species of Phialophora and Cladosporium which may produce this mycosis. Localization occurs in the skin, particularly of the lower extremities. Seldom does lymphatic spread occur and only exceptionally hematogenous dissemination, usually to the brain and meninges. Chronic verrucous, ulcerated and crusted lesions of the skin may result in considerable deformity of the extremities and invalidism. The mycosis is found in many tropical and subtropical countries, primarily in farm workers.*

Histologically, the corium shows microabscesses composed of numerous granulocytes and marginal granulation tissue containing giant cells (Fig. 16.11). Tuberculoid granuloma may also be produced. As in American blastomycosis, the overlying epidermis is hyperplastic. The brown, round fungus cells (Fig. 16.14) frequently are septate, have a diameter of 5–12 μ and often lie within giant cells.

Macroscopic: many similar skin lesions occur, particularly in the tropics.

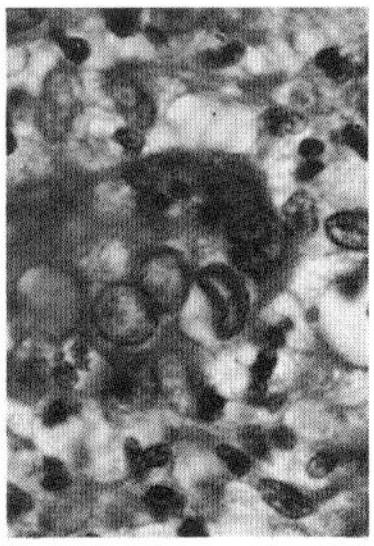

Fig. 16.14. Chromoblastomycosis. Giant cell containing three fungus bodies; H & E, 480×.

Coccidioidomycosis *(San Joaquin Valley fever)* (Figs. 16.12, 16.13 a, b, c). *The disease occurs most frequently in California and Arizona and certain parts of Central and South America, particularly where deserts exist. A large part of the population in an area may be infected.* Coccidioides immitis *occurs in dusty soil, attacks the lungs and mostly produces a benign disease. Much less frequently, spread occurs to internal organs, which is often fatal.* Figure 16.12 shows a pulmonary granuloma with numerous fungus cells which are phagocytosed in part by giant cells (×). The sporocysts contain endospores (→) or are empty. So-called coccidioidoma has been described, which shows extensive necrosis and, in contrast to histoplasmosis, only a slight tendency to calcification. Macroscopically, the lesions are similar to tuberculosis, which is true also of many other "deep" mycoses.

The fungus shows so-called dimorphism (as do *Histoplasma capsulatum, Blastomyces dermatitidis,* etc.), that is, it can grow in saprophytic form both in its natural habitat and in cultures grown at room temperature. The fungus also grows in parasitic form (as a mold with hyphae and arthrospores) in animals and humans (large spherules or sporocysts with numerous endospores which are expelled from the spherule or mother cell). The sporocysts (Fig. 16.13a) measure 30–60 μ in size and are round. The endospores are extravasated from the fungus cells (→ in Fig. 16.13b) and can attain the size of a white blood cell. Empty sporocysts (Fig. 16.13c →, × endospores) can be confused with *Blastomyces dermatitidis,* and endospores (Fig. 16.13b and c) with Histoplasma capsulatum and *Cryptococcus neoformans.*

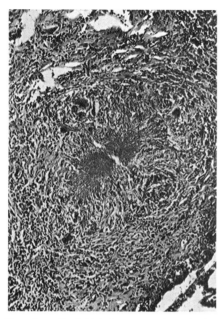

Fig. 16.15. Fresh histoplasma granuloma in the lung; H & E, 105×.

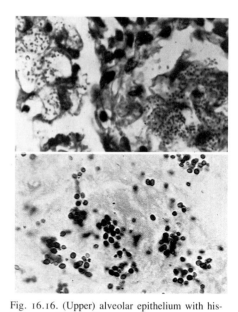

Fig. 16.16. (Upper) alveolar epithelium with his-toplasmas; H & E, 160×.
Fig. 16.17. (Lower) yeast form of *Histoplasma capsulatum;* Grocott stain, 320×.

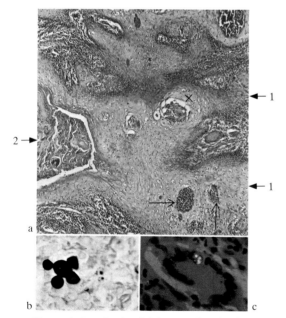

Fig. 16.18a. Paracoccidioidomycosis (South American blastomycosis) of the skin; H & E, 655×. b. Multiple budding of *Paracoccidioides brasiliensis* in tissue; Grocott stain, 520 ×. c. Fungal cell *(Parac. bras.)* in a giant cell, polarized light (so-called Maltese cross); H & E, 550×.

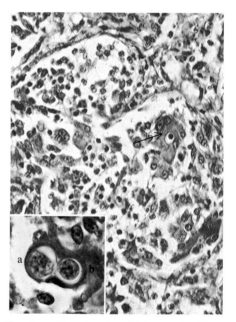

Fig. 16.19. North American blastomycosis of the lung; H & E, 525×. Inset: Solitary bud of Blasto-myces; a) mother cell; b) daughter cell; H & E, 1050×.

Histoplasmosis (Figs. 16.15, 16.16, 16.17). *Histoplasmosis is one of the most widely distributed mycoses. In the United States, it is estimated that more than 5 million persons have been infected. The clinical and pathological similarities to tuberculosis and the predominantly benign course prevented its recognition for a long time, with the result that most of the significant features of this mycosis have been recognized only in the past 30 years. Spontaneous cases are rare in Europe. The disease also occurs spontaneously in animals.*

Histoplasma capsulatum *(Darling) grows best in the soil of chicken houses, is spread apparently through the air and causes a primary lung infection. Most cases heal with a residue of focal calcification in the lung and hilar lymph nodes, where fungi can be demonstrated for a long time. Seldom, and only under special conditions, does the disease in the lung become generalized and have a fatal outcome particularly in children and adults over 40 years of age. In addition to the calcified residual foci in the lungs, cases are encountered with multiple scattered nodules, cavitation or histoplasmomas. Extrapulmonary histoplasmosis may involve any organ, the adrenals being affected frequently.*

Histologically, the lungs show histiocytic granulomas with central necrosis, an epithelioid cell type of granulation tissue and giant cells (Fig. 16.15). The tissue picture can be very similar to that of a tuberculous granuloma. In new infections the fungi are almost exclusively in the cytoplasm of histiocytes or alveolar epithelial cells (Fig. 16.16, small black granules). With hematoxylin and eosin stains, the fungi are not often recognized, but with the Grocott stain (Fig. 16.17), the organisms can be seen distinctly. There are also yeast-like forms $2-5$ μ in diameter.

Paracoccidioidomycosis *(South American blastomycosis,* Figs. 16.18 a, b, c). *As the name indicates, this disease occurs in South America. In Brazil, it is a major sanitary problem. Paracoccidioidomycosis is not encountered spontaneously in animals. In man, minor tissue changes attributed to the fungus have been seen in almost all organs.* It has a chronic course, commonly occurs with tuberculosis, and is the only deep mycosis that responds well to sulfonamide. After attacking the lung (portal of entry) it spreads especially to the skin and mucous membranes of the upper respiratory passages. Predominately attacks men over 40 in rural areas—as does blastomycosis. The habitat of *P. brasiliensis* is still not known.

Histologically, there is a combination of abscesses and granulation tissue. Calcification is rare. Figure 16.18 shows pseudoepitheliomatous hyperplasia of the epidermis with broad, deeply penetrating epidermal pegs ($\rightarrow$ 1, $\rightarrow$ 2 surface of the epidermis with keratin scales). Within the epidermis, there are numerous microabscesses ($\rightarrow$ in the picture) as well as granulomas ($\times$). The diagnosis rests on demonstration of large yeast-like fungi showing multiple budding (Fig. 16.18b). Frequently, the granulomas contain giant cells with enclosed fungi appearing as Maltese crosses in polarized light (Fig. 16.18c). Dead fungus cells of all sorts decompose leaving behind large dust-like masses of Grocott-positive particles, but surviving fungus cells are needed for diagnosis.

North American blastomycosis (Fig. 16.19) *occurs practically only in North America, but recently has been seen in Africa. Frequently, secondary skin lesions appear first. The lungs are the portal of entry for the fungus and from there hematogenous dissemination occurs. Spontaneous animal infections occur (dogs).* The microscopic changes are similar to those seen in South American blastomycosis. Figure 16.19 shows granulocytes in a lung alveolus as well as a giant cell which has phagocytized a fungus cell ($\rightarrow$). In tissues, the round, yeast-like fungi produce single daughter cells only (solitary budding). Figure 16.19. mother cell (a), daughter cell (b) in a giant cell.

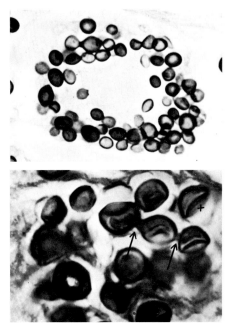

Fig. 16.20 (above). African histoplasmosis; Grocott stain, 700×.
Fig. 16.21 (below). Lobomycosis, skin; Grocott stain, 900×.

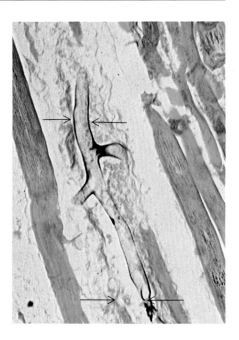

Fig. 16.22. Phycomycosis. Broad non-septated hyphae in skeletal muscle; Grocott stain, 800×.

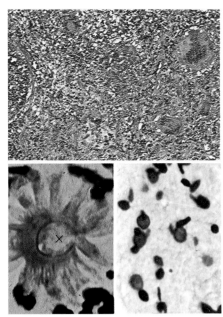

Fig. 16.23 (above). Sporotrichosis of the skin; H & E, 240×.
Fig. 16.24 (below, left). Asteroid bodies; H & E, 950×.
Fig. 16.25 (below, right). Pleomorphic yeast-like form of *Sporotrichum schencki* in rat tissue (post-innoculation); Grocott stain, 1150×.

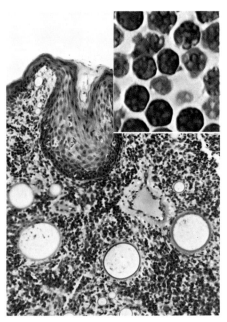

Fig. 16.26. Rhinosporidosis of nasal mucosa. Cystic fungus cells containing endospores; H & E, 140×. Inset: endospores in cystic fungus cells of *Rhinosporidium seeberi;* H & E, 920×.

African Histoplasmosis (Fig. 16.20). In addition to this special form of histoplasmosis, that until now was only known to occur in man and primates in Africa, there is also American histoplasmosis caused by *Histoplasma capsulatum* (Darling). African histoplasmosis differs from the American variety in several essential ways. The causative agent, *Histoplasma duboisi,* is found in tissues in its typical large form—about three times larger than *H. caps.* —often in large giant cells (Fig. 16.20). These large yeast cells must be differentiated from those of that other deep mycosis, *Blastomycosis dermatitidis,* that are similar but have only one nucleus. As a rule the nuclei of fungus cells are difficult to make out in routine sections. In addition to large yeast cells, small forms occur in tissues (similar to *H. caps.*). This characteristic without a doubt makes the diagnosis of the disease more difficult. Skin and bones are chiefly attacked. The portal of entry is the lung where the disease may be inconspicuous—as it is in American histoplasmosis. The incidence of the disease at the present is not certain for so far only those cases seen in academic institutions have been reported.

Lobomycosis (Fig. 16.21) This is a deep mycosis limited to the skin, also called keloid blastomycosis, first described in the Amazon in 1931 by J. Lobo. It has a limited geographical distribution—from northern Brazil into Surinam, Venezuela, Columbia and as far as Central America. It is still considered by many to belong to the paracoccidioidomycoses, although the grounds for this are not clear. The causative agent is now usually called *Loboa loboi*. In tissues the large yeast cells increase by budding, are typically arranged in chains ($\rightarrow$) and often have depressions ($\times$, Fig. 16.21).

Phycomycosis (Fig. 16.22). Absidia, mucor and rhizopus, as well as some other fungi grouped together under this term, are an important deep mycosis of worldwide distribution. It was at one time called mucormycosis. The characteristic finding in tissues is the presence of broad, nonseptated fungal elements ($\rightarrow$ in figure) or fragments of these that stain faintly with Grocott stain (Fig. 16.22). In H & E preparations the fungi frequently lie parallel to muscle and nerve fibers with which they may be confused. Hyphae of Candida and Aspergillus have a different arrangement and other structural pecularities. They penetrate the walls of blood vessels, destroy them and cause thrombosis. It is an opportunistic infection.

Sporotrichosis (Figs. 16.23, 16.24, 16.25) is a worldwide, relatively common deep mycosis of the skin. Only a few cases are known to become generalized or to have pulmonary involvement—from inhalation. *Sporotrichum schencki* causes tissue abscesses and a granulomatous reaction (Fig. 16.23, above). The small, round or elongated yeast forms of *Sp. schencki* are only rarely met with in human tissues. In contrast, after innoculation into animal tissues they multiply well and are easily recognized (Fig. 16.24). The finding of yeast cells containing asteroid bodies ($\times$, Fig. 16.25) is helpful in making a histological diagnosis.

Rhinosporidiosis (Fig. 16.26) *Rhinosporidium seeberi* is easily recognized in tissues. The fungus cells (sporanges) are large and cystic and have many small endospores (Fig. 16.26). Occasionally numerous globular bodies are seen in the endospores (Fig. 16.26, inset). The fungus cells resemble *C. immitis* (see Fig. 16.12). A nonspecific inflammation is the usual reaction and occasionally a foreign body reaction.

The disease occurs sporadically and universally; it is widespread in Asia, Ceylon and South America. Besides the nasal mucosa, the skin of the face and the mucous membranes of the facial cavities, particularly the conjunctiva, are affected.

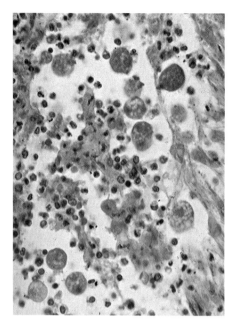

Fig. 16.27. Amebae in the submucosa of the large intestine (amebic dysentery); PAS-hematoxylin stains, 700×.

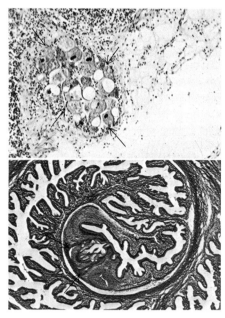

Fig. 16.28 (above). Balantidium dysentery; H & E, 168×.

Fig. 16.29 (below). Cysticercus; H & E, 105×.

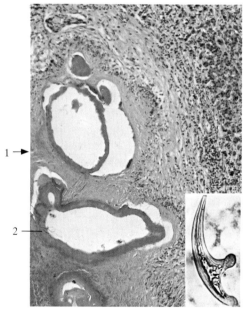

Fig. 16.30. Echinococcus cyst of the liver; H & E, 8×.

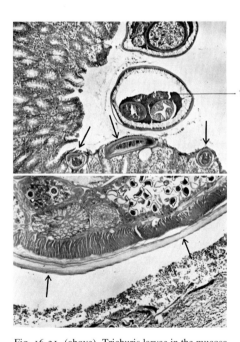

Fig. 16.31. (above). Trichuris larvae in the mucosa of the appendix; H & E, 310×.

Fig. 16.32 (below). Ascaris in bile duct; H & E, 72×.

Amebic dysentery (Fig. 16.27). *Amebic dysentery occurs chiefly in warm climates. Of the various types occurring in man, only the vegetative form of Entamoeba histolytica is seen in tissues. The existence of cysts and vegetative forms in the intestinal contents does not of itself signify disease.*

The intestinal lesions are usually confined to the colon. Ameba actively penetrate the intestinal wall and have both cytological and histolytical effects. At first, there is extensive necrosis of tissue, with formation of crater-like ulcers with undermined margins (similar to p. 124). **Histologically,** the base of the ulcers shows fibrin, necrotic tissue and many granulocytes. Careful inspection is necessary to discover the amebae in the submucosa of the large intestine. They appear as round cells with an eccentrically placed nucleus (Fig. 16.27). The cytoplasm is distinctly red with PAS-stain; with H & E, the protozoans can be easily overlooked or confused with reticulum cells, macrophages or ganglion cells. Figure 16.27 shows, in addition, infiltration of tissues with round cells and granulocytes.
Peritonitis from perforation is a frequent complication, along with dissemination of the ameba through the portal vein to the liver and other organs, where abscesses may form.

Balantidium dysentery (Fig. 16.28). Balantidium coli *occurs in man and animals independently of climatic influence.* The pathological changes in the tissues are similar to those of amebic dysentery. The living etiological agent has no histolytical effect. Inflammation is produced primarily by the presence of a large number of dead Balantidia as is perhaps also true in amebic dysentery. The disease is commonly accompanied by bacterial infection. Figure 16.28 shows Balantidia (→) in a lymph vessel in the periphery of a lymph node in the mesocolon.

Cysticercosis (Fig. 16.29). *This implies the seeding of larva* (Cysticercus cellulosae) *of the swine tapeworm* (Taenia solium) *in the various organs of man or swine after oral ingestion of eggs. Cysticercus is found in eastern Europe, Asia, South America and Central America. The larva are found predominantly in the central nervous system, eyes and skeletal muscles.* **Histologically,** the larvae are found enclosed in a vesicle arising from invagination. Often, the head end with hooks is visible (→). The diameter of a Cysticercus seldom is larger than 1.5 cm. The shape is variable. After the worm dies, a foreign body reaction occurs. Secondary calcification (x-ray) and the development of epilepsy, if the central nervous system is involved, provide clues for clinical diagnosis.

Echinococcosis (Fig. 16.30). *The larvae of* Taenia echinococcus *(dog tapeworm) pass through the portal vein into the liver, where they form cysts (hydatid cysts).* The figure shows cysts the wall of which consists of a ring of collagenous fibrous tissue (→ 1) on which rests a homogeneous, lamellar red chitinous layer (cuticle → 2). Scolices are often seen near the cuticle. The inset in the lower right in Figure 16.30 shows a single hook. The adjacent liver shows atrophy and lymphocytic infiltration.

Macroscopic: Either a large unilocular cyst or several cysts filled with daughter cysts. They are especially common in the right lobe of the liver. Echinococcus alveolaris (2% in humans): multiple small cysts bounded by a capsule of connective tissue (60% liver, 30% lung).

Intestinal worms (Figs. 16.31, 16.32). In tropical countries, *Ascaris* and *Trichuris trichiura* frequently are found in the lumen of the intestine. Hookworm *(Ancylostoma duodenale* and *Necator americanus)* causes severe anemia and wasting, which often leads to death in children. Larvae of *Trichuris trichiura* (Fig. 16.31) occasionally penetrate into the mucous membrane of the intestine. In Figure 16.31, two larvae are seen covered by a layer of intestinal epithelium (→). A transversely sectioned worm in the intestinal lumen contains numerous eggs (→ 1). *Ascaris lumbricoides* (Fig. 16.32) sometimes causes severe disease with eventual ileus or intestinal perforation and can also lodge in other organs. Figure 16.32 shows a longitudinally sectioned ascaris (→ cuticle) in a bile duct. The duct wall is inflamed and the worm contains ascaris eggs (→) some of which are outside the worm (→ 2). This patient died of multiple liver abscesses.

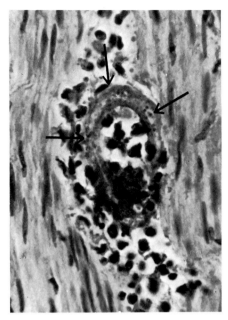

Fig. 16.33. Larva migrans and cellular reaction in the intestinal musculature; H & E, 630×.

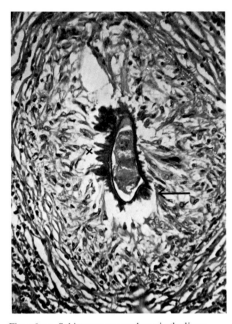

Fig. 16.34. Schistosoma granuloma in the liver; H & E, 300×.

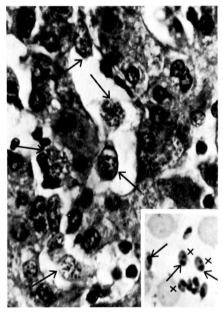

Fig. 16.35. Kala-azar (liver);
H & E, 450×.
Inset: *L. donovani* in peritoneal exudate (hamster);
Giemsa stain, 1.150×.

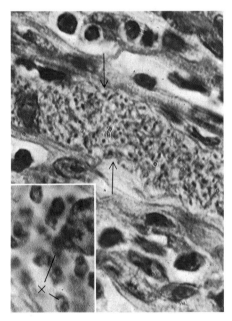

Fig. 16.36. Acute Chagas myocarditis (child);
H & E, 980×.
Inset: *Tr. cruzi* in Chagas encephalitis; H & E,
1,500×.

Larva migrans (Fig. 16.33). *This includes all conditions in which larvae and microfilaria, especially of nematodes such as strongyloides, ancylostoma, ascaris and toxocara canis and cati invade the skin and internal organs. The disease occurs mostly in children and causes symptoms of a general infection with fever and, in addition, shows blood eosinophilia. The larvae are found most particularly in infections with* **Strongyloides, Ancylostoma,** *Ascaris lumbricoides suum* as well as *Toxocara canis* and *cati.* In the last-named disease, man is a secondary host and the disease is known as visceral larva migrans. The larvae elicit a tissue reaction consisting of eosinophils and granulomas. The parasites are not ordinarily detected in the tissue (→). In most cases, exact classification is difficult.

The microfilarias (→), morphology of which does not easily lend itself to ordinary classification are distinguished from tissue fibers by their stippling (Fig. 16.33); difficult to recognize in cross section. They elicit an eosinophilic reaction (not always) and eosinophilic granulomas which in the tropics occur chiefly in internal organs. Microfilaria are frequently not found.

Schistosomiasis *(Bilharziasis,* Fig. 16.34). *Schistosoma belong to the* **trematodes.** *Three types are found in man.* **Schistosoma haematobium** *occurs in Africa and bordering countries.* **Schistosoma mansoni** *in Africa and South America and* **Schistosoma japonicum** *in Asia. The worm spends its youth in the outside world. Snails act as the intermediate host. Infection is the result of contact with infected water. Adult Schistosoma are found in the paravesicular tissues* (Schistosoma haematobium) *and mesenteric veins* (Schistosoma haematobium) *and* (japonicum). *The tissue changes and symptoms of the disease are caused by the eggs of the Schistosoma, which have characteristic structures that allow diagnosis of the type of parasite causing the infection. In* Schistosoma hematobium, *the eggs are found in the liver, ureter and genital organs (occasionally rectum and lungs)* Schistosoma mansoni *and* japonicum *eggs occur particularly in the walls of the intestines and liver.*

The eggs of trematodes cause a granulocytic or eosinophilic reaction in the earliest stages. Later, a typical granuloma forms which heals with calcification and connective tissue scarring. Complications are carcinoma of the urinary bladder, hepatic cirrhosis, cor pulmonale and, in the central nervous system, focal symptoms, depending upon the site. Figure 16.34 shows a Schistosoma granuloma in the liver. In the center, there is a *Sch. mansoni* egg with a lateral, pointed spine (→), which has important diagnostic significance. Externally, particularly on the other long side, the egg has a layer of prickly material that stains red with H & E (×). This is protein formed by the host and indicates an immune reaction (Hoeppli-Splendore phenomenon). Such a tissue reaction may also be caused by other microorganisms.

Kala-azar (visceral leishmaniasis, Fig. 16.35). *The name comes from India and means "black disease." It occurs also in Asia, Africa, southern Europe and South America. The protozoan* Leishmania donovani *produces visceral changes, as opposed to* Leishmania tropica *and* brasiliensis, *which produce only skin and mucous membrane lesions (mucocutaneous Leishmaniasis). Natural infection occurs in dogs, foxes and jackals, and the etiological agent is transmitted by Phlebotomus (sand fly).* Clinically, there is hepatosplenomegaly with fever, pancytopenia and increase of plasma globulins. The cytoplasm of cells of the reticuloendothelial system contains the causative organisms, $2-5 \mu$ in size. In Figure 16.35 numerous Leishmaniae are seen in the Kupfer cells of the liver. The typical Leishmaniae blepharoplasts are difficult to see in tissue, but are conspicuous in smears (Fig. 16.35, smear: → nucleus, × blepharoplast). Diagnostically knowledge of the organ involved is important since the organisms of Chagas disease and of mucocutaneous Leishmaniasis look alike in tissues. Histoplasmas, which resemble Leishmania in H & E stains (cf. Fig. 16.16) can be differentiated with Grocott stain.

Chagas disease (American trypanosomiasis, Fig. 16.36). The causative agent, *Trypanosoma cruzi,* is transmitted by the barbeiro (Triatoma and related Reduvüdae) and is found only in blood. In tissue they lose their flagella and look like Leishmaniae. They occur chiefly in heart muscle fibers in the form of nonencapsulated nests (→). In routine tissue sections blepharoplasts are hard to see. In the inset of Figure 16.36 (Chagas encephalitis) they appear as rod shaped structures within the Leishmaniae (×).

Involvement of heart muscle causes myocarditis. In acute cases the nests of parasites can be found and the diagnosis is relatively easy. In chronic myocarditis the organisms are found only rarely. If they are not found these chronic cases present a diagnostic problem since the cardiac hypertrophy and parietal thrombosis is similar to that found in Fiedler's idiopathic myocarditis or in viral myocarditis. Investigators in Brazil suggest that parasitic infection of the vegetative nervous system may lead to development of large organs.

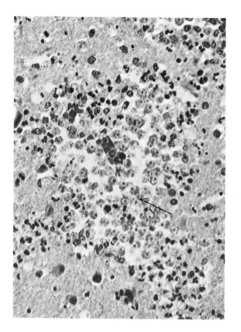

Fig. 16.37. Acanthoamoebiasis. Numerous Hartmanella amoeba in brain; H & E, 240×.

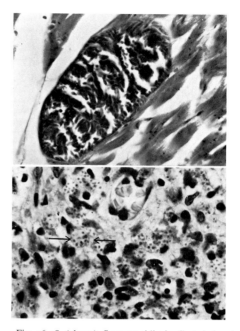

Fig. 16.38. (above). Sarcosporidiosis. Cysts in heart muscle (beef); H & E, 320×.
Fig. 16.39. (Below). Mucosal Leishmaniasis. Numerous, predominately intracellular *L. braziliensis;* H & E, 420×.

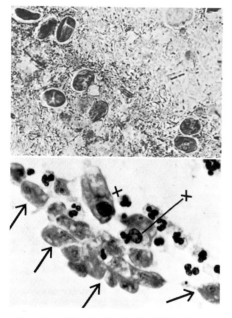

Fig. 16.40 (above). *Giardia lamblia* in fecal smear (child); H & E, 240×.
Fig. 16.41 (below). Trichomonas in vaginal smear. Papanicolaou stain; 320×.

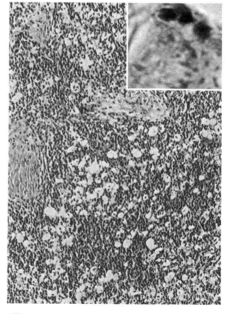

Fig. 16.42. Rhinoscleroma. Numerous pale Mikulicz cells; H & E, 130×.
Inset: *K. rhinoscleromatis* in Mikulicz cells: Giemsa stain, 1800×.

Acanthoamoebiasis (Fig. 16.37). In recent years infections due chiefly to acanthoamoeba have appeared in Europe, America and Australia. The amebae ascend through the nasal passages, along the fibers of the olfactory nerve and cause purulent meningoencephalitis. Most patients contract the disease from swimming pools.

The amebae of this group have a different structure than *E. histolytica*. They are round, vesicular ($\rightarrow$) and do not stain with PAS or Grocott stains (Fig. 16.37). The pathogenesis has been established in animals. After hematogenous dissemination the organisms die in other organs without eliciting a tissue reaction.

Macroscopic: purulent basal meningoencephalitis with abscesses.

Sarcosporidiosis (Fig. 16.38). Infection with the various forms of sarcocystus is of minor significance. It is more frequent in animals than in humans *(S. lindemanni)* and affects skeletal and cardiac muscle fibers, largely without an inflammatory reaction. The parasitic cysts are easily recognized in heart muscle in H & E stains. The comma shaped trophozoites are easily differentiated from *T. gondi* and the leishmania of *Tr. cruzi*.

Cutaneous and Mucocutaneous Leishmaniasis (Fig. 16.39). In Asia and Africa the lesions occur only in the skin and are caused by *L. tropica* and are called oriental boil. In South America in addition to the skin the facial mucous membranes are attacked. The pathogenesis of the latter is not entirely clear. Apparently it develops from a skin lesion (which may be completely healed) to secondary hematogenous spread to mucous membranes. Organism and disease are named according to the country of occurrence. Infection with *L. brasiliensis* is the most common. Figure 16.39 is not typical in that so many intracellular organisms are seen only exceptionally. In most cases the diagnosis must be based on the quite characteristic tissue reaction—without evident organisms. A granulomatous reaction, often only hinted at and without a necrotic tuberculoid granuloma, points to the diagnosis. Other infections must be differentiated by the use of special stains. Skin lesions may also occur in Kala-azar.

Macroscopic: nodular thickening, frequently ulceration only.

Giardiasis (Fig. 16.40). *Giardia lamblia,* a flagellate, is a very common inhabitant of the small intestine in all tropical countries, particularly in children. It causes mild intestinal disturbances. The organisms apparently occasionally penetrate the upper mucosal layers but elicit practically no tissue reaction. They are Grocott positive and scanty in routine sections, but are easily seen in smears (Fig. 16.40). The paired flagellae are not recognizable.

Trichomoniasis (Fig. 16.41). is a worldwide infection which causes vaginitis, urethritis, prostatitis and vesiculitis. The Grocott positive causative agents are often found in routine smears of exfoliative cytology (Fig. 16.41). They must be differentiated from epithelial cells ($\times$) and granulocytes. The nuclei and flagellae, however, are not easily seen. Infection may cause epithelial cell atypia, but has no causal relationship to cancer.

Rhinoscleroma (Fig. 16.42). Because lesions not only may occur in the nose, but also in the mucous membranes of the bronchi this disease is sometimes called "scleroma." It occurs in East Europe, Africa, Asia and South America, but nowadays chiefly only in tropical regions. The histological diagnosis is simple: in addition to plasma cells with Russel bodies there are numerous typical pale, so-called Mikulicz cells (Fig. 16.42). The fresh bacilli *(Klebsiella rhinoscleromatis)* are seen only occasionally (insert, Fig. 16.42). The pale Mikulicz cells, however, must be differentiated by special stains from those of other infections. Treatment is still unsatisfactory.

Macroscopic: firm, nodular or diffuse thickening of the mucous membranes of the upper respiratory passages which may result in stenosis.

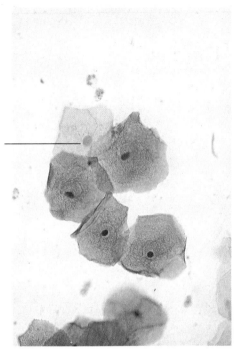

Fig. 17.1. Papanicolaou stain (vaginal smear, proliferative phase), 800×.

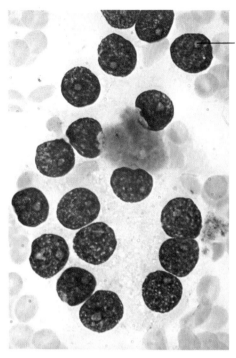

Fig. 17.2. May-Grunewald-Giemsa stain (normal thyroid epithelium); 800×.

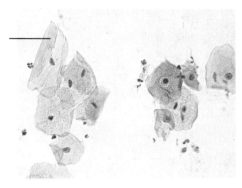

Fig. 17.3. Secretory phase (vaginal smear); Pap. stain, 200×.

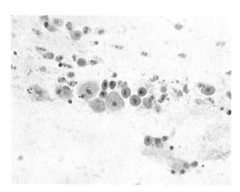

Fig. 17.4. Senile involution of mucosa (vaginal smear); Pap. stain, 200×.

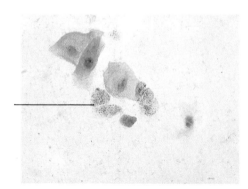

Fig. 17.5. Trichomonas in vaginal smear; Pap. stain, 320×.

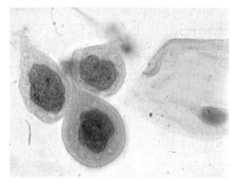

Fig. 17.6. Dyskeratosis in cervical smear; Pap. stain, 800×.

17. Cytodiagnosis

Cytodiagnosis is an investigative method which is employed ever more commonly particularly for the separation of tumors from inflammatory or degenerative lesions. The advantages of this method lie chiefly in the ease of obtaining material (ambulatory patients without anesthesia), the saving of time, the little technical equipment required and the ease of execution (smear → staining → report). These advantages also permit repeated control investigations of a large patient population, e.g., in cancer detection. With suitable experience and good technique cytodiagnosis has a high degree of reliability.

Material suitable for cytodiagnosis is of two sorts: 1. **Exfoliated cells** that have detached themselves or been scraped from the surface of an organ with the help of an instrument (wooden spatula). Exfoliated cells may also be obtained from effusions (e.g., ascites) or secretions (e.g., sputum or urine). 2. **Needle biopsy,** which involves sampling a solid or cystic mass with a cannula. Cell fragments are loosened from the tissue being sampled and are aspirated.

Cytologic technique. Material obtained from exfoliation or by needle biopsy is smeared on a microscopic slide. Preparations for *Papanicolaou staining* are fixed with alcohol (spray). Smears for *May-Grünwald-Giemsa staining* are air fixed.

Papanicolaou stain (Pap. stain., Fig. 17.1) is to be preferred when cytoplasmic structures need to be clearly shown. Figure 17.1 shows a cervical smear from a sexually mature woman **(proliferative phase of menstrual cycle)** with predominantly *superficial cells* that have acidophilic cytoplasm and pyknotic nuclei. The single *intermediate cell* from the midlayers of the mucosa has basophilic (greenish) cytoplasm and a vesicular nucleus (→).

May-Grünwald-Giemsa stain (MGG stain., Fig. 17.2) gives good rendition of nuclear details such as chromatin structure and nucleoli. Figure 17.2 shows a group of normal thyroid epithelial cells with finely lumpy chromatin and a rather small nucleolus (→).

Cervical cytology (Figs. 17.3–17.6) is chiefly concerned with the exfoliated squamous epithelial cells obtained from the external cervix and the cylindrical cells from the cervical canal (endocervix). It permits diagnosis of the status of the sexual hormones *(functional diagnosis: menstrual cycle and hormone activity)*, of the vaginal flora *(identification of the causative organisms of inflammations)*, of precursors of cancer *(dysplasia, carcinoma in situ)* and of malignant tumors *(squamous cell carcinoma)*.

Fig. 17.3 shows a smear from a sexually mature woman **(secretory phase)**. The arrangement of superficial intermediate cells with distinct cytoplasmic folding (→) in small groups is typical. With age **mucosal involution** occurs (Fig. 17.4). There are epithelial cells from the deeper cell layers. The cells are essentially smaller (cf. Fig. 17.3, taken at the same magnification).

Cytological examination frequently reveals the causative agent of an inflammation. In this case it is **Trichomonas** (Fig. 17.5) which show the characteristic reddish granules (→). Below the organisms there are basophilic intermediate cells and granulocytes.

Dyskeratosis (Fig. 17.6). Cells with large, hyperchromatic and polymorphic nuclei and still preserved cytoplasmic structure. Their presence suggests the early stages of dysplasia, carcinoma in situ or precancer. This finding must be confirmed by further diagnostic and therapeutic means, e.g., by cervical conization. In the field of cancer detection, preventive cytology has led to reduction in frequency of cervical carcinoma which today is less frequent than corpus carcinoma.

On the basis of cytology the following classification of cervical lesions has been proposed by Papanicolaou: Pap. Groups I and II are nonsuspicious, Group III doubtful, Group IV comprises dysplasia and carcinoma in situ and Group V invasive carcinoma.

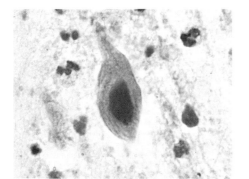

Fig. 17.7. Squamous carcinoma cell (sputum); H & E, 800×.

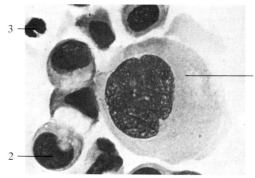

Fig. 17.8. Carcinoma cell in ascitic sediment; MGG stain, 800×.

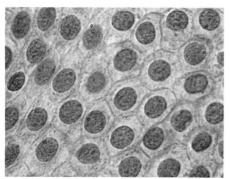

Fig. 17.9. Normal prostate; Pap. stain, 800×.

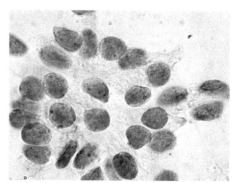

Fig. 17.10. Well differentiated prostatic carcinoma; Pap. stain, 800×.

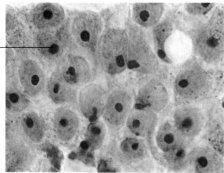

Fig. 17.11. Moderately well differentiated prostatic carcinoma; Pap. stain, 800×.

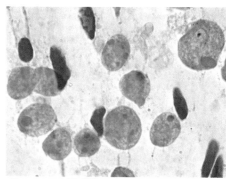

Fig. 17.12. Undifferentiated prostatic carcinoma; Pap. stain, 800×.

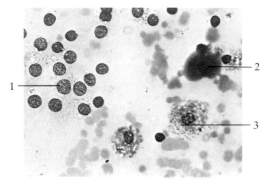

Fig. 17.13. Colloid goiter with cystic change; MGG stain, 320×.

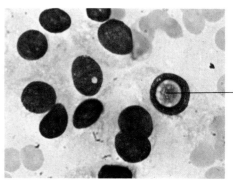

Fig. 17.14. Thyroid carcinoma (papillary type); MGG, 800×.

Sputum cytology (Fig. 17.7). Cytological investigation of sputum is of great value in the diagnosis of bronchogenic carcinoma. It makes possible detection of centrally placed tumors with a high degree of accuracy. Figure 17.7 shows a **tumor cell from a squamous cell carcinoma.** The nucleus is especially large and hyperchromatic. The nucleus/cytoplasm ratio is shifted in favor of the nucleus.

Exfoliative cytology of effusions (Fig. 17.8). The etiology of an effusion is a common clinical question – is it or is it not from a malignant tumor? Figure 17.8 shows a **carcinoma cell** ($\rightarrow$ 1) recovered from the sediment of ascitic fluid. The size and structure of the nucleus of the carcinoma cell distinguishes it from benign cells of the peritoneal lining ($\rightarrow$ 2) and from leucocytes ($\rightarrow$ 3).

Cytology of prostatic needle biopsy (Figs. 17.9–17.12). The diagnostic value of this is well recognized today, particularly in surveys of large groups of patients (early cancer detection). Transrectal aspiration biopsy with a thin needle (obtaining a sample from multiple sites in the prostate) commonly achieves a higher rate of correct diagnoses than is attained with histological examination of a single punch biopsy. Cytological investigation of a prostatic carcinoma also allows assessment of the grade of the tumor which is important for treatment.

Figure 17.9 shows a smear from **normal prostate.** The cells and nuclei are of uniform size and have distinct cell boundaries — signs of a benign nature *(so-called beehive structure:* occurs also in adenomyomatosis). In **well differentiated prostatic carcinoma** there are so-called *microadenomatous structures* (Fig. 17.10): a circular arrangement of cells showing essentially no nuclear changes but having faded, indistinct cell borders. In **moderately well differentiated prostatic carcinoma** (Fig. 17.11) nuclear changes are dominant. The nuclei are of different sizes, overlap one another and have large nucleoli ($\rightarrow$). In **undifferentiated prostatic carcinoma** (Fig. 17.12) the cells are isolated and *cellular dissociation and polymorphism predominate* and the nuclei show distinct variations in size.

Needle biopsy of the thyroid (Figs. 17.2, 17.13 and 17.14). Cytological study of the thyroid permits separation of a colloid goiter from inflammation or the different sorts of carcinomas. It contributes to clarification of "cold nodules" discovered by scintillation detectors. In Figure 17.13 (**goiter showing degenerative cystic changes**) there are typical thyroid cells ($\rightarrow$ 1, cf. also Fig. 17.2), a fragment of colloid ($\rightarrow$ 2), that is uniformly dark blue with MGG stain, and macrophages ($\rightarrow$ 3). Figure 17.14 shows **tumor cells from a papillary adenocarcinoma** of the thyroid in which can be seen the typical intranuclear cytoplasmic invagination.

Exfoliative and needle biopsy cytology are also of value in other organs, e.g. the gastrointestinal tract. By taking the sample with a brush, large areas of a suspicious organ can be examined. By combining these investigational methods with histological gastric suction or snip biopsies it is possible to attain nearly 100% accuracy of diagnosis. Needle biopsy of the breast also is highly reliable particularly when it is used in conjunction with mammography. It permits not only separation of benign and malignant tumors but also grading of a tumor.

Selected References

The following references are either review articles (indicated by *) which contain additional references or original papers of historical interest or special significance for the subject under discussion.
Many of the references in German or other foreign languages have been omitted from the English edition, since many English-speaking readers would find difficulty in reading them. The complete bibliography is, of course, contained in the 7th German edition of *Histopathologie* which is available in many libraries. Where serious omissions occurred because of deletion of German papers, comparable papers written in English have been substituted. – Ed.

Staining

Humason, G. L.: Animal Tissue Techniques (San Francisco: W. H. Freeman Company, 1972).*
Lillie, R. D., H. M. Fullmer: Histopathologic Technic and Practical Histochemistry (4th ed.; New York: McGraw-Hill Book Company, Inc., 1976).*
Pearse, A. G. E.: Histochemistry (London: J. & A. Churchill, Ltd., 1968).*

General and Special Pathology

Anderson, W. A. D., J. M. Kissane: Pathology (7th ed.; St. Louis: C. V. Mosby Company, Inc., 1977).*
Anderson, J. R.: Muir's Textbook of Pathology (10th ed.; Chicago, Year Book Medical Publishers, Inc., 1976).*
De Duve, C.: Lysosomes (New York: Ronald Press Co., 1959), p. 128.*
Dumont, A.: Lab. Invest. 14:2034 (1965).
Florey, H. W.: General Pathology (4th ed.; Philadelphia: W. B. Saunders Company, 1970).*
Gieseking, R.: Mesenchymal Gewebe und ihre Reaktionsformen im elektronenoptischen Bild (Stuttgart: G. Fischer, 1966).*
Gusek, W.: Submikroskopische Untersuchungen zur Feinstruktur aktiver Bindegewebszellen. Veröffentl. aus der morphologischen Pathologic (Stuttgart: G. Fischer, 1962).*
Henke, F., O. Lubarsch: Handbuch der speziellen pathologischen Anatomie und Histologie (Berlin: Springer-Verlag, 1931).*
La Via, M. F., R. B. Hill: Principles of Pathology (New York: Oxford University Press, 1975.
Majno, G., G. E. Palade: J. Biophys. Biochem. Cytol. 11: 571 (1961).
Robbins, S. L.: Pathologic Basis of Disease (Philadelphia: W. B. Saunders Company, 1974).
Sandritter, W., Beneke, G.: Allgemeine Pathologie, Schattauer, Stuttgart, 1974.
Sandritter, W., Thomas, C., Kirsten, W. H.: Macropathology (3d. ed.; Chicago: Year Book Medical Publishers, Inc., 1979.)
Schäfer, A., R. Bässler: Frankfurt. Ztschr. Path. 75: 37 (1966).
Smith, D. E., ed.: Survey of Pathology in Medicine and Surgery. Baltimore: The Williams & Wilkins Company (Bimonthly review).
Trump, B. F., J. L. Ericsson: In Zweifach, B. W., Grant, L., and McCluskey, R. T.: The Inflammatory Process p. 35 (New York: Academic Press, Inc., 1965).
Wartman, W. B.: Evaluation of Biopsy Diagnosis, Am. J. Clin. Path. 32: 207 (1959).
Carone, F. A. and Conn, R. B., ed.: Year Book of Pathology and Clinical Pathology. Chicago; Year Book Medical Publishers, Inc. (annual review).
Weissmann, G.: New England J. Med. 273: 1084 (1965).
Wessel, W., P. Gedigk: Virchows Arch. path. Anat. 332: 508 (1959).

Histology

Bloom, W., D. W. Fawcett: A Textbook of Histology (10th ed.; Philadelphia: W. B. Saunders Company, 1975).*
Karlson, P.: Introduction to Modern Biochemistry (4th ed.; New York and London: Academic Press, Inc., 1975). (Good correlation of biochemistry and morphology.)
Porter, K. R.: Fine Structure of Cells and Tissues, K. R. Porter and M. A. Bonneville (eds.) (4th ed.; Philadelphia: Lea & Febiger, 1973).*

Heart

General
Farrer-Brown, G.: Color Atlas of Cardiac Pathology (Chicago: Year Book Medical Publishers, Inc., 1977).
Gould, S. F.: Pathology of the Heart (2d ed.; Springfield, Ill.: Charles C Thomas, Publisher, 1960).*
Hudson, R. E.: Cardiovascular Pathology (Baltimore: The Williams & Wilkins Company, 1970).

Hypertrophy
Sandritter, W., G. Scommazoni, G.: Nature 202: 100 (1964).
Wartmann, W. B. and Hill, W. T.: In Gould, S. E.: Pathology of the Heart, 2nd ed.; Springfield, Ill.: Charles C Thomas, 1960.

Atrophy
Hellerstein, D., Santiago-Stevenson: Circulation 1: 93 (1950).

Myocardial Infarct—Coronary Insufficiency
Büchner, F.: Die Coronarinsuffizienz (Dresden, Leipzig: Steinkopff, 1939).*
Cushing, E. H., H. S. Feil, E. S. Stanton, W. B. Wartman: Infarction of the Cardiac Auricles. Brit. Heart J. 6: 115 (1944).
Galen, R. S. Progress in Human Pathology 6: 141 (1975).
Jennings, R. B., J. H. Baum, P. B. Herdson: Arch. Path. 79: 135 (1965).
Mallory, G. K., P. D. White, J. Salcedo-Salgar: Am. Heart J. 18: 647 (1939).
Mitchell, J. R. A., C. J. Schwartz: Arterial Disease (Oxford: Blackwell Scientific Publications, 1965).*
Sommers, H. M., R. B. Jennings: Lab. Invest. 13: 1491 (1964).
Wartman, W. B.: Definition of Myocardial Infarction, in: The Etiology of Myocardial Infarction, T. N. James and J. W. Keyes (cds.) (Boston: Little, Brown & Company, 1961).
Wartman, W. B., H. K. Hellerstein: Incidence of Heart Disease. Ann. Int. Med. 28: 41 (1948).

Myocarditis
Blankenhorn, M. A., E. A. Gall: Circulation 13: 217 (1956).*
Salfelder, K. H., W. Sandritter: Frankfurt Z. Path. 62: 88 (1951).
Saphir, O.: Arch. Path. 32: 1000 (1941).
Saphir, O.: Bull. Soc. int. Chir. 19: 463 (1960).

Endocarditis
Mittermayer, C., A. Waldthaler, W. Vogel, W. Sandritter: Beitr. Path. 143: 29 (1971).
Wartman, W. B.: Research in Burns. 9: 6 (1962).

Rheumatic Fever
Aschoff, L.: Verhandl. deutsch. Gesellsch. Path. 8: 46 (1904).

Pericarditis
Schorn, J.: In: Das Herz des Menschen (Stuttgart: Georg Thieme, 1956).*

Blood Vessels

Arteriosclerosis
Rokitansky, C.: Über einige der wichtigsten Krankheiten der Arterien (Wien: Hof- u. Staatsdruckerei, 1852).
Wartman, W. B.: Hemorrhage into the Arterial Wall. Am. Heart J. 39: 79 (1950).
Wissler, R. W., J. C. Geer: The Pathogenesis of Arteriosclerosis (Baltimore: The Williams & Wilkins Company, 1972).

Coronary Arteriosclerosis
Enos, F., R. H. Holmes, J. Beyer: J. A. M. A. 152: 1090 (1953).
Fulton, W. F. M.: The Coronary Arteries (Springfield, Ill.: Charles C Thomas, Publisher, 1965).*

Klemperer, P.: Am. J. Cardiol. 5: 94 (1960).
Fleckenstein, A., J. Janke, H. J. Doring, O. Leder: In Recent Adv. in Studies on Cardiac Structure and Metab. 6:22 (Baltimc.e: University Park Press, 1975).

Inflammation
Buerger, L.: Am. J. M. Sc. 136: 567 (1908).
Lewis, T.: Clin. Sc. 3: 287 (1938). (Raynaud's disease.)

Thrombosis
Rodman, N. F., Jr., R. G. Mason, K. M. Brinkhous: Fed. Proc. 22: 1356 (1963).
Rodman, N. F., Jr., J. C. Painter, N. B. McDevitt: J. Cell Biol. 16: 225 (1963).
Sandritter, W.: Behringwerk-Mitteilungen 41: 37 (1962).
Sandritter, W., G. Beneke: In E. Kaufmann and M. Staemmler: Lehrbuch der speziellen pathologischen Anatomie (Berlin: W. de Gruyter, 1965).*
Zahn, W.: Int. Beitr. wissensch. Med. 2: 199 (1891).

Lung

General
Bowden, D. H.: Current Topics in Pathology: 55: 1 (1971) (congestion).
Laurell, C. B., S. Eriksson: Scand. J. Clin. Lab. Invest. 15: 132 (1963) (emphysema).
Schultz, H.: Die submikroskopische Anatomie und Pathologie der Lunge (Berlin: Springer-Verlag, 1959).*
Spencer, H.: Pathology of the Lung (Oxford: Pergamon Press, 1962).*

Fat Embolism
Sevitt, S.: Fat Embolism (London: Butterworth & Co., 1962).*

Asthma
Dunnil, M. S.: J. Clin. Path. 13: 27 (1960).

Interstitial Pneumonia
Hamman, L., A. R. Rich: Bull. Johns Hopkins Hosp. 74: 177 (1944).

Anthracosis
Anderson, R. B., F. D. Gunn: Am. J. Path. 26: 735 (1950).

Tuberculosis
Diagnostic Standards and Classification of Tuberculosis. National Tuberculosis Association, New York, 1961.*
Koch, R.: Berl. klin. Wchnschr. 1882: 221.
Langhans, Th.: Virchows Arch. path. Anat. 42: 382 (1868).

Shock
Sandritter, W., H. G. Lasch: Methods and Achievements in Experimental Pathology (Basel: S. Karger, 1966).
Thal, A. P.: Shock: A Physiologic Basis for Treatment (Chicago: Year Book Medical Publishers, Inc., 1971).

Alimentary Tract

General
Bockus, H. L.: Gastroenterology (3d ed.; Philadelphia: W. B. Saunders Company, 1974).*
Sheehy, T. W., M. H. Floch: The Small Intestine (New York: Hoeber Medical Division, Harper & Row, Publishers, 1964).*

Fungal Infections
Emmons, C. W., C. H. Binford, J. P. Utz, K. J. Kwon-Chung: Medical Mycology (3d ed. Philadelphia: Lea & Febiger, 1977).*

Gastritis
Oehlert, W.: Z. Allg. Med. 1974: 8–96.
Palmer, E. D.: Medicine 33: 199 (1954).*

Gastric Ulcer
Illingworth, C. F. W.: Peptic Ulcer (Edinburgh: E. & S. Livingstone, Ltd., 1953).*

Typhoid Fever
Huckstep, R. L.: Typhoid Fever and Other Salmonella Infections (Edinburgh: E. & S. Livingstone, Ltd., 1962).*

Appendix
Aschoff, L.: Appendicitis (trans.) (London: G. C. Pether, 1932).

Enterocolitis
Broberger, O., P. Perlmann: J. Exper. Med. 110: 657 (1959).
Kroneberg, G., W. Sandritter: Ztschr. ges. exper. Med. 120: 329 (1953).
Mohr, H. J.: Chemotherapia 6: 1 (1963).
Sandritter, W., H. G. Lasch: Pathologic Aspects of Shock, in: Methods and Achievements in Experimental Pathology (Basel: S. Karger AG., 1966).*
Takeuchi, A., Sprinz, H., LaBrec, E. H. Formal, S. B.: Am. J. Path. 47: 1011 (1965).

Regional Ileitis
Crohn, B. B., L. Ginzburg, G. D. Oppenheimer, J. A. M. A. 99: 1923 (1932).

Whipple's Disease
Chears, W. C., C. T. Ashworth: Gastroenterology 41: 129 (1961).
Kjaerheim, A., Midtevdt, T., Skrede, E., Gjowe, E.: Acta path. microbiol. scand. 66: 135 (1966).
Whipple, G. H.: Bull. Johns Hopkins Hosp. 18: 382 (1907).

Mucoviscidosis
Anderson, D. H.: Ann. New York Acad. Sc. 93: 500 (1962).

Liver

General
Popper, H., F. Schaffner: Liver: Structure and Function (New York: McGraw-Hill Book Company, Inc., 1957).*
Rappaport, A. M., Z. J. Borowy, W. M. Lougheed, W. H. Lotto: Anat. Rec. 119: 11 (1954).

Amyloidosis
Teilum, G.: Acta path. Scandinav. 61: 21 (1964).

Eclampsia
Black-Schaffer, B., D. S. Johnson, W. G. Gobbel: Am. J. Path. 26: 397 (1950).
Dexter, L., S. Weiss, F. W. Haynes, H. S. Sise: J. A. M. A. 122: 145 (1943).

Cirrhosis
Sherlock, S.: Diseases of the Liver and Biliary System (5th ed.; St. Louis: C. V. Mosby Co., Inc., 1975).*
Steiner, P. E., J. Higginson: Acta Un. internat. contra cancrum 17: 581 (1961).
Thaler, H. Beitr: Allg. Path. 112: 173 (1952).

Erythroblastosis
Allen, F. H., L. K. Diamond: Erythroblastosis Fetalis (Boston: Little, Brown & Company, 1957).
Potter, E. L.: Arch. Path. 41: 223 (1946).

Hepatitis
Dienhardt, F., A. Holmes, R. Capps, H. Popper: J. Exp. Med. 125: 673, 1967

Electron Microscopy
Ashworth, C. T., D. J. Werner, M. D. Glass, N. J. Arnol: Am. J. Path. 47: 917 (1965).
Biava, C.: Lab. Invest. 13: 301 (1964).
Biava, C.: Lab. Invest. 13: 1099 (1964).
Biava, C., M. Muklova-Montiel: Am. J. Path. 46: 775 (1965).
Herdson, P. B., J. P. Kaltenbach: J. Cell Biol. 25: 485 (1965).
Mallory, K. G.: Lab. Invest. 9: 132 (1960).
Reynolds, E. S.: J. Cell Biol. 19: 139 (1963).

Kidney

General
Allen, A. C.: The Kidney (2d ed.; New York: Grune & Stratton, Inc., 1962).*
Bell, E. T.: Renal Diseases (Philadelphia: Lea & Febiger, 1950).*
Black, D. A. K., N. F. Jones: Renal Disease (4th ed.; St. Louis, C. V. Mosby Co., Inc., 1978).
Heptinstall, R. H.: Pathology of the Kidney (Boston: Little, Brown & Co., 1966).
Potter, E.: Normal and Abnormal Development of the Kidney (Chicago: Year Book Medical Publishers, Inc., 1972).
Volhard, F., Th. Fahr: Die Brightsche Nierenkrankheit (Berlin: Springer-Verlag, 1914).*

Nephrosis
Earle, D. P., R. B. Jennings, M. Bernik: Prog. Cardiovas. Dis. 4: 148 (1961).

Arterio-Arteriolosclerosis
Smith, J. P.: J. Path. Bact. 69: 147 (1955).

Kimmelstiel-Wilson's Glomerulosclerosis
Kimmelstiel, P., C. Wilson: Am. J. Path. 12: 83 (1936).

Glomerulonephritis
Ellis, A.: Lancet 1: 1 (1942).
Herdson, P. B., R. B. Jennings, D. P. Earle: Arch. Path. 81: 117 (1966).
Jennings, R. B., D. P. Earle: J. Clin. Invest. 40: 1525 (1961).
Masugi, M., Y. Sato: Virchows Arch. path. Anat. 293: 615 (1934).
Pfeiffer, E. F., W. Sandritter, K. Schöffling, G. Treser, E. Kraus, W. Menk, M. Herrmann: Ztschr. ges. exper. Med. 132: 436 (1960).
Sandritter, W., E. F. Pfeiffer: Verhandl. deutsch. Gesellsch. Path. 43: 213 (1959).

Pyelonephritis
Quinn, E. L., E. H. Kass: Biology of Pyelonephritis (Boston: Little, Brown & Company, 1960).*

Cysts
Osathanondh, V., E. L. Potter: Arch. Path. 77: 459 (1964).

Electron Microscopy
Dalton, A. J., F. Haguenau, ed.: Ultrastructure of the Kidney, New York—London: Academic Press, 1967.
Miller, F., G. E. Palade: J. Cell Biol. 23: 519 (1964).
Thoenes, W.: Zwanglose Abhandlung aus dem Gebiet der normalen und pathologischen Anatomie (Stuttgart: George Thieme, 1964).*
Totović, V.: Virchows Arch. path. Anat. 340: 251 (1966).
Wachstein, M., M. Besen: Am. J. Path. 44: 383 (1964).

Genitalia-Pregnancy

Testicle
Pugh, R. C. B.: Pathology of the Testis (Oxford: Blackwell Scientific Publications, 1976).

Prostate
Staehler, W., H. Ziegler, D. Völter, G. E. Schubert, W. B. Wartman: Color Atlas of Cytodiagnosis of the Prostate (Chicago: Year Book Medical Publishers, Inc. 1977).

Female Genitalia
Haines, M., C. W. Taylor: Gynecological Pathology (London: J. & A. Churchill, Ltd. 1975).
Novak, E. R., J. D. Woodruff: Gynecologic and Obstetric Pathology (7th ed., Philadelphia: W. B. Saunders Company, 1974).

Endocrine Glands

Bloodworth, J. M. B.: Endocrine Pathology (Baltimore: The Williams & Wilkins Company, 1968).
Kuppermann, H. S.: Human Endocrinology (London: Blackwell Scientific Publications, 1963).*

Adrenals
Sherwin, R. P., V. J. Rosen: Am. J. Clin. Path. 43: 200 (1965).

Hypophysis
Adams, C. W. M., K. V. Swettenham: J. Path. Bact. 74: 95 (1958).
Schönemann, A.: Virchows Arch. path Anat. 129: 310 (1892).

Pancreatic Islet Cells
Gepts, W.: Diabetes 14: 619, 1965

Skin—Breast

Diseases of the Skin
Clark, W. H., L. From, E. A. Bernardino, et al.: The histogenesis and biologic behavior of primary human malignant melanomas of the skin, Cancer Res. 29: 705 (1969).
Lever, W. F., G. Schaumberg-Lever: Histopathology of the Skin (5th ed.; Philadelphia: J. B. Lippincott Company, 1975).
Milne, J. A.: An Introduction to the Diagnostic Histopathology of the Skin (London: Edward Arnold & Co., 1972).*
Percival, G. H., G. L. Montgomery, T. C. Dodds: Atlas of Histopathology of the Skin (Edinburgh: E. & S. Livingston, Ltd., 1962).

Diseases of Breast
Cutler, S. J., M. M. Black, I. S. Goldberg: Prognostic factors in cancer of the female breast, Cancer 16: 1589 (1963).
Haagensen, C. D.: Diseases of the Breast (Philadelphia: W. B. Saunders Company, 1971).
Thomas, C.: in M. Schwalger, Ch. Herfarth: Klinik der Frauenheilkunde und Geburtshilfe (München: Urban & Schwartzenberg, 1977).

Muscles

Adams, R. D., D. Denny-Brown, C. M. Pearson: Diseases of Muscle (3d ed.; New York: Hoeber Medical Division, Harper & Row, Publishers, 1975).*
Greenfield, J. G., G. M. Shy, E. C. Alvord, L. Berg: An Atlas of Muscle Pathology in Neuromuscular Diseases (Edinburgh: E. & S. Livingstone, Ltd., 1957).*

Spleen and Lymph Nodes

Spleen
Blaustein, A.: The Spleen (New York: McGraw-Hill Book Company, Inc., 1963).*

Amyloid
Benditt, E. P., N. Eriksen: Proc. Nat. Acad. Sc. 55: 308 (1966).
Boeré, H., L. Ruinen, J. H. Scholten: J. Lab. & Clin. Med. 66: 943 (1965).

Caesar, R.: Path. et microbiol. (Basel) 24: 387 (1961).
Cohen, A. S., E. Gross, T. Shirahama: Am. J. Path. 47: 1079 (1965).
Glenner, G. G.: Acta path. microbiol. scand. Section A. 80 Suppl. 233: 144 (1972).
Glenner, G. G., W. D. Terry: Ann. Rev. Med. 25: 131 (1974).
Puchtler, H., F. Sweat, M. Levine: J. Histochem. 10: 355 (1962).
Puchtler, H., F. Sweat: J. Histochem. 13: 693 (1965).
Schneider, G.: Ergebn. allg. Path. u. Path. Anat. 46: 1 (1964).*
Teilum, G.: Am. J. Path. 32: 945 (1956).

Lymph Nodes
Lukes, R. J., J. J. Butler: Cancer Res. 26: 1063 (1966).
Marshall, A. H. E.: An Outline of the Cytology and Pathology of the Reticular Tissue (London: Oliver
    & Boyd, Ltd., 1956).*
Masshoff, W.: Deutsche med. Wchnschr. 87: 915 (1962).
Piringer-Kuchinka, A.: Verhandl. deutsch. Gesellsch. Path. 36: 352 (1953).
Piringer-Kuchinka, A., I. Martin, O. Thalhammer: Arch. Path. Anat. 331: 522 (1958).
Wartman, W. B.: Sinus Cell Hyperplasia of Lymph Nodes. Brit. J. Cancer. 13: 389 (1959).

Boeck's Disease
Freiman, D. G.: New England J. Med. 239: 664, 709, 742 (1948).
Scadding, J. G.: Sarcoidosis (London: Eyre & Spottiswoode, 1967).

Hodgkin's Disease
Fresen, O.: Ann. New York Acad. Sc. 73 (1958).
Hoster, H. A., M. B. Dratman, L. F. Craver, H. A. Rolnick: Cancer Res. 8: 17 (1948).*
Kaplan, H. S.: Hodgkin's Disease (Cambridge, Mass.: Harvard University Press, 1972).*
Lukes, R. J., and Butler, J. J.: Cancer Res. 26: 1063, 1966.

Blood and Bone Marrow
Thompson, R. B.: Disorders of the Blood (London: J. & A. Churchill, Ltd., 1977).*
Wintrobe, M. M., G. R. Lee, D. R. Boggs, T. C. Bithell, J. R. Athens, J. Foerster: Clinical Hematol-
    ogy (7th ed.; Philadelphia, Lea & Febiger, 1974).*

Bones and Joints

Ackerman, L. V., H. J. Spjut, M. R. Abell: Bones and Joints (Baltimore: The Williams & Wilkins
    Company, 1976).
Harrison, C. V.: Diseases of Bone, Chapter IX in Recent Advances in Pathology (7th ed.; London: J. &
    A. Churchill, Ltd., 1960).
Jaffe, H. L.: Tumours and Tumorous Conditions of the Bones and Joints (London: Henry Kimpton,
    1958).*
Lichtenstein, L.: Bone Tumors (St. Louis: The C. V. Mosby Company, Inc. 1959).*
Paget, J.: Med. Chir. Tr., London 60: 37 (1877).

Brain and Spinal Cord

General
Blackwood, W., J. A. N. Corsellis: Greenfield's Neuropathology (3d ed.; Chicago: Year Book Medi-
    cal Publishers, Inc., 1976).
Wartman, W. B.: Pathology of Epidemic Typhus. Arch. Path. 56: 397, 512 (1953).

Tumors

Reviews
Ambrose, E. J., F. J. Roe: The Biology of Cancer (London: D. van Nostrand, 1963).
Atlas of Tumor Pathology. Armed Forces Institute, Washington, D. C., 1953.*
Bernhard, W., N. Granboulan: Exper. Cell. Res., suppl. 9, 1963.
Busch, H.: Biochemistry of the Cancer Cell (New York: Academic Press, Inc., 1962).*

Denoix, P.: Mechanism of Invasion in Cancer (U.I.C.C. Monograph, vol. 6. Heidelberg: Springer, 1967).

International Histological Classification of Tumours. WHO, Geneva, 1969–1977.

Hamperl, H., L. V. Ackermann: Illustrated Tumor Nomenclature (New York: Springer Verlag, 1969).

Homburger, F.: The Physiopathology of Cancer (New York: Hoeber Medical Division, Harper & Row, Publishers, 1953).*

Potter, V. R.: Cancer Res. 24: 1085 (1964).*

Willis, R. A.: Pathology of Tumours (London: Butterworth & Co., Ltd., 1960).*

Carcinogenesis
Ciba Foundation Symposium on Carcinogenesis (London: J. & A. Churchill, Ltd., 1959).*

Electron Microscopy
Bernhard, W.: Cancer Res. 20: 712 (1960).*

Bernhard, W.: Verhandl. deutsch. Gesellsch. Path. 1961, S. & G. Fischer, Stuttgart.*

Burkitt, D.: Brit. J. Surg. 46: 218 (1958).

Ozzello, L.: Cancer 26: 1186 (1970).

Parry, E. W., F. N. Ghadially: Cancer 18: 1026 (1965).

Stewart, S. E.: Tr. New York Acad. Sc. 28: 290 (1966).

Thomas, C., H. J. Steinhardt, K. Kuchemann, D. Maas, U. Riede: Current Topics in Pathology (1977).

Tumors of Skin and Mucosae
Dukes, C. E.: J. Path. & Bact. 50: 527 (1940).

MacKee, G. M., A. C. Cipollaro: Am. J. Cancer, 1937.*

Stout, A. P.: Tumors of the Stomach. Atlas of Tumor Pathology. Bd. VI/21. Armed Forces Institute of Pathology, Washington, D.C., 1953.*

Mammary Tumors
Bonser, G. M., I. A. Dosse, I. W. Jull: Human and Experimental Breast Cancer (London: Pitman, 1961).*

Muir, R.: J. Path. & Bact. 42: 155 (1941).

Ovarian Tumors
Barzilai, G.: Atlas of Ovarian Tumors (New York: Grune & Stratton, Inc., 1949).*

Enge, L. A.: Am. J. Obst. & Gynec. 68: 348 (1954).

Basalioma
Albertini, A.: Schweiz. med. Wchnschr. 1941: 992.

Krompecher, E.: Beitr. path. Anat. 28: 1 (1900).

Assor, D.: Cancer 20: 2125 (1967).

Hypernephroma
King, Stanton: Renal Neoplasia. (Boston: Little, Brown & Company, 1967.)

Carcinoma In Situ
Hamperl, H.: In Cancer of the Cervix, Ciba Foundation Study Group, No. 3 (London: J. & A. Churchill, Ltd., 1959).

Sandritter, W.: In A. Linke: Früherkennung des Krebses. S. 43 (Stuttgart: F. K. Schattauer, 1962).

Sandritter, W.: Verhandl. deutsch. Gesellsch. Path. 48: 34 (1964).

Paget's Carcinoma
Paget, J.: Bartholomew's Hosp. Rep. X (1874).

Metastasis
Walther, H. E.: Krebsmetastasen (Basel: B. Schwabe, 1948).*

Willis, R. A.: The Spread of Tumors in the Human Body (2d ed.; London: Butterworth & Co., Ltd., 1952).*

345

Chorionepithelioma
Ahlström, C. G.: Acta path. Scandinav. 8: 213 (1931).

Fibroma
Capell, D. F., G. L. Montgomery: J. Path. & Bact. 44: 517 (1937).
Stout, A. P.: Bull. Hosp. Joint Dis. (N. Y.) 12: 126 (1951).
Stout, A. P.: Cancer 7: 953 (1954).

Keloid
Garb, J., M. J. Stone: Am. J. Surg. 58: 315 (1942).

Myxoma
Stout, A. P.: Ann. Surg. 127: 706 (1948).

Hemangioma
McCarthy, W. D., G. T. Pack: Surg., Gynec. & Obst. 91: 465 (1950).
Stout, A. P.: Cancer 2: 1027 (1949).

Sarcoma
Stout, A. P.: Cancer 1: 30 (1948).

Fibrosarcoma
Stout, A. P.: Tumors of the Soft Tissues. Atlas of Tumor Pathology. II/5. Armed Forces Institute of Pathology, Washington, D.C., 1953.

Neurinoma, Neurofibroma
Recklinghausen, F. D. von: Festschrift für Rudolf Virchow. S. 138 (Berlin: Hirschwald, 1882).

Brain Tumors
Russel, D., L. J. Rubinstein: Pathology of Tumors of the Nervous System (4th ed.; Baltimore, The Williams & Wilkins Company, 1977).*

Pigmented Nevus, Melanoma
Affleck, D. H.: Am. J. Cancer 27: 120 (1936).
Klauder, J. V., H. Beermann: Arch. Dermat. 71: 2 (1955).
Masson, P.: Am. J. Path. 8: 367 (1932).

Cytodiagnosis
Graham, R. M.: The Cytologic Diagnosis of Cancer (2d ed.; Philadelphia: W. B. Saunders Company, 1963).*
Koss, L. G., G. R. Durfee: Diagnostic Cytology and Its Histopathologic Bases (London: Pitman, 1961).*
Papanicolaou, G. N.: Atlas of Exfoliative Cytology (Cambridge, Mass.: Harvard University Press, 1954).*
Staehler, W., H. Ziegler, D. Völter, G. F. Schubert, W. B. Wartman: Color Atlas of Cytodiagnosis of the Prostate (Chicago: Year Book Medical Publishers, Inc., 1977).

Fungi—Parasites

General
Ash, J. E., S. Spitz: Pathology of Tropical Diseases (Philadelphia: W. B. Saunders Company, 1947).*
Emmons, C. W., C. H. Binford, J. P. Utz, K. J. Kwon-Chung: Medical Mycology (3d ed.; Philadelphia: Lea & Febinger, 1977).*
Faust, E. C., P. F. Russell, R. C. Jung: Craig and Faust's Clinical Parasitology (8th ed.; Philadelphia: Lea & Febiger, 1970).*
Marcial-Rojas, R. A.: Pathology of Protozoal and Helminthic Diseases (Baltimore: The Williams & Wilkins Company, 1971).

Salfelder, K., M. De Mendelovici, J. Schwartz: Multiple Deep Fungus Infections: Curr. Top. Path. 57: 123 (1973).

Technic
Coons, A. H., M. H. Kaplan: J. Exper. Med. 91: 1 (1950).
Gridley, M. F.: Am. J. Clin. Path. 23: 303 (1953).
Grocott, R. G.: Am. J. Clin. Path. 25: 975, 1955.
Salfelder, K., T. R. De Liscano, St. Stefanko: Mykosen 11: 679 (1968).

Amebic Dysentery
Faust, E. C.: Amebiasis (Springfield, Ill.: Charles C Thomas, Publisher, 1954).*

Cystocercosis
Dixon, H. B. F., F. M. Lipscomb: Med. Res. Council Ser. No. 292, London, 1961.*

Kala-Azar
Donovan, C.: Brit. M. J. 1903: 79.
Leishman, W. B.: Brit. M. J. 1903: 1252.

Chagas' Disease
Chagas, C.: Mem. Inst. Oswaldo Cruz, 2: 159 (1909).
Gould, S. E.: Am. J. Path. 36: 533 (1960).

Larva Migrans
Beaver, P. C.: Exper. Parasitol. 5: 587 (1956).*

Pneumocystis
Carini, A.: Com. Soc. Med. São Paulo, p. 204, August 16, 1910.
Henderson, D. W., et al.: Pathology 6: 235 (1974).
Salfelder, K., et al.: Neumocistosis (Merida, Venezuela: University de Los Andes, 1965).
Walzer, P. D., et al.: Ann. Int. Med. 80: 83 (1974).

Candidiasis
Lodder, J., N. J. W. Kreger-Van Rij: The Yeasts (Amsterdam: North-Holland Publishing Company, 1952).*
Salfelder, K., et al.: Curr. Top. Path. (1976).

Aspergillosis
Salfelder, K.: Arch Gewebpath. Gewerbehyg. 18: 233 (1960).
Schwarz, J.: Path. Ann. 8: 81 (1973).

Actinomycosis
Peabody, J. W., J. H. Seabury: Am. J. Med: 28: 99 (1960).
Slack, J. M.: Actinomycetacea, in Bergey's Manual of Determinative Bacteriology, R. E. Buchanan and N. E. Gibbons (eds.) (8th ed.; Baltimore: The Williams & Wilkins Company, 1974).
Weed, L. A., A. H. Baggenstoss: Am. J. Clin. Path. 19: 201 (1949).

Nocardiosis
Gonzales-Ochoa, A.: Systemic Mycoses, CIBA Found. Sympos. (Boston: Little, Brown and Company, 1967).

Cryptococcosis
Littman, M. L., L. E. Zimmermann; Cryptococcosis (New York: Grune & Stratton, Inc., 1956).*

Chromomycosis
Carrion, A. L.: Internat. J. Dermat. 14: 27 (1975).

Coccidioidomycosis

Ajello, L.: Coccidioidomycosis (Tucson, Ariz.: Univ. Arizona Press, 1967).
Fiese, M. J.: Coccidioidomycosis (Springfield, Ill.: Charles C Thomas, Publisher, 1958).*
Smith, L. E.: Coccidioidomycosis. H. A. Christian, Oxford Medicine, Vol. V/XIV-B. 1943.*

Histoplasmosis

Binford, C. H.: Am. J. Clin. Path. 25: 25 (1955).
Darling, S. T.: J. A. M. A. 46: 1283 (1906).
Emmons, C. W.: Pub. Health Rep. 64: 892 (1949).
Straub, M., J. Schwarz: Am. J. Clin. Path. 25: 727 (1955).
Straub, M., J. Schwarz: J. Path. et Microbiol. (Basel) 25: 421 (1962).
Sweany, H. C.: Histoplasmosis (Springfield, Ill.: Charles C Thomas, Publisher, 1960).*

Blastomycosis

Gilchrist, T. C.: Rep. Johns Hopkins Hosp. 1: 269 (1896).
Movat, H. Z., N. V. P. Fernando: Lab. Invest. 12: 895 (1963).
Nelson, E., K. Blinzinger, H. Hager: J. Neuropath. & Exper. Neurol. 21: 155 (1962).
Prose, P. H., L. Lee, S. D. Balk: Am. J. Path. 47: 403 (1965).
Samorajsky, T., J. M. Ordy, J. R. Keefe: J. Cell Biol. 26: 779 (1965).
Schwarz, J., G. L. Baum: Am. J. Clin. Path. 21: 999 (1951).
Steiner, J. W., A. Jézéquel, M. J. Phillips, K. Miyai, K. Arakawa: Progress in Liver Diseases (New York: Grune & Stratton, Inc., 1965).*
Wiener, J., D. Spiro, R. G. Lattes: Am. J. Path. 47: 457 (1965).

Rhinosporidiosis

Karunaratne, W. A. E.: Rhinosporidiosis in Man (London:Athlone Press, 1964).*

Acanthoamebiasis

Carter, R. F.: Trans. Roy. Soc. Trop. Med. & Hyg. 66: 193 (1972).

Sarcosporidiosis

Mandour, A. M.: Trans. Roy. Soc. Trop. Med. & Hyg. 59: 432 (1965).

Mucocutaneous Leishmaniasis

Gernham, P. C. C.: Bull. Wld. Hlth. Org. 44: 477 (1971).

Giardiasis

Faust, E. C., L. Gonzales-Mugaburu: Am. J. Trop. Med. & Hyg. 14: 276 (1965).

Trichomoniasis

Crowley, E.: J. Urol. 91: 302 (1964).
Donne, A.: C. R. Acad. Sci. (Paris) 3: 385 (1836).

Cytomegalie

Horsfall, F. L., Jr., I. Tamm: Viral and Rickettsial Infections of Man (Philadelphia: J. B. Lippincott Company, 1965).

Cytodiagnosis

Graham, R. M.: The Cytologic Diagnosis of Cancer (Philadelphia: W. B. Saunders Company, 1963).*
Koss, L. G., G. R. Durfee: Diagnostic Cytology and Its Histopathologic Basis (London: Pitman Medical Publishing Company, 1961).*
Papanicolaou, G. N.: Atlas of Exfoliative Cytology (Cambridge, Mass.: Harvard University Press, 1954).*
Staehler, W. H., H. Ziegler, D. Völter, G. F. Schubert, W. B. Wartman: Color Atlas of Cytodiagnosis of the Prostate (Chicago: Year Book Medical Publishers, Inc., 1977).

Index